Handbook of Experimental Pharmacology

Volume 205

For further volumes:
http://www.springer.com/series/164

Hannsjörg W. Seyberth · Anders Rane
Matthias Schwab
Editors

Pediatric Clinical Pharmacology

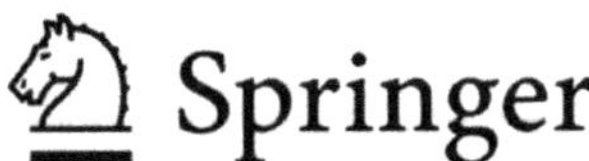 Springer

Editors
Prof. em. Dr. Hannsjörg W. Seyberth
Klinik für Kinder- und Jugendmedizin
Philipps-Universität Marburg
Baldingerstraße
35043 Marburg, Germany

Present address:
Lazarettgarten 23
76829 Landau
Germany
seyberth@staff.uni-marburg.de

Prof. Dr. Matthias Schwab
Dr. Margarete Fischer-Bosch-
Institut für Klinische Pharmakologie (IKP)
Auerbachstrasse 112
70376 Stuttgart
Germany

Department of Clinical Pharmacology
Institute of Experimental and Clinical
Pharmacology and Toxicology
University Hospital
Tübingen
Germany
matthias.schwab@ikpstuttgart.de

Prof. Dr. Anders Rane
Karolinska University Hospital
Karolinska Institutet
Dept. Laboratory Medicine
Div. Clinical Pharmacology
Stockholm
Sweden
anders.rane@ki.se

ISSN 0171-2004   e-ISSN 1865-0325
ISBN 978-3-642-20194-3   e-ISBN 978-3-642-20195-0
DOI 10.1007/978-3-642-20195-0
Springer Heidelberg Dordrecht London New York

Library of Congress Control Number: 2011937023

Preface

Historical development of pediatric pharmacology started at the very beginning of pharmacology and pediatrics in the mid-nineteenth century. Actually, in many places both medical disciplines stem from the same origin, the urban polyclinics or ambulances.

Already in the first therapeutic textbooks in pediatrics, often written by pharmacologists, it was stated that children are not small adults as demonstrated by the fact that the volume of distribution (Vd) for many drugs is larger in infants and drug reactions can be quite different in young children as seen with opiates, aspirin, and caffeine.

Unfortunately with the entry into a more scientific area at the beginning of the twentieth century pharmacology and pediatrics took up different paths. On the one hand, the pharmacologists became more and more fascinated by the options of learning more about the autonomic nervous system from studies with experimental animals, and on the other hand, the pediatricians discovered the enormous impact of microbiology for the prevention and treatment of infectious diseases and impact of biochemistry for the development of age appropriate nutrition, especially for infants. At the same time with losing interest in pediatric pharmacology pediatric teachers have started to propagate pharmacotherapeutic nihilism, especially for newborns and infants with the arguments of (a) lack of appropriate pediatric formulations and age appropriate posology, (b) unpredictable effects of maturation and development on pharmacokinetics and pharmacodynamics and vice versa, (c) effects of drugs on maturation and development, and (d) last but not least of missing verbal communication with very young children, which considerably reduced the options of assessing drug efficacy and tolerance in this young pediatric population.

With this history in mind, it is not at all surprising that in the 1970s when several modern pediatrics subspecialties like oncology, neonatal intensive care, cardiology, and transplantation with the need of extensive drug treatment appeared on the scene, the orphan drug status became more and more obvious. Many pediatricians and pediatric scientists in academic institutions and in pharmaceutical industry have lost or even never gained interest and professional competence in pediatric pharmacotherapeutics. This has led to a widespread off label use of highly potent but also precarious modern medicines especially in the very young and very sick pediatric population.

The objective of this volume is to overcome in part some of these gaps by giving an overview of the present state of the art of pediatric clinical pharmacology including developmental physiology, pediatric-specific pathology, special tools and methods for development of drugs for children (assessment of efficacy, toxicity, long-term safety, etc.) as well as regulatory and ethical knowledge and skills. In the future, structural and educational changes have to lead back to a closer cooperation and interaction of pediatrics with (clinical) pharmacology and pharmacy. Medical faculties and learned societies might consider establishing a tenure track system for well-trained pediatric pharmacologists. Moreover, the young general pediatrician needs to be better trained in the basics of pediatric drug treatment. Hopefully, pediatric pharmacology will not end with better knowledge and medical service for children in high-industrial countries only but will also help to improve drug treatment especially for those children in the developing countries. Intense international networking initiatives could be very helpful to come closer to achieve the goal of better medicines for all children worldwide.

Truly the time should be over, in which drug treatment was everybody's business with the consequence that this everybody's business is frequently nobody's business (Shirkey 1975).

Marburg, Germany	Hannsjörg W. Seyberth
Stockholm, Sweden	Anders Rane
Stuttgart/Tübingen, Germany	Matthias Schwab

Contents

Part III   Specific Pediatric Pharmacology

Contributors

Maurice J. Ahsman Department of Clinical Pharmacy, Erasmus MC, Rotterdam, The Netherlands

Dina Battino Department of Neurophysiopathology and Epilepsy Centre, IRCCS Foundation Carlo Besta, Neurological Institute, Milan, Italy

Joachim Boos Klinik und Poliklinik für Kinder- und Jugendmedizin, Westfälische Wilhems-Universität, 48149 Münster, Germany

Jörg Breitkreutz Institut für Pharmazeutische Technologie und Biopharmazie, Heinrich-Heine-Universität Düsseldorf, Universitätsstraße 1, 40225 Düsseldorf, Germany
joerg.breitkreutz@uni-duesseldorf.de

Patricia Bright U.S. Department of Health and Human Services, Food and Drug Administration, Office of the Commissioner, Office of Pediatric Therapeutics, Silver Spring, MD 2011, USA

Oscar Della Pasqua Division of Pharmacology, Amsterdam Center for Drug Research, Leiden University, Einsteinweg 55, P.O. Box 9503, 2300 RA Leiden, The Netherlands; Clinical Pharmacology & Discovery Medicine, GlaxoSmithKline R&D, Stockley Park, Uxbridge, UB11 1BT, United Kingdom
odp72514@gsk.com

Saskia N. de Wildt Intensive Care and Department of Pediatric Surgery, Erasmus MC Sophia Children's Hospital, Dr. Molewaterplein 60, 3015 GJ Rotterdam, The Netherlands
s.dewildt@erasmusmc.nl

Abdelbasset Elzagallaai Division of Clinical Pharmacology and Toxicology, Hospital for Sick Children, University Avenue 555, Toronto M5G 1X8, ON, Canada

Fatma Etwel Division of Clinical Pharmacology and Toxicology, Hospital for Sick Children, University Avenue 555, Toronto M5G 1X8, ON, Canada

Jason Gerson U.S. Department of Health and Human Services, Food and Drug Administration, Office of the Commissioner, Office of Pediatric Therapeutics, Silver Spring, MD 2011, USA

Ulrich Heininger Universitäts-Kinderspital beider Basel (UKBB), Postfach, CH-4005 Basel, Switzerland
Ulrich.Heininger@ukbb.ch

Steven Hirschfeld National Children's Study Eunice Kennedy Shriver, National Institute of Child Health and Human Development, 31 Center Drive, Room 2A03, MSC 2425, Bethesda, MD 20892, USA
hirschfs@mail.nih.gov

Hans V. Hogerzeil Essential Medicines and Pharmaceutical Policies, World Health Organization, 1211 Geneva 27, Switzerland

Kalle Hoppu Poison Information Centre, Helsinki University Central Hospital and Hospital for Children and Adolescents, Institute for Clinical Sciences, University of Helsinki, P.O. Box 790 (Tukholmankatu 17), 00029 HUS (Helsinki), Finland
kalle.hoppu@hus.fi

Evelyne Jacqz-Aigrain Department of Pediatric Pharmacology and Pharmacogenetics, Clinical Investigation Center, CIC Inserm 9202, French network of Pediatric Investigation Centers (CICPaed), Hôpital Robert Debré, 48 Boulevard Sérurier, 75935 Paris, France
evelyne.jacqz-aigrain@rdb.aphp.fr

Ralph E. Kauffman Division of Clinical Pharmacology and Medical Toxicology, The Children's Mercy Hospitals and Clinics, University of Missouri at Kansas City, 2401 Gillham Road, Kansas City, MO 64108, USA

Gregory L. Kearns Division of Pediatric Pharmacology and Medical Toxicology, Department of Medical Research, Children's Mercy Hospital, Kansas City, MO, USA

Gideon Koren The Motherisk Program, Division of Clinical Pharmacology and Toxicology, Hospital for Sick Children, University Avenue 555, Toronto M5G 1X8, ON, Canada
gidiup_2000@yahoo.com

Stephanie Läer Department of Clinical Pharmacy and Pharmacotherapy, Heinrich-Heine-University of Düsseldorf, Universitätsstrasse 1, 40225 Düsseldorf, Germany
stephanie.laeer@uni-duesseldorf.de

Pirjo Laitinen-Parkkonen Health Care and Social Services, City of Hyvinkää, Suutarinkatu 2 C, 05801 Hyvinkää, Finland

Catherine S. Lee U.S. Department of Health and Human Services, Food and Drug Administration, Office of the Commissioner, Office of Pediatric Therapeutics, Silver Spring, MD 2011, USA

Ron A.A. Mathot Department of Clinical Pharmacy, Erasmus MC, Rotterdam, The Netherlands

Bernd Meibohm College of Pharmacy, University of Tennessee Health Science Center, 874 Union Avenue, Rm. 5p, Memphis, TN 38163, USA

Dirk Mentzer Paul-Ehrlich-Institut, Referate Arzneimittelsicherheit, Paul-Ehrlich-Str. 51-59, 63225 Langen, Germany

Robert M. Nelson U.S. Department of Health and Human Services, Food and Drug Administration, Office of the Commissioner, Office of Pediatric Therapeutics, Silver Spring, MD 2011, USA
Robert.Nelson@fda.hhs.gov

Martin Offringa Department of Paediatric Clinical Epidemiology, Emma Children's Hospital, Academic Medical Centre, University of Amsterdam, Meibergdreef 9, 1105 AZ Amsterdam, The Netherlands
m.offringa@amc.uva.nl

Klaus Rose klausrose Consulting Pediatric Drug Development & More, Birsstrasse 16, 4052 Basel, Switzerland
rose@granzer.biz

Michelle Roth-Cline U.S. Department of Health and Human Services, Food and Drug Administration, Office of the Commissioner, Office of Pediatric Therapeutics, Silver Spring, MD 2011, USA

Agnes Saint-Raymond Scientific Advice, Paediatrics, and Orphan Drug Sector, European Medicines Agency, 7 Westferry Circus, Canary Wharf, London E14 4HB, United Kingdom

Matthias Schwab Dr. Margarete Fischer-Bosch-Institute of Clinical Pharmacology, Auerbachstrasse 112, 70376 Stuttgart, Germany; Department of Clinical Pharmacology, Institute of Experimental and Clinical Pharmacology and Toxicology, University Hospital, Tübingen, Germany

Hannsjörg W. Seyberth Klinik für Kinder- und Jugendmedizin, Philipps-Universität Marburg, Baldingerstraße, 35043 Marburg, Germany; Present address: Lazarettgarten 23, 76829 Landau, Germany
seyberth@staff.uni-marburg.de

Dick Tibboel Intensive Care and Department of Pediatric Surgery, Erasmus MC Sophia Children's Hospital, Dr. Molewaterplein 60, 3015 GJ Rotterdam, The Netherlands

Torbjörn Tomson Department of Clinical Neuroscience, Karolinska Institutet, S-171 76 Stockholm, Sweden
torbjorn.tomson@karolinska.se

Johannes N. van den Anker Division of Pediatric Clinical Pharmacology, Department of Pediatrics, Children's National Medical Center, 111 Michigan Avenue, NW, Washington, DC 20010, USA
jvandena@cnmc.org

Hanneke van der Lee Department of Paediatric Clinical Epidemiology, Emma Children's Hospital, Academic Medical Centre, University of Amsterdam, Meibergdreef 9, 1105 AZ Amsterdam, The Netherlands

Vera Vlahović-Palčevski Department for Clinical Pharmacology, University of Rijeka Medical School, University Hospital Center Rijeka, Krešimirova 42, 51000 Rijeka, Croatia
vvlahovic@inet.hr

Siri Wang Norwegian Medicines Agency, Tønsberg Hospital Pharmacy, Sven Oftedalsvei 6, N-0950 Oslo, Norway
siri.wang@noma.no

Magnus Westgren Division of Obstetrics and Gynecology, Department of Clinical Science, Intervention and Technology, Centre for Fetal Medicine, Karolinska University Hospital, Karolinska Institutet, S-141 86 Stockholm, Sweden
magnus.westgren@ki.se

Wei Zhao Department of Pediatric Pharmacology and Pharmacogenetics, Clinical Investigation Center, CIC Inserm 9202, French network of Pediatric Investigation Centers (CICPaed), Hôpital Robert Debré, 48 Boulevard Sérurier, 75935 Paris, France

Part I
General Considerations and Methodological Aspects

Basics and Dynamics of Neonatal and Pediatric Pharmacology

Hannsjörg W. Seyberth and Ralph E. Kauffman

Contents

Abstract Understanding the role of ontogeny in the disposition and actions of medicines is the most fundamental prerequisite for safe and effective pharmacotherapeutics in the pediatric population. The maturational process represents a continuum of growth, differentiation, and development, which extends from the very small preterm newborn infant through childhood, adolescence, and to young adulthood.

H.W. Seyberth (✉)
Klinik fur Kinder- und Jugendmedizin, Philipps-Universität Marburg, Baldingerstraße,
35043 Marburg, Germany

Present address:
Lazarettgarten 23, 76829 Landau, Germany
e-mail: seyberth@staff.uni-marburg.de

R.E. Kauffman
Division of Clinical Pharmacology and Medical Toxicology, The Children's Mercy Hospitals and
Clinics, University of Missouri at Kansas City, 2401 Gillham Road, Kansas City, MO 64108, USA

H.W. Seyberth et al. (eds.), *Pediatric Clinical Pharmacology*,
Handbook of Experimental Pharmacology 205,
DOI 10.1007/978-3-642-20195-0_1, © Springer-Verlag Berlin Heidelberg 2011

Developmental changes in physiology and, consequently, in pharmacology influence the efficacy, toxicity, and dosing regimen of medicines. Relevant periods of development are characterized by changes in body composition and proportion, developmental changes of physiology with pathophysiology, exposure to unique safety hazards, changes in drug disposition by major organs of metabolism and elimination, ontogeny of drug targets (e.g., enzymes, transporters, receptors, and channels), and environmental influences. These developmental components that result in critical windows of development of immature organ systems that may lead to permanent effects later in life interact in a complex, nonlinear fashion.

The ontogeny of these physiologic processes provides the key to understanding the added dimension of development that defines the essential differences between children and adults. A basic understanding of the developmental dynamics in pediatric pharmacology is also essential to delineating the future directions and priority areas of pediatric drug research and development.

Keywords Ontogeny • Pediatric population • Classification • Maturation • Developmental changes • Pharmacokinetics • Pharmacodynamics • Neonatal pharmacology • Pediatric pharmacotherapeutics • Long-term safety

Abbreviations

ADHD	Attention-deficit/hyperactivity disorder
ACE	Angiotensin-converting enzyme
ACh	Acetylcholine
AN	Anorexia nervosa
ATR	Angiotensin receptor
BN	Bulimia nervosa
CDL	Chronic lung disease
Clsys	Systemic clearance
CYP	CytochromeP450
DCT	Distal convoluted tubule
GABA	Gamma-aminobutyric acid
GnRH	Gonadotropin-releasing hormone
HPG	Hypothalamic–pituitary–gonadal
KCC2	Potassium-chloride cotransporter type 2
nAChRs	Nicotine acetylcholine receptors
NAT	N-Acetyltransferase
NEC	Necrotizing enterocolitis
NCCT	Sodium-chloride cotransporter
NKCC1	Sodium-potassium-2-chloride cotransporter type 1
PDA	Patent ductus arteriosus
PDE	Phosphodiesterase
P-gp	P-glycoprotein

RDS	Respiratory distress syndrome
ROP	Retinopathy of prematurity
SIDS	Sudden infant death syndrome
SLT	Salt-losing tubular disorder
SSRI's	Selective serotonin reuptake inhibitors
TDM	Therapeutic drug level monitoring
UGT	Uridine diphosphate glucuronosyltransferase
V(d)	Volume of distribution

1 Introduction

A safe and effective medication for children requires a fundamental understanding and integration of the role of ontogeny in the disposition and actions of medicines. As the most fundamental prerequisite, one has to consider the basic principle that children are not small adults!

The German-American and father of American pediatrics, Abraham Jacobi (1830–1919), recognized the importance of and the need for age-appropriate pharmacotherapy when he emphasized: *"Pediatrics does not deal with miniature men and women, with reduced doses and the same class of disease in smaller bodies, but … has its own independent range and horizon"* (Kearns et al. 2003). Along that line of argumentation some years later the German pioneer of pediatric pharmacology, Rudolf Fischl (1862–1942), wrote: *"Die Therapie des Kindesalters bedeutet nicht lediglich eine Restriktion der Behandlung der Erwachsenen, sondern baut sich auf genaue Kenntnisse der Physiologie dieser Lebensepoche auf"* (Fischl 1902). Moreover, he stated: *"Viel Unglück hat schon die Mathematik in der Medizin angerichtet, und eine einfache Berechnung der sogenannten refrakten Dosen für das Kindesalter aus der Gewichtsdifferenz können leicht ebenfalls ein solches anrichten"* (Fischl 1902). Harry Shirkey (1916–1995), the well-known American pharmacist and pediatrician, wrote in his textbook on Pediatric Therapy with other words: *"The long list of dosage rules based on age, body weight or surface and their respective authors is testimony that no rule is entirely satisfactory in producing an exact fraction of the known adult dose that is applicable to a particular child"* (Shirkey 1975). This fundamental knowledge of determining the pediatric dosage of a medicine is even today – 100 years later – often ignored. Thus, as the first step for a successful approach to pediatric therapeutics, one must appreciate the differences among pediatric subpopulations with their typical features and health problems and the nonlinear and dynamic process of maturation. The ontogeny of basic physiologic processes provides guideposts for understanding the mechanisms underlying differences between different developmental stages within the pediatric and adult populations.

2   Classification of the Pediatric Population

The pediatric population represents a continuum of growth and development, which extends from the very small preterm newborn infant through childhood, adolescence, and to young adulthood (Fig. 1). The internationally agreed (Food and Drug Administration 2000), and to some extent arbitrary, classification of the pediatric population is as follows:

- Preterm infants (<37 weeks gestation)
- Term newborn infants (0–28 days)
- Infants and toddlers (>28 days to 23 months)
- Children (2–11 years)
- Adolescents (12 to 16–18 years, depending on the region)

Substantial changes in body composition and proportions accompany growth and development. Embedded within this continuum of growth and development is substantial individual variation. Developmental changes in physiology and, consequently, in pharmacology influence the efficacy, toxicity, and dosing regimen of medicines (posology) used in children. It is, therefore, important to review characteristics of the relevant periods of development from birth, through adolescence, to adulthood.

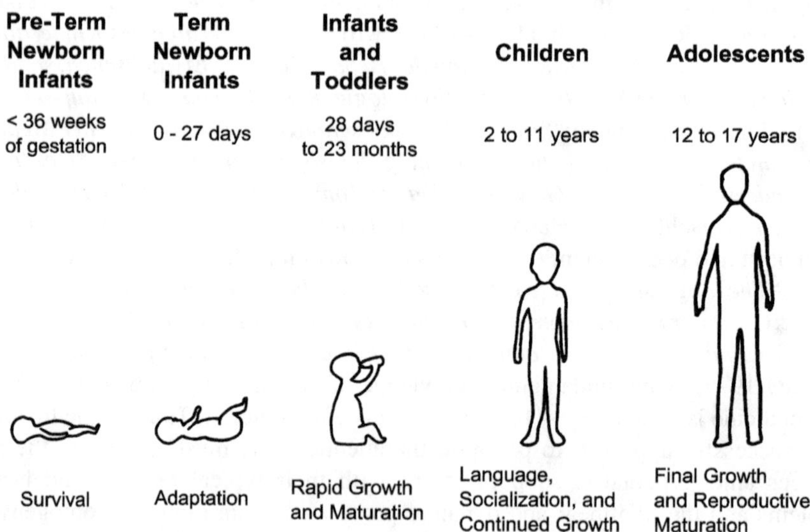

Fig. 1 Five stages of development. The pediatric population extends from the preterm and term newborn infant through childhood, and adolescence, or even to young adulthood. Each period of development has its own very specific characteristics, such as period of survival, period of adaptation, period of rapid growth and physiological maturation, period of language, socialization, and continued growth, and period of final growth and reproductive maturation

3 Description of the Five Relevant Periods of Development, Their Typical Features, Common Health Problems, and the Impact on Pediatric Pharmacotherapy

3.1 The Preterm Newborn: Period of Survival

3.1.1 Body Composition and Proportion

Body composition correlates with both gestational and postnatal age, and it continues to change significantly during the first year of life (Ahmad et al. 2010; Ellis 2000; Fomon and Nelson 2002). High body water content and extracellular/intracellular water ratio as well as very low body fat and muscle mass in the preterm infant are important contributors to altered volumes of distribution (V(d)) of hydrophilic and lipophilic medicines or highly tissue-bound drugs such as the cardiac glycosides. For example, the larger total body water content of the newborn infant (approximately 80% as compared with 60% of body weight by 5 months of age) results in a larger mg/kg-loading dose of water-soluble medicines, such as the aminoglycosides (Pacifici 2009).

The relatively large head circumference and cranial volume is the leading characteristic of the body proportion from the very preterm newborn to the older infant and toddler. Relatively large brain weight and cerebral blood flow, limited plasma protein binding capacity, as well as increased blood–brain barrier permeability all predispose the CNS to higher concentrations of administered medicines than later in life (Strolin Benedetti et al. 2005).

Likewise, increased skin permeability needs to be considered whenever a medicine is applied on the skin. Increased dermal absorption may increase risk of adverse effects as with antibacterial agents such as alcohol and hexachlorophene solution (Stewart and Hampton 1987) or provide an option for painless and noninvasive transdermal drug delivery in preterm newborns as with caffeine for apnea (Barrett and Rutter 1994).

3.1.2 Developmental Changes of Physiology with Their Pathophysiology and Safety Hazards

The Very Preterm Newborn (<30 Weeks of Gestation)

The very (extremely) preterm newborn around the 22–23 weeks of gestation is at the limit of viability because the incompletely developed complex pulmonary–cardiovascular system is not prepared to function well in the extrauterine environment, even with intensive support. The multiple hazards are as follows:

- *Respiratory distress syndrome (RDS)*
  Before primitive alveoli have formed and surfactant production has begun, the lung cannot adequately function as an organ of gas exchange. At an early and intermediate stage of pulmonary maturation, the very preterm newborn requires administration of exogenous surfactant and prolonged mechanical ventilation to prevent and/or treat severe RDS. These treatments, along with lung immaturity, are commonly associated with development of chronic lung disease of prematurity (Stevens et al. 2007).
- *Persistent fetal circulation*
  In this condition, the transitional from fetal to neonatal circulation is characterized by pulmonary hypertension and patent ductus arteriosus (PDA), which are responsible for marked right to left circulatory shunting and hypoxia.
- *Incomplete cerebral autoregulation*
  Impaired or completely missing cerebral autoregulation is a risk factor for intraventricular hemorrhage with parenchymal brain injury and posthemorrhagic complications later in life such as cerebral palsy, hydrocephalus, and cognitive deficits (Szabó et al. 2009).
- *Necrotizing enterocolitis (NEC)*
  Immaturity of the gastrointestinal tract and immune system predisposes the very preterm infant to NEC with life-threatening complications including fulminate septic shock (Neu 2007; Thompson and Bizzarro 2008).

The Late Preterm Newborn (31–36 Weeks of Gestation)

At this stage, the infant is rarely in a life-threatening situation, but still is at risk for a series of serious health problems related to immaturity of several organ systems. These include:

- *Transient tachypnea*
  Lack of clearance of lung fluid and relative deficiency of pulmonary surfactant may cause transient tachypnea and RDS (Raju et al. 2006).
- *Relapse into fetal circulation*
  Partial relapse into fetal circulation may lead to pulmonary hypertension of the newborn. This condition may be associated with sepsis or sometimes with maternal use of selective serotonin reuptake inhibitors (SSRIs) (Konduri and Kim 2009; Koren and Boucher 2009; Ramachandrappa and Jain 2009).
- *Temparature instability and apnea*
  CNS immaturity may lead to poor temperature control (Raju et al. 2006) and failure of respiratory control with central apnea (Hunt 2006).
- *Peristaltic dysfunction*
  Immaturity of the gastrointestinal tract may lead to feeding problems related to peristaltic dysfunction and failure of sphincter control in the esophagus, stomach, and intestines (Lebenthal and Lebenthal 1999; Neu 2007).

- *Jaundice and hypoglycemia*
  Prolonged hyperbilirubinemia and hypoglycemia are risk factors for brain injury (Raju et al. 2006).
- *Susceptibility to infection*
  An incompetent (naïve) immune system increases susceptibility to infection and predisposes the infant to sepsis (Clapp 2006).

3.1.3 Major Organs of Metabolism and Elimination

Developmental immaturity has a major impact on drug disposition in preterm infants. Changes in the V(d) have already been mentioned in the context of body composition. The next most important pharmacokinetic factor for pediatric dosing is reduced systemic clearance (Cl_{sys}) due to immaturity of the liver and kidneys, the most important organs involved in the process of drug metabolism and elimination. The relatively large V_d and reduced Cl_{sys} in neonates commonly require a higher loading dose and lower maintenance dose of many drugs (Bartelink et al. 2006). The gray baby syndrome, a fatal cardiovascular collapse, is a frequently cited historical example of drug toxicity on the basis of immature hepatic glucuronidation of chloramphenicol leading to supratherapeutic systemic concentrations when infants were given doses used in older children (Asmar and Abdel-Haq 2005).

Hepatic Metabolism

Because of quantitative and qualitative differences in hepatic drug metabolism, medicines that are primarily metabolized by the liver may need to be administered in reduced doses until the age of about 2 months (Alcorn and McNamara 2002; Allegaert et al. 2007; Anderson and Lynn 2009; Bartelink et al. 2006). Enzymes most commonly involved in drug metabolism are those of the cytochrome P450 (CYP) family (phase I reactions) and the uridine diphosphate glucuronosyltransferase (UGT), sulfotransferase, glutathione-*S*-transferase, and *N*-acetyltransferase (NAT) families (phase II reactions). Each of the specific isozymes within a family matures at different rates during the first several years of life. The effect on metabolism of a specific medication depends on the dominant enzymatic pathway(s) responsible for metabolism of the drug. Several studies have been performed with medicines, which are frequently used in neonatology. Indomethacin is a substrate for CYP2C9 (Koukouritaki et al. 2004; Rodrigues AD 2005); phenobarbital is also a substrate for CYP2C9 in addition to CYP2C19 (Goto et al. 2007; Löscher et al. 2009); caffeine is metabolized by CYP1A2 and NAT2 (Pons et al. 1989); and morphine is a specific substrate for UGT2B7 (Coffman et al. 1997). These medicines function as markers for hepatic metabolic activity, which is low relative to older children and adults, leading to reduced total clearance of these drugs during the neonatal period (al-Alaiyan et al. 2001; Battino et al. 1995; Hartley et al. 1994; Yaffe et al. 1980).

A qualitative difference in hepatic drug metabolism is exemplified by the different metabolite profile of theophylline in newborns with the attendant risk of caffeine toxicity (Bory et al. 1979; Lowry et al. 2001). Theophylline and caffeine are frequenty used to treat apnea of prematurity. In contrast to adults, in preterm newborns caffeine is a biotransformation product of theophylline and may accumulate to toxic levels with chronic theophylline dosing. To avoid this complication, caffeine is the preferred methylxanthine to treat apnea of prematurity. This reduces the risk of methylxanthine toxicity and avoids the need for routine therapeutic drug level monitoring (TDM) (Charles et al. 2008; Natarajan et al. 2007; Steer and Henderson-Smart 2000).

Renal Elimination

At birth renal function is rather low, with a GFR down to 1 ml/min/kg, and does not approach adult levels before the age of 6–12 months (Alcorn and McNamara 2002). Tubular secretion matures more slowly and full renal function is reached at approximately 2–3 years of age (Fawer et al. 1979; Fettermann et al. 1965). Delayed maturation of tubular reabsorption leads to glomerulotubular imbalance with the risk of salt and water wasting (Alcorn and McNamara 2002; Bartelink et al. 2006; Celsi and Aperia 1993). On the positive side, the decreased ability to concentrate aminoglycosides in the tubular epithelium contributes to decreased nephrotoxicity of aminoglycosides in newborns (Fleck and Bräunlich 1995; McCracken 1986).

Thus, it is not surprising that furosemide, which is mainly excreted as a substrate of the PAH transport pathway unchanged in the urine, has a prolonged plasma half-life (often exceeding 24 h) and a very low renal clearance particularly in the very preterm newborns (Mirochnick et al. 1988; Peterson et al. 1980). Similarly, weak organic acids such as penicillins and cephalorins, which are frequently used in newborns, also have very low total clearances in preterm infants. The kidney almost exclusively excretes these medicines by an active tubular organic anion transport system, which has 20–30% of adult capacity at birth and approaches adult capacity at approximately 7–8 months (Alcorn and McNamara 2002).

3.1.4 Ontogeny of Drug Targets in the Perinatal Period

During the perinatal period many fundamental changes take place, which are unique to the newborn and are not observed again during infancy, childhood, and adolescence. To describe all these changes, which certainly have an impact on drug targets, would be far beyond the scope of this subsection. Thus, only selected aspects, where substantive progress is relevant to pediatric pharmacology, including molecular pharmacodynamics and pharmacogenetics, are discussed.

Receptors/Binding Sites

– *Adrenergic receptors*
  The ontogeny of drug–receptor interactions, particularly of the adrenergic and cholinergic systems, has been of long-standing interest to pediatric pharmacologists (Boréus 1972). However, methods for isolation of homogeneous cells from organs of the fetus or the newborn ensuring that the cells and receptors have not been altered during isolation and purification have not been adequately developed (Whitsett et al. 1982). Nevertheless, there is ample direct and indirect experimental evidence of ontogenic regulation of receptor number and function. In the newborn rat brain, there are an increased number of β-adrenergic receptors during the first weeks of life, while at the same time the number of α-adrenergic receptors is declining after an initial rise in the rat brain shortly after birth (Whitsett et al. 1982). Unfortunately, due to methodological reasons, similar data in human tissue are often missing. Thus, more readily accessible circulating nucleated blood cells, e.g., leukocytes, have been used with the assumption that they may reflect the status of adrenergic receptors in the actual target organ of interest (Fraser et al. 1981). Decreased β-adrenergic receptor sites have been described in human cord blood neutrophils (PMN) of infants vaginally delivered at term (Roan and Galant 1982). These findings may reflect ontogenic differences between the neonatal and adult PMN. However, the effect of increasing catecholamine secretion during the stress of delivery resulting in downregulation of the β-adrenergic receptors cannot be ruled out.
  More recent molecular pharmacology studies in the postnatal rat devoted to the ontogenesis of β-adrenergic signaling indicate that, in contrast to the receptor downregulation and desensitization of β-adrenergic receptors observed in the adult, the numbers and responsiveness of β-adrenergic receptors increase in most tissues of the immature organism in response to prolonged treatment with betamimetics during the postnatal period. This developmental stage of the rat approximately correlates with the mid-to-late second and early third trimester of human gestation (Slotkin et al. 2003). The process of downregulation and desensitization are not inherent properties, but rather acquired during the above-mentioned vulnerable time interval when pregnant women may be treated with betamimetics for preterm labor. Thus, intrauterine overstimulation with betamimetics during this critical period of prenatal development can induce a permanent shift in the balance of adrenergic-to-cholinergic tone with the risk of inducing functional and behavioral teratogenesis. This is a currently offered working hypothesis in an attempt to explain the association of prolonged (3–4 weeks) betamimetic treatment for tocolysis and bronchodilatation of the mother with increases in functional and behavioral disorders, including psychiatric disorders (e.g., autism), poor cognitive and motor function, and school performance as well as changes in blood pressure (e.g., hypertension) in the offspring (Witter et al. 2009).

– *Prostanoid receptors*
  Prostanoids are abundantly generated throughout the perinatal period. They are thought to be key players in the regulation of ductus arteriosus tone and in the

autoregulation of blood flow to the brain and retina as well as to the renal and splanchnic vascular beds (Seyberth and Kühl 1988; Smith 1998; Wright et al. 2001). The rapid changes in vascular physiology during postnatal life are not only accomplished by rapid changes of the synthesis and metabolism of these autacoids, but also by rapid adjustments in the turnover of prostanoid receptor expression. This has been particularly well studied in the regulation of ductus arteriosus tone (Smith 1998).

In utero, the main factors maintaining patency of the ductus arteriosus are low oxygen tension and high levels of PGE_2 and PGI_2 (Fig. 2), which are acting through prostanoid EP_4 and IP receptors (Smith 1998; Smith and McGrath 1994; Leonhardt et al. 2003; Wright et al. 2001). Both receptors are coupled to adenylate cyclase (Boie et al. 1994; Honda et al. 1993). cAMP generated by this enzyme is considered to be the main intracellular second messenger involved in smooth muscle relaxation, which is consistent with the potent vasodilator effect PGE_2 and PGI_2 on the ductus. After birth, increased ductal oxygen tension and a fall of prostanoid levels, which is accompanied by a marked reduction of

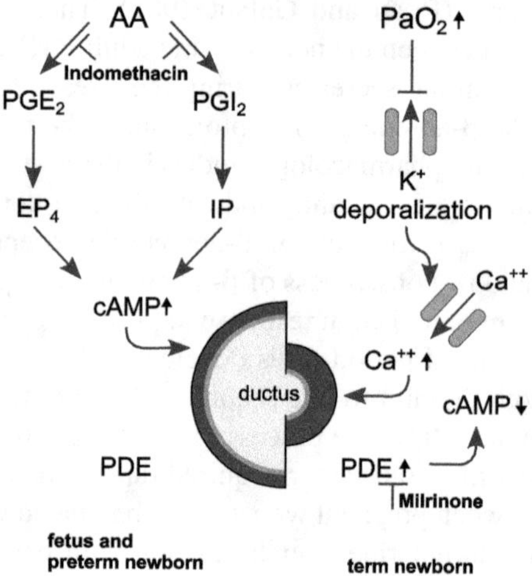

Fig. 2 Perinatal switch of ductus arteiosus from vasodilation to vasoconstriction. In utero, and to some extent in the pretem newborn, patency of the ductus arteriosus is maintained by high levels of PGE_2 and PGI_2 in addition to low oxygen tension. The potent vasodilator effect PGE_2 and PGI_2 on the ductus is mediated through PGE_2 and PGI_2 receptors, EP_4 and IP, respectively, by increasing cAMP. cAMP is considered to be the main intracellular second messenger involved in smooth muscle relaxation of the ductus. Postnatal increase in arterial PaO_2 plays an important role in functional closure of the ductus, which starts with oxygen-induced inhibition of O_2-sensitive potassium channels. This leads to smooth muscle cell depolarization and consequently to increased calcium influx through voltage-dependent L-type calcium channels. In parallel with advancing gestation, smooth muscle phosphodiesterase (PDE) isoforms in the ductus are increasingly expressed leading to decreased intracellular cAMP, thus supporting the shift from dilatation to constriction of the ductus arteriosus. PDE inhibitors such as milrinone, however, can prevent this shift

prostanoid receptor expression, induces closure, thus promoting contraction of the ductus arteriosus (Bouayad et al. 2001; Smith et al. 2001; Wright et al. 2001).

Preterm infants with RDS and mechanically ventilated lungs are prone to develop a symptomatic PDA on the basis of persistent PGE_2 and PGI_2 release probably from the ventilated lung (Smith 1998; Seyberth et al. 1984). Thus, at the present time the most appropriate pharmacological intervention is the treatment with prostaglandin synthesis inhibitors (Fig. 2), such as indomethacin (Hammerman et al. 2008; Leonhardt and Seyberth 2003; Ohlsson et al. 2008). However, this systemic inhibition of endogenous prostanoid synthesis has some negative consequences. Firstly, all prostanoid effects are inhibited including those of TxA_2 and $PGF_{2\alpha}$, which do have additional vasoconstrictor potential via specific receptors on the ductus. Secondly, inhibition of all endogenously synthesized prostanoids has negative effects on a variety of physiological and protective functions of blood cells and organs such as platelets, kidney, and intestinal tract (Seyberth and Kühl 1988; Smith 1998; Wright et al. 2001). A potent and selective EP_4 receptor antagonist might be a more appropriate alternative for pharmacologically induced ductal closure (Momma et al. 2005b; Smith 1998; Wright et al. 2001). A selective EP_4 receptor agonist, on the other hand, could be an ideal tool in maintaining the ductus open in newborns with ductus-dependent congenital obstructive heart malformations (Momma et al. 2005a; Leonhardt et al. 2003; Smith 1998).

During experimental studies, predominately with fetal lambs, another important aspect of clinical relevance has become apparent. With increasing gestational age, and, certainly after birth, before irreversible anatomic remodeling of the ductus takes place there is a decreasing ductal sensitivity to vasodilatory prostanoids. This desensitization is not only accomplished by a reduction of PGE_2 receptor density but also by inhibition of the receptor-coupled mechanism, which leads to lower intracellular cAMP concentrations (Waleh et al. 2004). With advancing gestation, smooth muscle phosphodiesterase (PDE) isoforms in the ductus are increasingly expressed leading to increased cAMP degradation and decreased intracellular cAMP, thus inducing a shift from dilatation to constriction of the ductus arteriosus (Liu et al. 2008). This crucial role of these phosphodiesterases in the regulation of ductal tone needs to be considered when proposing use of PDE inhibitors such as milrinone for treatment of cardiac failure in preterm infants (Toyoshima et al. 2006) (Fig. 2). There is good experimental and clinical evidence that PDE 3 inhibitors prevent closure of the ductus arteriosus in preterm newborns, thus antagonizing the positive inotropic effect of these drugs in these infants (Paradisis et al. 2009; Toyoshima et al. 2006).

Channels and Transporters

– *Channel maturation and regulation of ductal tone during the perinatal period*
  Developmental changes of channel activities have been studied during rapid physiological changes around birth. Besides the prostanoid system complex,

non-PG procontractile pathways are involved in the oxygen-induced functional closure of the ductus arteriosus. The postnatal increase in arterial PaO_2 plays an important role in active ductal constriction (Fig. 2). This functional closure of the ductus starts with oxygen-induced inhibition of O_2-sensitive potassium channels, which leads to smooth muscle cell depolarization and consequently to increased calcium influx through voltage-dependent L-type calcium channels (Nakanishi et al. 1993; Thébaud et al. 2004; Waleh et al. 2009). In preparation for extrauterine life, the expression of the calcium channels starts to increase during late gestation, while the inhibitory effect of the potassium channels declines (Clyman et al. 2007; Waleh et al. 2009). Thus, in preterm infants this maturation of active ductal vasoconstriction has not been fully completed, which contributes to persistent ductal patency. Since changes in membrane potential clearly play a critical role in regulating ductal tone, compounds acting at O_2-sensitive potassium channels are promising candidates for pharmacomanipulation of the ductus arteriosus after birth in both term and preterm infants (Smith 1998).

This understanding of the ontogenetic changes in tuning the muscular wall of the ductus is essential to understanding the mechanism by which chronic in utero inhibition of prostanoid synthesis is associated with temporary delay or even prevention of postnatal ductal closure. At the same time, when synthesis of relaxing prostanoids is inhibited, the expression of the O_2-sensitive potassium channel and calcium L-channel genes in the ductus wall is also reduced. In other words, the capability of O_2-induced ductal constriction has been weakened or even abolished (Momma et al. 2009; Reese et al. 2009). These experimental findings have been corroborated by clinical observations. The so-called paradoxical failure of ductal closure can be induced either after prenatal administration of indomethacin for preterm labor or after indomethacin treatment immediately after birth for prevention of patent ductus (Hammerman et al. 1998; Momma et al. 2009; Norton et al. 1993).

– *Channels and transporters involved in transepithelial electrolyte transport*
Another field, in which channels and transporters play an important role, is the transepithelial electrolyte transport in the developing kidney. Tubular reabsorption of salt and water begins maturing with very dynamic changes during the perinatal and early postnatal period (Alcorn and McNamara 2002). The so-called pharmacotyping of inherited hypokalemic salt-losing tubular disorders (SLT) associated with secondary hyperaldosteronism was extremely helpful in identifying common targets for mutations and developing interventions by pharmacologists (Reinalter et al. 2004) (Fig. 3). The furosemide-like SLT with a loop disorder and the thiazide-like SLT with a distal convoluted tubule (DCT) disorder are the two major types of SLT (Seyberth 2008). The phenotypes of the two genetic and the pharmacologically distinct "human knockouts" – defects of NKCC2 and NCCT – are almost identical, which include, in addition to hypokalemic alkalosis in both of them, polyuria, isosthenuria, and hypercalciuria for the furosemide type and hypomagnesemia and hypocalciuria for the thiazide type (Jeck et al. 2005; Peters et al. 2002). Moreover, patients with a loop disorder

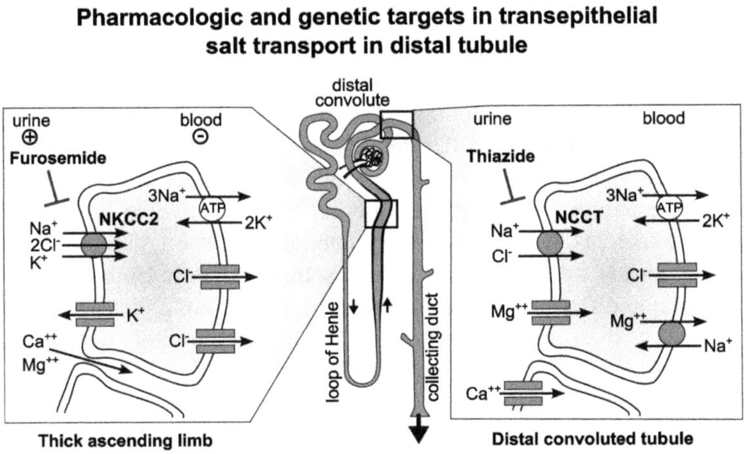

Fig. 3 Pharmacologic and genetic targets in transepithelial salt transport in distal tubule. Inherited hypokalemic salt-losing tubular disorders (SLT) associated with secondary hyperaldosteronism have common targets for mutations and pharmacological interventions such as the furosemide-sensitive sodium-potassium-chloride cotransporter (NKCC2) and the thiazide-sensitive sodium-chloride cotransporter (NCCT). The furosemide-like SLT is primarily a polyuric and hypercalciuric loop disorder, while the thiazide-like SLT is a distal convoluted tubule (DCT) disorder, which is characterized by persistent hypomagnesemia and hypocalciuria

do not respond to furosemide but do respond, as expected, to thiazide treatment (Köckerling et al. 1996). In contrast, the diuretic response in patients with a DCT defect is just the opposite (Colussi et al. 2007). The time of clinical presentation is another major difference between the two tubular disorders (Peters et al. 2002). While the loop defect presents in utero with fetal polyuria associated with the development of polyhydramnios and premature birth, the thiazide-like DCT defect rarely becomes symptomatic before late infancy with hypokalemic alkalosis as a consequence of a relatively mild salt and water diuresis.

From these experiments of nature one can predict that, in contrast to loop diuretics, thiazide diuretics are not going to be very efficacious in preterm infants. The NCCT in the DCT probably is not active and/or not expressed at that early stage of development. This hypothesis might be supported by the results of a well-controlled drug study with preterm infants (Green et al. 1983). While infants receiving furosemide clearly exhibited diuretic activity, *the response in those given chlorothiazide* (20 mg/kg/d) *was no different from patients not given diuretics*. Immunohistological studies with renal tissue of very preterm infants need to be done to prove this hypothesis directly.

Endocrine/Paracrine System and Renal Function

Complex endocrine/paracrine interactions of the renin-angiotensin and the renal prostanoid system are critically involved in the protection and maintenance of adequate renal blood perfusion and function. The extreme low blood pressure of the preterm infant with a mean arterial pressure of about 30 mm Hg makes an effective filtration pressure highly dependent on the activity of vasoconstrictive angiotensin II on the one hand and on vasodilatory renal prostanoids on the other hand (Evans and Moorcraft 1992; Guignard 2002; Prevot et al. 2002; Seyberth et al. 1991). This well-coordinated vasoconstriction and vasodilatation of the afferent and efferent glomerular vasculature renders renal function oversensitive to any angiotensin-converting enzyme (ACE) inhibitor or angiotensin receptor (ATR) antagonist and prostanoid synthesis inhibitor. Thus, besides their intrinsic potency one cannot expect any major differences in renal toxicity among ACE inhibitors and ATR antagonists as well as among prostanoid synthesis inhibitors (FitzGerald and Patrono 2001; Frölich 1997; Guignard 2002; Prevot et al. 2002). As long as one avoids a prolonged ineffective circulatory volume created by extreme fluid restriction, unnecessary furosemide treatment, and failure of ductal closure (all are additional stimuli for the renin-angiotensin system), no major renal damage to the preterm newborn is to be expected (Leonhardt et al. 2004; Seyberth et al. 1983). Under this condition, even a 10- to 100-fold overdose of indomethacin, caused by medication error, does not lead to significant deterioration of renal function (Narayanan et al. 1999; Schuster et al. 1990).

3.1.5 Environment and Critical Windows/Periods of Development of Immature Organ Systems with Resulting Permanent Effects on Phenotype

A classical pediatric example of this phenomenon – also sometimes called "programming" – is congenital hypothyroidism. If this condition remains undetected and untreated shortly after birth, it gives rise to lifelong phenotypic changes and learning difficulties. There is no comparable condition in adulthood because although hypothyroidism occurs in later life, the central nervous system has ceased developing. Now we discuss similar effects due to postnatally applied environmental and/or pharmacological factors.

Pathophysiology of Retinopathy of Prematurity

Retinopathy of prematurity (ROP) is an instructive model to study the long-term consequences of an interruption of a complex maturation process by premature birth, particularly if it happens in the middle of a critical time window of development. In addition, the course of this vascular disease can be followed under clinical conditions by repeated inspections of the retina.

ROP remains an important cause of morbidity in the extremely preterm infant. The significantly improved survival of very premature infants due to advances in neonatal intensive care during the last decades has decreased mortality of the most immature newborns, but has not diminished the incidence of ROP worldwide

(Holmström et al. 2007; Wheatley et al. 2002). ROP is a multifactorial disease of the developing retinal vasculature under environmental, nutritional, and genetic influence. The postnatal interruption of a very vulnerable ongoing development around 26 weeks of gestation is a major trigger of this biphasic ocular disease (Hellström et al. 2009; Kermorvant-Duchemin et al. 2010). During the first ischemic phase after birth, premature exposure of the retina to hyperoxia induces an arrest in vascular development with a degeneration of already existing blood vessels. In the second, vasoproliferative phase the avascular and ischemic retina triggers a compensatory release of proangiogenic factors. This leads to abnormal, upregulated extraretinal neovascularization, which may progress to retinal detachment and finally to blindness. Basically, ROP is the result of an unbalanced activity of various proangiogenic (such as VEGF and IGF1) and antiangiogenic (such as thrombospondin-1) factors, interacting with protective effects of nutritional factors (such as docosahexaenoic acid), and cytotoxic effects of oxidative and nitro-oxidative stress-dependent mediators generated from interaction of *trans*-arachidonic acid with the nitrogen dioxide radical or its precursors (Balazy and Chemtob 2008; Kermorvant-Duchemin et al. 2010). This more complex view on the pathophysiology of ROP, however, poses new challenges for more rational pharmacologic interventions in the future. Presently, ROP-induced blindness in children, adolescents, and young adults has to be considered as a major cause of all visual disorders.

Postnatal Dexamethasone Treatment and Neurological Outcome

Over the past 20 years, corticosteroid use in the preterm infant has fallen in and out of favor. Steroids were introduced in the 1980s as a mode of preventing and treating chronic (inflammatory) lung disease (CLD) in the preterm infant population. This use has been targeted toward low birth weight infants who cannot be weaned off the ventilator. Dose, duration, and timing of treatment with dexamethasone, the steroid typically used in NICUs, have varied. Corticosteroids given postnatally are potentially neurotoxic when given in high dose or when used in the first 96 h of life. The mechanism by which they cause central nervous system damage is unknown, but may be related to increased risk of periventricular leukomalacia (Levene 2007). Unfortunately, there is still a need for long-term follow-up and reporting of late neurological and developmental outcomes, especially among surviving infants, in those who participated in randomized trials of early postnatal corticosteroid treatment and who have already been sent to school (Doyle et al. 2010).

3.2 The Newborn Term Infant: Period of Adaptation

3.2.1 Body Composition and Proportion

Body water content and extra/intracellular water ratio remain high as compared to infants and children. However, with each week of gestational age body fat content increases when compared with preterm newborns (Ahmad et al. 2010; Ellis 2000; Fomon and Nelson 2002). Besides relatively large body surface area and head circumference as well as high permeability of blood–brain barrier and skin, rapid weight gain is a typical feature during this period of growth and development (Strolin Benedetti et al. 2005). Greater vulnerability to CNS drug toxicity (e.g., local anesthetic agents and opioids) is in part the consequence of the decreased blood–brain barrier (Latasch and Freye 2002)

3.2.2 Developmental Changes of Physiology with Their Pathophysiology and Safety Hazards

Although the term newborn is in a much more mature stage of development than the preterm newborn, they share several health problems with each other.

Drug Risk of Kernicterus

Icterus neonatorum (physiological jaundice) is certainly a safety hazard for both the term and preterm newborn. It is the result of increased bilirubin production following postnatal breakdown of fetal red blood cells combined with transient limitation in the conjugation of bilirubin by the liver. Excess circulating unconjugated bilirubin is bound to high-affinity acidic binding sites on plasma albumin, from where it can be displaced by highly bound acidic drugs, such as sulfisoxazole and ibuprofen, thereby increasing the concentration of free unconjugated bilirubin that may diffuse into the CNS. This increases the risk of kernicterus in newborn infants (Ahlfors 2004; Gal et al. 2006).

Metabolic Risk During Adaptation

Metabolic instability during the adaptation period shortly after birth may cause symptomatic hypoglycemia and hypocalcemia with seizures. This adaptive instability is often an endocrine/metabolic emergency situation leading to hospital admission (No authors listed 2004). Besides prematurity and intrauterine growth retardation, gestational diabetes is the most common cause for this neonatal complication (Jain et al. 2008a, b).

Immature Immune System

Immaturity of innate and adaptive immune responses in the perinatal period predisposes the neonate to increased infectious morbidity and mortality, the most common complications for all newborns (No authors listed 2004; Satwani et al. 2005).

Increased Susceptibility to Seizure

In addition to the anatomical and metabolic causes of seizures, the newborn brain is inherently prone to seizures as a consequence of incomplete neuronal maturation processes. The first months of postnatal life are critical for brain development (Ben-Ari and Holmes 2006; Dubois et al. 2008). At this age cerebral growth and maturation are intense and are influenced by multiple external stimuli encountered after birth. Besides dendritic growth and synaptic overproduction (in the gray matter), which is followed by synaptic pruning, myelination in white matter is essential for fast impulse conduction and for the structure maturation of functional networks (Ben-Ari and Holmes 2006; Dubois et al. 2008; Holopainen 2008). It is thought that at this stage the excitatory activity is enhanced and might contribute to the developing brain's greater capacity for activity-dependent plasticity. Myelination is a long nonlinear process that runs from the last trimester of gestation through the second decade of life with a peak in the first postnatal year. Besides these structural changes, complex changes in development and function of neurotransmitter systems also occur including the postnatal excitatory-to-inhibitory switch in gamma-aminobutyric acid (GABA) signaling. These functional changes are described in more detail in "Neurotransmitters, Transporters, and Channels".

3.2.3 Drug Disposition

Enteral Drug Absorption

Ongoing changes in growth, function, and differentiation of the gastrointestinal tract occur during adaptation to normal postnatal life. These changes may have significant effects on systemic delivery of medicines taken by the oral route. Obviously enteral drug absorption and bioavailability of medicines, which are administered by mouth, become quite important, as oral dosing is the most common and convenient route of administration.

In the first hours and days after birth, the intestinal weight and the mucosal mass almost double to accommodate the change from umbilical cord to oral feeding, which is similar to the change from parenteral to oral feeding (Commare and Tappenden 2007). This rapid intestinal growth and functional development is stimulated by feeding of colostrum, which is rich on peptide growth factors such as EGF, TGF alpha, and IGF-1. The large amount of secretory IgA in colostrum, which has a high systemic bioavailability, may also play a role in intestinal development in addition to providing immunologic protection (Commare and Tappenden 2007).

Several important examples illustrate the spectrum of dynamic developmental changes of the gastrointestinal tract during early infancy. These include altered gastric acid secretion, gastrointestinal transit time, and biliary and pancreatic exocrine function, all of which can significantly affect drug absorption and bioavailability of orally administered medicines in the first weeks of life.

Although parietal cells are well developed at term, the gastric pH is neutral at birth. Decreased capacity for hydrogen ion secretion persists throughout infancy, particularly represented by decreased acid production following pentogastrin stimulation (Anderson and Lynn 2009; Stewart and Hampton 1987; Strolin Benedetti et al. 2005). In addition, gastric contents are buffered by frequent feedings and gastric emptying is delayed. Altogether, these factors significantly influence the time course of drug absorption and bioavailability of acid-labile proteins and medicines such as growth factors and penicillins, respectively (Strolin Benedetti et al. 2005). Gastrointestinal absorption may also be facilitated for macromolecules such as lactalbumin from human milk or for aminoglycosides in early infancy as a consequence of the immature gastrointestinal mucosal barrier with increased permeability (Axelsson et al. 1989; Bhat and Meny 1984). In contrast, there are also examples of decreased absorption, such as the absorption of fat-soluble vitamins (vitamins D and E) in newborn infants probably because of the inadequate bile salt concentration in the ileum (Strolin Benedetti et al. 2005) or poor lipase hydrolysis of orally administered esters of a prodrug such as the palmitate ester of chloramphenicol (Shankaran and Kauffman 1984). Similarly, one step beyond intestinal absorption and hepatic uptake, the ester prodrug oseltamivir is only partially hydrolyzed to the active oseltamivir carboxylate by human carboxylasases. As the activity of these enzymes is not fully developed in fetuses and young children (Yang et al. 2009), one has to expect a low systemic bioavailability of the active metabolite and a low efficacy of this neuraminidase inhibitor in newborn infants and young children.

Little information regarding the clinical effects of ontogenetic changes of cytochrome P450 enzymes and transporter proteins such as P-glycoprotein (P-gp) in the small bowel is available (Johnson and Thomson 2008). Many oral medicines used in pediatrics are major substrates for intestinal forms of CYP3A. In duodenal biopsy specimens from pediatric patients aged 2 weeks to 17 years, CYP3A4 expression and function were continuously increased with age (Johnson et al. 2001). CYP3A4 was practically absent in the fetal duodenum and was expressed at relatively low levels in the newborn, indicating a low first-pass metabolism of pediatric medicines such as erythromycin (Johnson and Thomson 2008). There is also some evidence that expression of the transporter protein P-gp is very low in the intestines of term infants as compared to young adults (Miki et al. 2005).

Reduced expression of CYP3A and P-pg in newborns and young children can result in increased bioavailability of medicines. For example, a study on oral midazolam in preterm infants showed a higher bioavailability of 49% compared to 27–36% in children (de Wildt et al. 2002; Johnson and Thomson 2008). However, the effect of reduced intestinal and hepatic first-pass metabolism on bioavailability can offset several other bioavailability reducing factors such as altered gut physiology (see above), intraluminal pH, reduced gastric emptying, or intestinal transit time.

Major Organs of Metabolism and Elimination

Decreased systemic clearances for most medicines are mainly related to immaturity of hepatic and renal function (Alcorn and McNamara 2002; Rane 2005). Under normal conditions, parturition triggers the dramatic development of hepatic metabolism and renal function of the newborn term infant. However, there is marked variability in the various maturation processes among the individual drug-metabolizing enzymes and renal excretory functions, which often last over the whole first year of life. Thus, this situation is a rapidly changing transitional phase between the state of a newborn and that of an infant and a toddler (Alcorn and McNamara 2002; Bartelink et al. 2006; Strolin Benedetti et al. 2005). Clearly, at that early stage of development both genetic polymorphisms and ontogeny have a major impact on individualized pharmacotherapy (Allegaert et al. 2007).

The Breast-Fed Infant

Under certain circumstances, breast-feeding and maternal pharmacotherapy can become a neonatal risk. This has been demonstrated by fatal opioid poisoning in neonates, whose breast-feeding mothers are ultrarapid metabolizers of codeine to morphine (Madadi et al. 2009). In this situation, the high maternal morphine levels in breast milk can deliver an excessive morphine load to the low metabolizing infant, resulting in pharmacologically significant opioid levels. However, in general with a few exceptions such as bromocriptine, cocaine, ergotamine, or lithium most maternal medicines are relatively safe for nursing infants (Berlin 2005; Berlin et al. 2009).

3.2.4 Ontogeny of Drug Targets in the Neonatal and Postnatal Periods

Receptors/Binding Sites

Opioid receptors are not fully developed in the newborn rat – one of the most appropriate animal models to study the human species – and mature into adulthood (Freye 1996; Latasch and Freye 2002). A phenomenal increase in opioid binding sites occurs during maturation. Receptor density varies by brain region, with earlier development of caudal and later development in rostral parts of the CNS. Earlier development of opioid receptors in the medulla and pons, where the respiratory center is located, is consistent with the clinical observations that the mean plasma concentration of morphine that induces respiratory depression is in all pediatric age groups including the newborns in the same range, while the mean blood level to suppress pain is – with some overlap – about four to five times higher in newborns and young infants as compared to older infants and children (Bouwmeester et al. 2003; Lynn et al. 1993; Olkkola et al. 1988). These pharmacological differences of opioids in newborns, if neglected, may be a source of adverse drug reactions (e.g., respiratory depression) when attempting to provide rapidly effective opioid analgesia in newborns.

Neurotransmitters, Transporters, and Channels

The present understanding of seizures in the developing brain is derived from animal models. Experimental models provide only a limited view of the complexity of clinical data; however, the electrophysiological, molecular, and anatomical features of seizures in the developing brain can usually transcend interspecies differences (Ben-Ari and Holmes 2006). In addition, during the early postnatal period, a time when the immature brain is highly susceptible to seizures, GABA exerts a paradoxical excitatory action in all animal species, including primates.

The mechanism of increased excitability of the immature brain is basically described as follows (Ben-Ari and Holmes 2006; Ben-Ari et al. 2007): During the early postnatal period, at a time when the immature brain is highly susceptible to seizures, GABA, which in the adult brain is the primary inhibitory neurotransmitter, exerts paradoxical excitatory action. GABA is initially excitatory because of a larger intracellular concentration of chloride in immature neurons compared to mature neurons. The shift from a depolarizing to a hyperpolarizing chloride current is mediated by an active sodium-potassium-2-chloride cotransporter type 1 (NKCC1) that facilitates the accumulation of chloride in neurons and by a delayed expression of a neuron-specific potassium-chloride cotransporter type 2 (KCC2) that extrudes chloride to establish adult concentrations of intracellular chloride. The depolarization by GABA of immature neurons is sufficient to generate sodium action potentials and to activate voltage-dependent calcium channels, leading to a large influx of calcium that in turn triggers long-term changes of synaptic efficacy. The synergistic action of GABA and calcium channels is unique to the developing brain and has many consequences on the impact of GABAergic synapses, such as seizure susceptibility. In addition, agents that interfere with the transport of chloride exert an antiepileptogenic action. With maturation, there is increasing function of KCC2 and decreasing function of NKCC1, which explain the declining strength of depolarization with age. For the clinical consequences of these ontogenetic changes in early infancy, see "Seizures".

3.2.5 Environment and Critical Periods/Windows of Development of Immature Organ Systems with Resulting Permanent Effects

Two examples that demonstrate the sensitivity of time windows of the brain maturation and neuronal plasticity are presented.

Neonatal Painful Injuries and Their Long-Term Effects on Pain Response Later in Life is an Appropriate Example in This Context

The evidence that untreated or insufficiently treated pain in neonates and infants results in long-term adverse consequences (e.g., hyperalgesia) stems from several well-planned studies such as the randomized clinical trial on the effect of neonatal circumcision with and without a topical local anesthetic on pain response during subsequent vaccination 4–6 months later (Taddio et al. 1997). Even in extremely preterm infants, painful procedures during intensive care and surgery have an impact on somatosensory perception later in life (Walker et al. 2009; Hohmeister et al. 2010). Thus, the immature CNS is a challenge when managing pain treatment in infants with an emphasis on the need for a longer term view (Fitzgerald and Walker 2009).

Inappropriate Treatment of Neonatal Seizures Also Has Long-Term Effects on Brain Development and Function

Microcephaly, postnatal epilepsy, developmental delay, cerebral palsy, and behavioral problems are commonly associated with repeated or prolonged and electroencephalographically proven neonatal seizures (Glass and Wirrell 2009; Holmes 2009). While separating the consequences of seizure from consequences of the underlying etiology is clinically quite difficult, there is a considerable body of evidence from animal studies, which support the hypothesis that neonatal seizures can adversely interfere with the highly regulated developmental processes of the brain (Holmes 2009; Holopainen 2008). These animal data indicate that neonatal seizures, in contrast to seizures in a mature stage of the brain with fixed circuitry, are followed by long-lasting and persistent sequelae. These detrimental consequences are caused by alterations of developmental programs rather than by neuronal cell death, as occurs in adults. Decreases in neurogenesis and sprouting of mossy fibers, long-standing changes in signaling, and finally failure to construct efficient networks are the consequences of these alterations. These anatomic and physiologic changes correlate well with behavioral dysfunction and permanent handicaps later in life (Holmes 2009; Holopainen 2008).

All these reports provide good evidence for the need to prevent seizures in neonates. However, highly effective and safe anticonvulsive medicines for neonatal seizures with appropriate target- and age-specificity are not currently available, although some promising drug targets for the immature brain have been proposed (Glass and Wirrell 2009; Sankar and Painter 2005). The most commonly used first-line anticonvulsants, phenobarbital and phenytoin, are borderline effective and potentially neurotoxic for the developing brain (Bittigau et al. 2003).

3.3 The Infant and Toddler: Period of Rapid Growth and Physiological Maturation

3.3.1 Body Composition and Proportion

At this stage of development young children are still rapidly growing. Body weight typically doubles by 5 months of age and triples by 1 year. By the first birthday, body length and surface area increase by 50 and 200%, respectively. During this period of rapid growth, accumulation of fat is remarkably rapid during the first 6 months of age. In contrast, body water content, particularly the extracellular/intracellular ratio, continues to decrease throughout infancy (Fomon and Nelson 2002). From the drug disposition point of view, it is notable that the weight of liver and kidney relative to total body weight reaches maximum in the 1- to 2-year-old child, at the period of life when capacity for drug metabolism and elimination also tends to be greatest (Kauffman 2005; Murry et al. 1995)

3.3.2 Developmental Changes of Physiology with Their Pathophysiology and Typical Disorders with Their Health Problems

Respiratory Tract Infections

During the stage of intense lung growth and airway remodeling, small airway size predisposes the child to acute obstructive lower airway diseases, e.g., bronchiolitis (see also "Receptors/Binding Sites"), as well as to upper respiratory tract infections. These infections probably lead to edema and dysfunction of the Eustachian tube, which frequently contributes to middle ear infection (otitis media) (Kerschner 2007).

General Susceptibility to Infectious Diseases

Postnatal maturation of the immune system is not yet complete during early childhood, similar to the respiratory system (Holt et al. 2005). The reduced capability to express a sustained immune response predisposes young children to infectious diseases. In addition, this concurrent maturation of immunologic and respiratory functions may have implications for programming of long-term response patterns to exogenous inflammatory stimuli within the immune and respiratory systems (Holt et al. 2005).

Seizures

As already mentioned in "Increased Susceptibility to Seizure" and "Neurotransmitters, Transporters, and Channels", this period of maturation is associated with the highest tendency for seizure activity of anytime in life. A large number of pathological processes may lead to seizures, including birth trauma and hypoxic–ischemic insults immediately after birth, systemic infections and metabolic imbalances in neonates, or fever in febrile seizures, which typically happen in infants and young children (Ben-Ari and Holmes 2006). The high excitatory state of the immature brain may also have some impact on the paradoxical effects of midazolam in the very young (Tobin 2008).

Neoplastic Diseases

Embryonic tumors such as neuroblastoma, nephroblastoma (Wilms tumor), and retinoblastoma are most common during the first year of life. These tumors are much less common in older children and adults after cell differentiation processes have slowed considerably (Kadan-Lottick 2007).

3.3.3 Major Organs of Metabolism and Elimination

Frequently but not always, older infants, toddlers, and young children (see also "Functional and Physiological Processes with Their Pathophysiology and Typical Disorders and Their Health Problems") exhibit the greatest overall drug clearance, which is the result of the high metabolic and excretory function of liver and kidney. For example, the half-life of diazepam is shortest in infants and longest in preterm newborns and the elderly, with the magnitude of differences being more than threefold (Coffey et al. 1983; Kauffman 2005; Mandelli et al. 1978). This "toddler overshoot" may lead to therapeutic failure in cases where insufficient dose for age is administered (Anderson and Lynn 2009; Chen et al. 2006; Läer et al. 2005). (For more clinically relevant examples, see "Major Organs of Metabolism and Elimination".)

3.3.4 Ontogeny of Drug Targets

Receptors/Binding Sites

Obstructive bronchiolitis responds poorly to β-adrenergic agonists (betamimetics) due, at least in part, to reduced β-adrenergic receptor sites in the bronchial tree of the wheezing toddler (Chavasse et al. 2002; Gadomski and Bhasale 2006; Lenney and Milner 1978; Schindler 2002). Lack of betamimetic response may also be due to small airways, mucus secretion, and to vasodilatation with mucosal edema of the bronchial wall in bronchiolitis. Betamimetics probably have minimal effect on airway edema as opposed to bronchial smooth muscle contraction. Thus, the most likely explanation of this inconsistency or even failure of a bronchodilator response is the heterogeneity of causes for infantile wheezing (Barr et al. 2000; Subbarao and Ratjen 2006).

Mediators

More recently, another mediator system has been discussed that might be involved in hyperresponsiveness of the tracheal–bronchial system of an infant or toddler. In a well-established guinea pig maturational model that utilizes tracheal strips from infant, juvenile, and adult animals, the role of airway smooth muscle in immature airway hyperresponsiveness has been studied (Chitano et al. 2005). In contrast to the adult, the infantile airway smooth muscle characteristically has a prostanoid-mediated reduction of spontaneous relaxation during electric field stimulation (Wang et al. 2008). Inhibition of prostanoid synthesis abolishes this reduced relaxation and the age difference. A major role for leukotrienes was excluded. Thus, it was concluded that the reduced spontaneous relaxation in immature airway smooth muscle of the guinea pig and probably the airway hyperresponsiveness in the young is associated with and most likely causally related to increased release of contractile prostanoid ($PGF_{2\alpha}$, PGD_2, and TXA_2) (Wang et al. 2008). However, extrapolation of the animal data to infants and toddlers with obstructive airway disease has not yet been validated through well-designed efficacy and toxicity studies with prostanoid synthesis inhibitors. Such well-controlled clinical studies would be quite helpful in resolving the debate as whether ibuprofen is deleterious or protective in children with asthma-related symptoms (Kanabar et al. 2007; Kauffman and Lieh-Lai 2004).

Immune function

Another system, which is subjected to a variety of maturation processes, is the complex in vivo immune system. This complexity makes it extremely difficult to assess its activity quantitatively. Thus, an in vitro model with peripheral blood monocytes has been established, which enables the quantification of cellular pharmacodynamics of the immunosuppressant cyclosporine (Marshall and Kearns 1999). Two surrogate biomarkers of effect have been chosen: Cell proliferation as a functional, yet nonspecific, marker of lymphocyte response to antigen and IL-2 expression as a specific marker of CD4 + lymphocyte activation. As reflected by significant age dependence in the derived pharmacodynamic parameters of IC_{50} (cell proliferation) and IC_{90} (IL-2 expression), the cellular targets for cyclosporine action obtained from infants (<12 months of age) showed a twofold or respectively a sevenfold higher sensitivity to cyclosporine as compared with children, adolescents, and young adults (Marshall and Kearns 1999). This factor, if neglected, may be a source of iatrogenic risk during immunosuppressive therapy of an infant, e.g., after allograft transplantation.

Thermoregulation

In a PK/PD study with ibuprofen, a more favorable antipyretic response was observed for infants compared with older children, despite a pharmacokinetic profile whose parameter estimates were independent of age (Kauffman and Nelson 1992). A mechanism for this age-related difference in the antipyretic response is postulated as follows: Relative surface area in infants is 1.7 times of that in children (>6 years). The skin is the primary organ through which heat is emitted. So the patient with the greatest body surface area relative to the body mass will be most efficient at decreasing body temperature (Kauffman and Nelson 1992).

3.3.5 Environment and Critical Window of Development

Tobacco Exposure Contributes to Sudden Infant Death Syndrome

A critical window of vulnerability of the nicotinic acetylcholine receptors (nAChRs) is hypothesized (Cnattingius 2004; Dwyer et al. 2009; Kinney 2009).

Sudden infant death syndrome (SIDS) remains the leading cause of postnatal infant mortality. There is a major association between intrauterine exposure to cigarette smoking and postnatal environmental tobacco smoke and the risk for SIDS. Furthermore, this risk of death is positively correlated with daily cigarette use (Hunt and Hauck 2007). In searching for an underlying biological mechanism (s), the "brainstem hypothesis" was born (Kinney 2009), which appears to be quite logical as the brainstem is the key brain region that controls the autonomic nervous system including breathing, blood pressure, chemosensitivity, temperature, and upper airway reflexes.

Although SIDS most likely results from a complex interaction of several dysfunctional neurotransmitter systems in the brainstem, there is good evidence from the clinical literature and experimental animal models that the diverse effects of nicotine exposure interfere with the critical regulatory role of nAChRs during prenatal, early postnatal, and even adolescent brain maturation (Dwyer et al. 2009). Various maturational processes in the brain are physiologically regulated by acetylcholine (ACh) via activation of nAChRs, which are ligand-gated ion channels. In accordance with the key regulatory role of ACh throughout ontogenesis, there is a transient appearance and alteration in the subunit composition of nAChRs, particularly during critical periods when brain maturation is most sensitive to perturbation (Dwyer et al. 2009). This is consistent with the key regulatory role of ACh of nAChR ontogenesis. Thus, it is not surprising that this transmitter system can be perturbed by exogenous nicotine exposure during vulnerable developmental windows, leading to serious and persisting consequences.

Methods to assess the function of the autonomic nervous system in infants of mothers who smoked will be essential to investigating the longer term effects of nicotine exposure. So far, during passive repositioning (60° head-up tilt) nicotine-exposed infants exhibit persistent (up to 1 year) cardiovascular stress hyperreactivity with orthostatic dysregulation (Cohen et al. 2010). It remains to be explored, if this autonomic dysfunction in infants of smoking mothers leads to longer lasting "reprogramming" of infant blood pressure control mechanisms and eventually to hypertension. If this were found to be so, autonomic dysregulation in the infant would potentially be an early predictive test for long-term suseptibility to cardiovascular complications later in life.

3.4 The Child: Period of Language, Socialization, and Continued Growth

3.4.1 Body Composition and Proportion

This period is characterized by slower growth rate with slender figure, increasing muscular mass, and relative stable body habitus until the pubertal growth spurt. In general, the various composition compartments – except the extracellular water compartment – remain basically unchanged during this period of steady growth (Ellis 2000; Kauffman 2005).

3.4.2 Functional and Physiological Processes with Their Pathophysiology and Typical Disorders and Their Health Problems

Four Diseases with Immune Dysfunction

- *Rheumatic diseases* of childhood, including connective tissue and collagen diseases, are characterized by autoimmune activity of T- and B-lymphocytes. Typical systemic but nonspecific manifestations are arthralgia, weakness, and fever, which make it absolutely necessary to exclude infections and malignancies (Miller 2007).
- *Acute glomerulonephrits*, such as poststreptococcal glomerulonephritis, is mediated by nephritogenic immune complexes and activation of the complement system. It is most common in children aged 5–12 years and uncommon before the age of 3 years (Davis and Avner 2007).
- *Childhood asthma* represents the most common allergic disorder in children, with severe immune dysregulation and marked expansion of T helper type 2 (Th2) cells that secrete cytokines favoring IgE synthesis and eosinophilia (Leung 2007). Approximately 80% of all asthmatics report disease onset prior to 6 years of age (Liu et al. 2007).
- *Diabetes mellitus type 1* is the most common endocrine–metabolic disorder of childhood and adolescence with two peaks of presentation occurring at the age of 5–7 years and at the time of puberty. The first peak may correspond to the time of increased exposure to infectious agents coincident with the beginning of

school (Alemzadeh and Wyatt 2007). The pathogenesis of this disorder is considered to be an autoimmune destruction of pancreatic islet β-cells, which eventually leads to insulin deficiency.

Epilepsy

Childhood absence epilepsy is the most common form of pediatric seizures. This benign idiopathic generalized epilepsy in an otherwise apparently healthy child is characterized by daily frequent but brief spells. It is uncommon before the age of 5 years and typically goes into remission at the age of 10–12 years with a generally good prognosis (Guerrini 2006).

Neoplastic Diseases

The most common lymphohematopoietic neoplastic diseases, i.e., acute lymphoblastic leukemia and lymphomas, have a striking peak incidence between 2 and 6 years of age. In addition to this age relationship, genetic and environmental risk factors have been observed such as Down syndrome and ionizing radiation (Kadan-Lottick 2007; Tubergen and Bleyer 2007). It is of note that pediatric neoplastic diseases differ markedly from adult malignancies (predominately solid cancers) in prognosis, distribution, tumor site, and molecular biology.

Neurobehavioral Disorders

This period is characterized by increased intellectual performance, rapid language acquisition, socialization, and appearance of behavior disorders. The most common neurobehavioral disorder of childhood and one of the most prevalent chronic health conditions affecting school-aged children are the attention-deficit/hyperactivity disorders (ADHD). Multiple factors have been implicated in the etiology of ADHD, such as perinatal complications (e.g., toxemia and traumatic delivery), maternal smoking and alcohol use, and genetic disposition (Raishevich and Jensen 2007). Unfortunately, a childhood diagnosis of ADHD often leads to persistent ADHD throughout the life span. Besides psychosocial and behaviorally oriented treatment, psychostimulant medication is a therapeutic option. However, this last option is not without risk, particularly when carried out over an extended period of time (see "Ontogeny of Drug Targets").

Accidents

Intensified physical activity, practice of skills, and participation in competitive sports lead to increased risk of vehicular accidents and sports-related injuries at schools or playground, particularly among middle-school-aged children (6–11years of age). Upper extremity and head injuries are by far most common.

3.4.3 Major Organs of Metabolism and Elimination

The child at this stage of development is intermediate between the immature infant and the young adult (Kauffman 2005). The clearances of many hepatically metabolized medicines, such as theophylline (Hendeles and Weinberger 1983), omeprazole (Litalien et al. 2005), midazolam (Reed et al. 2001), and isoniazid (McIlleron et al. 2009) are increased in children (ages 2–11 years) compared with those of adults. This also applies to medicines, which are predominantly eliminated by the kidney, such as sotalol (Läer et al. 2005) and amikacin (Vogelstein et al. 1977). Consequently, higher doses are often required to achieve comparable therapeutic levels.

3.4.4 Ontogeny of Drug Targets

Glucose Metabolism

Recently, Hussain and coworkers reported hypoglycemia in children secondary to β-blocker treatment (Hussain et al. 2009). They presented five patients (1–5 years) out of 570 patients at their institution who were prescribed regular β-blockers over the same time period, who had severe hypoglycemic episodes while taking noncardioselective β-blockers (nadolol and propranolol) for prevention of arrhythmia. From these data, they estimated an overall risk of hypoglycemia to be around 1%. However, when only those children younger than six years of age were considered, they speculated that the hypoglycemic risk is threefold higher. Thus, at that age young children, who are per se prone to idiopathic ketotic hypoglycemia, have to be monitored very carefully when treated with β-blockers, which decreases glycogenolysis, gluconeogenesis, and lipolysis. At least two major possibilities for this instability of glucose homeostasis have to be considered: (1) maturational dysregulation in the adrenergic system, including particularly signal transduction via the β2-adrenergic receptors; or (2) some intrinsic hepatic weakness of glucose mobilization combined with some inappropriate feeding regimen during this phase of early childhood. Ongoing studies with propranolol for severe infantile hemangiomas may provide some additional data in a younger age group (Sans et al. 2009), which will be helpful to answer these questions.

Coagulation System

The age-dependent coagulation system can be described as an evolving and yet functional system in the young (Kuhle et al. 2003). For optimal prevention and diagnosis of hemostatic problems, reference ranges for children of all age groups have been established. However, information on the developmental and maturational changes in the pharmacodynamics of anticoagulants such as warfarin is very limited. Apparently, Japanese children (1–11 years) with low plasma concentrations of vitamin K-dependent coagulation factors possess increased sensitivity to the anticoagulant effect of warfarin (Takahashi et al. 2000). Although prepubertal and adult patients showed comparable mean plasma concentrations of warfarin, prepubertal children showed significant lower plasma concentrations of protein C and prothrombin fragments 1 and 2 and higher INR. This augmented response to warfarin in children, e.g., with congenital heart disease and valve replacement, should be considered when estimating the most appropriate warfarin dose for them.

3.4.5 Environment and Critical Windows of Development

In this prepubescent pediatric population, one has primarily to consider the long-term consequences of drug treatment of patients with chronic diseases or conditions known as the "new pediatric morbidity" such as childhood asthma, neurodevelopmental disorders, and cancer as well as obesity, arterial hypertension, and type 2 diabetes (Cox et al. 2008; Hausner et al. 2008). The latter disorders are the consequences of "modern lifestyle" in Western as well as in emerging countries, characterized by a decline in physical activity and an increased consumption of "fast" processed food with high salt and caloric content. Consequently, there is a growing need for antihypertensives, antihyperlipidemics, and type 2 antidiabetic drugs in children (Cox et al. 2008). The long-term consequences over the whole life span are as yet unknown.

Chemotherapy

While cancer as a cause of morbity and mortality is not new to the pediatric population, as the survival rate has dramatically improved for a variety of neoplastic diseases over the past several decades, the prevalence and duration of chemotherapy has increased. This success in cancer survival is not without long-term effects on later maturation processes, such as those of the reproductive, immunological, skeletal, neural, behavioral, and cardiovascular systems. For example, the anthracycline doxorubicin, a very effective chemotherapeutic agent for certain childhood malignancies, is associated with a delayed serious and potentially life-threatening cardiotoxicity. Even years after completion of medication, particularly when treatment occurred during infancy and early childhood, persistent myocardiocyte loss, myocardial fibrosis, and failure of myocardial growth are observed as sequelae of former doxorubicin treatment (Hausner et al. 2008). In a more recent study, it has been shown that the relative hazard of congestive heart failure, pericardial disease, and valvular abnormities in adult survivors of childhood and adolescent cancer treated with anthracyclines increased two to five times (Mulrooney et al. 2009).

Asthma-Controller Medication

The most common chronic medical condition of children is asthma. Accordingly, use of asthma-controller medication is the highest of all chronic medication use in children (Cox et al. 2008; Hausner et al. 2008). Unfortunately, the potentially negative effects of inhaled glucocorticoids on linear growth, even in the absence of hypothalamic–pituitary axis suppression, as well as long-term deleterious effects on the cardiovascular and pulmonary systems from early intervention with long-acting β-adrenergic receptor agonists are not sufficiently well studied Ducharme et al. 2010; Hausner et al. 2008).

ADHD Medication

In the treatment of ADHD, pharmacotherapy with psychostimulants is commonly employed in school-aged boys (less commonly in girls) to increase the ability to concentrate, improve overall school performance, and attenuate disturbing hyper-activity. With the marked increase in the prescription of these medicines, such as methylphenidate and amphetamines, the warnings about questionable cardiovascu-lar safety of these compounds have become more and more insistent (Nissen 2006). All these sympathomimetic psychostimulants substantially increase heart rate and blood pressure, potentially predisposing the child to serious cardiovascular effects or sudden death, particularly in subgroups of individuals at heightened risk, such as those with congenital heart disorders and/or increased blood pressure. In addition, these agents may have negative effects on sleep, appetite, and growth; effects that are certainly not irrelevant during childhood and adolescence. Thus, it is of utmost importance to carefully consider the benefit-to-risk when prescribing psychostimulant medications.

3.5 The Adolescent: Period of Final Growth and Reproductive Maturation

3.5.1 Body Composition and Proportion

Puberty is another extremely important phase in the physical and psychosocial development of the adolescent. The age of onset of puberty varies as a function of ethnicity, health status, genetics, nutrition, and activity level. Generally, puberty begins between 8 and 14 years and occurs almost two years earlier in females than males (Tanner and Davies 1985).

The main features of this maturation period are as follows: Pubertal growth spurt, which accounts for approximately 25% of final adult height, changes in the body habitus, and remodeling of the body over a relative short period of time with sexual maturation. This includes feminization with more fat content in females and masculinization with more muscular mass in males (Ellis 2000). Besides these changes in skeletal growth and alteration in body composition, cardiorespiratory changes take place such as doubling of the weight of the heart and rise in systolic blood pressure primarily in boys associated with increase in lung size and vital capacity and a drop in respiratory rate (Irwin 2003). Blood volume, red cell mass, and hematocrit increase throughout puberty in boys, while these parameters remain constant for girls. At the same time, dramatically increased levels of gonadal steroid hormones, which are secreted in a pulsatile manner, are involved in regulating plastic changes in neuronal structure and function. These modulation processes of brain circuits at puberty can have effects on changes in social behavior, risk-taking behaviors, and cognitive function at adolescence (Cameron 2004; Paus et al. 2008). Thus, it is not so surprising, when these processes are suboptimal in timing and/or magnitude that the risk of cognitive, affective, and addictive disorders increases (see below).

3.5.2 Functional and Physiological Processes and Their Pathophysiology and Typical Disorders and Their Health Problems

Growth Retardation

Growth retardation, also called stunting, may be a consequence of a variety of factors such as undernutrition, intestinal worm infections, vitamin D deficiency (rickets), chronic intoxication with arsenic and manganese (e.g., through household wells in South Asia), chronic and/or consumptive diseases, long-term drug-induced immunosuppression (e.g., posttransplantation), and premature pubertal development (precocious puberty). In general, optimal intrauterine, infant, and childhood growth is an important basis for satisfactory growth during adolescence.

Endocrine Dysfunctions

– *Precocious, markedly delayed, or absent puberty* are disorders of the hypothalamic–pituitary–gonadal (HPG) axis. Hormonal interventions are directed at both the acute and the long-term consequences of disturbed pubertal development, e.g., treatment of a patient with gonatropin-dependent early puberty (true precocious puberty) with gonadotropin-releasing hormone (GnRH) analogues to postpone pubertal maturation and to secure the pubertal growth spurt and final height by preventing premature closure of the long bone growth plates (Brämswig and

Dübbers 2009). In contrast, delayed pubertal development may be induced by substitution with gonadal steroid hormones in a teenager with absent puberty as a result of a gonadal disorder with hypergonatropic hypogonadism as seen in chromosomal anomalies, such as Ulrich–Turner syndrome.

- *Primary dysfunctional uterine bleeding and dysmenorrhea* remain leading reproductive complaints in menstruating female adolescents. This results from the immature HPG axis and painful prostaglandin-stimulated myometrial contraction, respectively. Thus, early longer term treatment with oral contraceptives and/or prostaglandin synthesis inhibitors appears to be justified (Moscicki 2003), although long-term consequences of this therapy on the reproductive system have not yet been studied.
- After the first peak of presentation in the early school age (see "Four Diseases with Immune Dysfunction"), *diabetes mellitus* type 1 has the second peak of disease onset. This is thought to be related to the pubertal growth spurt induced by gonadal steroids and growth hormone secretion, which antagonizes insulin (Alemzadeh and Wyatt 2007). In this context, it is of note that the second peak in onset occurs – as one would have expected – earlier in girls than in boys.

Malignancies

Malignancies, which are common in early adulthood, such as testicular and ovarian carcinoma, Hodgkin disease, the sarcomas such as osteosarcoma, Ewing sarcoma, and other soft-tissue sarcomas are the most common types of cancer in adolescence (Kadan-Lottick 2007).

Emotional Instability

It is believed that gonadal steroid hormones modulate the activity of a number of neurotransmitter systems, including cholinergic, serotonergic, noradrenergic, and dopaminergic neurons. These complex central nervous system pathways play central roles in regulating many higher order brain functions, including cognitive functions and emotional regulation (Cameron 2004). It is therefore not surprising that suicides, drug addiction, and risk-taking behavior are major health problems in adolescents.

- *Substance use and abuse* such as binge drinking and marijuana and cocaine use are quite common in the adolescent population particularly in the Western countries. Both cigarette use and alcohol use begin early in adolescence with a mean age of onset of about 12 years. Girls consistently report greater daily use of cigarettes than boys, whereas boys report greater use of alcohol than girls (Marcell and Irwin 2003a). Continued nicotine abuse in the female population into the childbearing years has grave implications for future pregnancies, including increased risk of fetal growth restriction, preterm births, still-births, placental abruption, and possibly also sudden infant death syndrome (Cnattingius 2004).

- *Unintentional injuries*, as the result of a high risk-taking behavior in combination with alcohol consumption, are the primary cause of premature mortality in adolescents, accounting for more than 50% of deaths in that age group. It is not surprising that the mortality rate in male teenagers is nearly twice that of girls. Acute traumatic injuries resulting from nonfatal accidents account for the largest number of hospital days and outpatient physician visits for both adolescent boys and girls (Marcell and Irwin 2003b).

Sexual Behavior

Adolescents continue to initiate sexual activity early in the second decade of life. Again age of menarche, ethnic origin, and social status may have a significant influence on the age of first sexual intercourse; but one can assume that more than 50% of middle teen adolescents will have this experience and are prone to sexually transmitted diseases and ectopic pregnancies (Marcell and Irwin 2003c; Dalton 2007).

- *Covariation of risk behaviors*
  As already mentioned above, there is a close association of alcohol and unintentional injury. There also appears to be a relationship between cigarette smoking and the use of illicit substances as well as failure to use effective contraception leading to unintended pregnancy (Marcell and Irwin 2003d). In the worst case, the sequence of progression can be as follows: alcohol and cigarettes precede marijuana use, which is followed by other illicit drugs (including psychedelics, cocaine, heroin, and prescribed and nonprescribed stimulants, sedatives, and tranquilizers), leading to a cumulative effect of all substances and sometimes to high-risk teenage pregnancies.

Mental Health Problems During Adolescence

- *Depression and suicide*
  Transient depressive feelings are common during adolescence. Among these patients, the risk of suicide is increased significantly. Presently, it is the third leading cause of death in adolescents (Boris and Dalton 2007). Rates of completed suicide increase steadily across the teen years, peaking in the early 20s. The male:female ratio for completed suicide is approximately 4:1. For every completed suicide, it is estimated that there are many more (about 50) suicide attempts with significant underreporting and female predominance. Most female suicide attempts involve drug ingestions or superficial cutting, whereas males use more lethal means such as firearms and hanging (Boris and Dalton 2007).

Although adolescent females are more at risk for depression compared to males, males are generally more aggressive and impulsive than females.

– *Eating disorders*

Anorexia nervosa (AN) and bulimia nervosa (BN) are common psychiatric disorders in adolescents and young adults with high rates of morbidity and mortality. The incidence of both disorders has increased in the general population over the last two decades and remains eight times higher in the female than male teenage population (Abraham and Stafford 2007).

Extreme feelings of dissatisfaction with weight and shape and fear of gaining weight are the main causes of these disorders, leading typically to amenorrhea and to a maintenance weight of 15% below the ideal body weight in AN. Other clinical manifestations of eating disorders include severe malnutrition, self-induced vomiting (particularly in BN with episodes of compulsive overeating), and use of laxatives and/or diuretics. This may lead to dehydration, peripheral vasoconstriction, hypothermia, bradycardia, severe electrolyte imbalance with cardiac arrhythmia, osteopenia with stress fractures, hypoproteinemia with peripheral edema, and decreased glomerular filtration. This complex clinical condition is associated with severe medical and psychiatric comorbidity for which pharmacotherapy has a limited role at the present time. Nevertheless, the drugs mainly used in the treatment of eating disorders are antidepressants such as SSRIs, tricyclics, and atypical antipsychotic agents (Powers and Bruty 2009). However, dosing, side-effect profile, and long-term effects of these medications in children and adolescents are not well studied (Hausner et al. 2008).

3.5.3 Major Organs of Metabolism and Elimination

Around the onset of puberty with increased growth hormone levels and activation of the reproductive axis, drug-metabolizing enzyme capacity begins gradually to decline. This decline continues throughout adolescence and concludes with attainment of adult capacity at the completion of pubertal development (Kennedy 2008). During this period of marked hormonal changes and fluctuation, an apparent inverse relationship between levels of growth and sex hormones and drug-metabolizing activity can be observed. For example, a Tanner stage-dependent decrease in CYP1A2-mediated caffeine clearance has been described in healthy adolescents (Lambert et al. 1986). A more direct demonstration of this relationship was observed among growth hormone-deficient prepubertal children in whom physiological growth hormone replacement was associated with a twofold increase in the half-life of amobarbital, a probe of hepatic microsomal drug metabolism (Redmond et al. 1978). At least in part, changes in body composition may also have an effect on the V(d) as illustrated by a highly significant positive correlation of Tanner stage with theophylline elimination half-life and lean body mass and between lean body mass and V(d) in adolescents with asthma (Cary et al. 1991).

Gender differences in drug disposition also become more apparent during puberty (Beierle et al. 1999; Kennedy 2008; Lambert et al. 1986).

Thus, the effects of rapid growth, sexual maturation, and the large amount of variability in the timing of these developmental events on pharmacokinetics must be considered during studies with teenagers. The concept of developmental rather than chronological age should be applied whenever it is possible (Cary et al. 1991; Finkelstein 1994; Kennedy 2008).

These ontogenetic and pharmacokinetic changes during this stage of growth and sexual maturation are especially important when treating common chronic illnesses of adolescence, such as asthma, diabetes, epilepsy, and depression. This complex hormonal and pharmacotherapeutic interplay can further be complicated by on and off oral contraceptive therapy, teenage pregnancy, smoking, self-medication, and illicit drug use.

With respect to renal elimination, it is of note that glomerular filtration and tubular absorption are not influenced by sexual maturation, in contrast to tubular secretion of medicines, e.g., tubular secretion of digoxin, which declines during adolescence to the level seen in adults (Linday et al. 1984; Linday et al. 1981). Methotrexate, which is excreted by the kidney via glomerular filtration and tubular secretion, also shows reduced clearance as a function of age through adolescence (Donelli et al. 1995).

3.5.4 Ontogeny of Drug Targets

The effects of physical growth and sexual maturation on the expression of important drug targets, such as receptors, transporters, and channels, remain essentially unexplored. This is in contrast to the available comprehensive knowledge about ontogenetic differences in pharmacodynamics in the perinatal period. A major obstacle (hurdle) may be greater difficulties in monitoring quantitatively the relevant clinical end points or appropriate surrogate markers of drug action, efficacy, and toxicity throughout the course of pubertal development and sexual maturation. Moreover, pediatricians have relatively neglected research in the area of adolescent medicine in the past.

3.5.5 Environment and Critical Windows of Development

Long-term safety of medicines and, even more so, the long-term consequences of addictive substances use and drug abuse are of major concern in this pediatric population, e.g., tobacco and alcohol consumption and doping with central stimulants or androgens (Dwyer et al. 2009; Hausner et al. 2008; Sjöqvist et al. 2008).

Nicotine as a Gateway Drug

There is ample experimental and some epidemiological evidence that tobacco or nicotine administration particularly during adolescence is a gateway drug that increases the likelihood of subsequent use of other addictive substances (Dwyer et al. 2009). The ability of nicotine to interfere via the AChRs directly or indirectly with various transmitter systems such as the acetycholinergic, dopaminergic, or serotonergic systems may play a role in subsequent addictive behavior. Although the functional role of nAChRs in adolescent maturational processes has not been fully explored, neurochemical and behavioral studies with experimental animals suggest that they may regulate limbic system circuitry that is undergoing critical experience-dependent reshaping during this period (Dwyer et al. 2009). Thus, adolescence may be a particularly vulnerable period, during which nicotine exposure might produce long-term changes in function of the limbic system. This system supports a variety of functions including emotion, behavior, and long-term memory and is hereby involved in addictive disorders.

Anabolic Androgenic Steroids

The misuse of performance-enhancing drugs such as anabolic androgenic steroids is another example of the potential for long-term effects when used during this vulnerable period of maturation. Unfortunately, use of performance enhancers is quite common in young sportspeople, both in high schools and in noncompeting amateurs with a high predominance of male students. The estimated percentage in this adolescent population is at least 3–5% (Sjöqvist et al. 2008). In early adolescents (age 10–13 years), a typical adverse effect with permanent long-term consequences from this kind of doping is premature closure of epiphysial growth plates with ultimate stunted linear growth. In middle and late adolescence testicular atrophy and gynecomastia in males and virilization and long-term amenorrhea in females dominate the endocrine effects. The major cardiovascular side effects are hypertrophic cardiomyopathy and hypertension. In addition, common neuropsychiatric side effects include mood changes, such as mania, hypermania, depression, and increased aggressive behavior (Sjöqvist et al. 2008). In combination with alcohol and central stimulants, anabolic androgenic steroids seem to be strongly synergistic in producing impulsive violent behavior or suicide and homicide, respectively. The whole spectrum of the long-lasting effects of these steroids in humans is not well studied, but at least the effects on muscular fibers last much longer than a couple of years.

Psychostimulants

The long-term risk of extended use and misuse of central stimulants as performance-enhancing drugs has already been mentioned and briefly discussed in

"ADHD Medication". These risks are particularly relevant for the male teenage population at secondary school, in which the diagnosis of ADHD is frequently made with a prevalence of about 8% as compared to only 2% in girls (Huss et al. 2008).

4 Future Directions

There is a permanent need to fill the gaps of our knowledge about the continuous developmental changes of therapeutic targets (e.g., enzymes, transporters, receptors, and channels) from the fetus to young adult. These gaps include following sections.

4.1 Appropriate Tools for Assessment of Drug Action

Development of age-appropriate methods and tools for the assessment of drug actions and effects in the pediatric population, such as intermediate end point or surrogate markers, biomarkers, functional tests, scores, scales, and PK/PD analyses.

4.2 Appropriate Animals and Cell Models

Development of appropriate and predictive animal models, cell systems, in vitro tests, and in silico simulation; all tools which are important and helpful to manage – at least in part – the delicate and ethically and legally complex situation of research in a very vulnerable population.

4.3 Appropriate Methods for Long-Term Safety Effects

Development of appropriate epidemiological methods for the evaluation of long-term safety and potential programming effects of pharmacological interventions at an early stage of development, assessment of predictive value of surrogate end points in predicting long-term efficacy and toxicity (particularly with chronic exposures), identification of vulnerable windows of developmentally immature organ systems (e.g., cardiovascular, neurological, immunological, and reproductive systems) that might be especially sensitive to pharmacological perturbation, and additional study to evaluate the impact of a disease state that is unique to children.

References

Abraham A, Stafford B (2007) Eating disorders. In: Kliegman RM, Behrman RE, Jenson HB, Stanton BF (eds) Nelson textbook of pediatrics, 18th edn. Saunders Elsevier, Philadelphia

Ahlfors CE (2004) Effect of ibuprofen on bilirubin–albumin binding. J Pediatr 144:386–388

Ahmad I, Nemet D, Eliakim A, Koeppel R, Grochow D, Coussens M, Gallitto S, Rich J, Pontello A, Leu SY, Cooper DM, Waffarn F (2010) Body composition and its components in preterm and term newborns: a cross-sectional, multimodal investigation. Am J Hum Biol 22:69–75

al-Alaiyan S, al-Rawithi S, Raines D, Yusuf A, Legayada E, Shoukri MM, el-Yazigi A (2001) Caffeine metabolism in premature infants. J Clin Pharmacol 41:620–627

Alcorn J, McNamara PJ (2002) Ontogeny of hepatic and renal systemic clearance pathways in infants: part II. Clin Pharmacokinet 41:1077–1094

Alemzadeh R, Wyatt DT (2007) Diabetes mellitus in children. In: Kliegman RM, Behrman RE, Jenson HB, Stanton BF (eds) Nelson textbook of pediatrics, 18th edn. Saunders Elsevier, Philadelphia

Allegaert K, van den Anker JN, Naulaers G, de Hoon J (2007) Determinants of drug metabolism in early neonatal life. Curr Clin Pharmacol 2:23–29

Anderson GD, Lynn AM (2009) Optimizing pediatric dosing: a developmental pharmacologic approach. Pharmacotherapy 29:680–690

Asmar BI, Abdel-Haq NM (2005) Macrolides, chloramphenicol, and tetracyclines. In: Yaffe SJ, Aranda JV (eds) Neonatal and pediatric pharmacology – therapeutic principles in practice, 3rd edn. Lippincott Williams & Wilkins, Philadelphia

Axelsson I, Jakobsson I, Lindberg T, Polberger S, Benediktsson B, Raiha N (1989) Macromolecular absorption in preterm and term infants. Acta Paediatr Scand 78:532–537

Balazy M, Chemtob S (2008) Trans-arachidonic acids: new mediators of nitro-oxidative stress. Pharmacol Ther 119:275–290

Barr FE, Patel NR, Newth CJ (2000) The pharmacologic mechanism by which inhaled epinephrine reduces airway obstruction in respiratory syncytial virus-associated bronchiolitis. J Pediatr 136:699–700

Barrett DA, Rutter N (1994) Transdermal delivery and the premature neonate. Crit Rev Ther Drug Carrier Syst 11:1–30

Bartelink IH, Rademaker CM, Schobben AF, van den Anker JN (2006) Guidelines on paediatric dosing on the basis of developmental physiology and pharmacokinetic considerations. Clin Pharmacokinet 45:1077–1097

Battino D, Estienne M, Avanzini G (1995) Clinical pharmacokinetics of antiepileptic drugs in paediatric patients. Part I: phenobarbital, primidone, valproic acid, ethosuximide and mesuximide. Clin Pharmacokinet 29:257–286

Beierle I, Meibohm B, Derendorf H (1999) Gender differences in pharmacokinetics and pharmacodynamics. Int J Clin Pharmacol Ther 37:529–547

Ben-Ari Y, Holmes GL (2006) Effects of seizures on developmental processes in the immature brain. Lancet Neurol 5:1055–1063

Ben-Ari Y, Gaiarsa JL, Tyzio R, Khazipov R (2007) GABA: a pioneer transmitter that excites immature neurons and generates primitive oscillations. Physiol Rev 87:1215–1284

Berlin CM Jr (2005) The excretion of drugs and chemicals in human milk. In: Yaffe SJ, Aranda JV (eds) Neonatal and pediatric pharmacology – therapeutic principles in practice, 3rd edn. Lippincott Williams & Wilkins, Philadelpha

Berlin CM Jr, Paul IM, Vesell ES (2009) Safety issues of maternal drug therapy during breastfeeding. Clin Pharmacol Ther 85:20–22

Bhat AM, Meny RG (1984) Alimentary absorption of gentamicin in preterm infants. Clin Pediatr (Phila) 23:683–685

Bittigau P, Sifringer M, Ikonomidou C (2003) Antiepileptic drugs and apoptosis in the developing brain. Ann NY Acad Sci 993:103–114

Boie Y, Rushmore TH, rmon-Goodwin A, Grygorczyk R, Slipetz DM, Metters KM, Abramovitz M (1994) Cloning and expression of a cDNA for the human prostanoid IP receptor. J Biol Chem 269:12173–12178

Boréus LO (1972) Fetal pharmacology. Raven Press, New York

Boris NW, Dalton R (2007) Suicide and attempted suicide. In: Kliegman RM, Behrman RE, Jenson HB, Stanton BF (eds) Nelson textbook of pediatrics, 18th edn. Saunders Elsevier, Philadelphia

Bory C, Baltassat P, Porthault M, Bethenod M, Frederich A, Aranda JV (1979) Metabolism of theophylline to caffeine in premature newborn infants. J Pediatr 94:988–993

Bouayad A, Kajino H, Waleh N, Fouron JC, Andelfinger G, Varma DR, Skoll A, Vazquez A, Gobeil F Jr, Clyman RI, Chemtob S (2001) Characterization of PGE2 receptors in fetal and newborn lamb ductus arteriosus. Am J Physiol Heart Circ Physiol 280:H2342–H2349

Bouwmeester NJ, van den Anker JN, Hop WC, Anand KJ, Tibboel D (2003) Age- and therapy-related effects on morphine requirements and plasma concentrations of morphine and its metabolites in postoperative infants. Br J Anaesth 90:642–652

Brämswig J, Dübbers A (2009) Disorders of pubertal development. Dtsch Arztebl Int 106:295–303

Cameron JL (2004) Interrelationships between hormones, behavior, and affect during adolescence: understanding hormonal, physical, and brain changes occurring in association with pubertal activation of the reproductive axis. Introduction to part III. Ann N Y Acad Sci 1021:110–123

Cary J, Hein K, Dell R (1991) Theophylline disposition in adolescents with asthma. Ther Drug Monit 13:309–313

Celsi G, Aperia A (1993) Sodium, chloride, and water. In: Holliday MA, Barratt TM, Evner ED (eds) Pediatric nephrology. Lippincott Williams & Wilkins, Philadelphia

Charles BG, Townsend SR, Steer PA, Flenady VJ, Gray PH, Shearman A (2008) Caffeine citrate treatment for extremely premature infants with apnea: population pharmacokinetics, absolute bioavailability, and implications for therapeutic drug monitoring. Ther Drug Monit 30:709–716

Chavasse R, Seddon P, Bara A, McKean M (2002) Short acting beta agonists for recurrent wheeze in children under 2 years of age. Cochrane Database Syst Rev: CD002873

Chen N, Aleksa K, Woodland C, Rieder M, Koren G (2006) Ontogeny of drug elimination by the human kidney. Pediatr Nephrol 21:160–168

Chitano P, Wang L, Murphy TM (2005) Mechanisms of airway smooth muscle relaxation during maturation. Can J Physiol Pharmacol 83:833–840

Clapp DW (2006) Developmental regulation of the immune system. Semin Perinatol 30:69–72

Clyman RI, Waleh N, Kajino H, Roman C, Mauray F (2007) Calcium-dependent and calcium-sensitizing pathways in the mature and immature ductus arteriosus. Am J Physiol Regul Integr Comp Physiol 293:R1650–R1656

Cnattingius S (2004) The epidemiology of smoking during pregnancy: smoking prevalence, maternal characteristics, and pregnancy outcomes. Nicotine Tob Res 6(Suppl 2):S125–S140

Coffey B, Shader RI, Greenblatt DJ (1983) Pharmacokinetics of benzodiazepines and psychostimulants in children. J Clin Psychopharmacol 3:217–225

Coffman BL, Rios GR, King CD, Tephly TR (1997) Human UGT2B7 catalyzes morphine glucuronidation. Drug Metab Dispos 25:1–4

Cohen G, Jeffery H, Lagercrantz H, Katz-Salamon M (2010) Long-term reprogramming of cardiovascular function in infants of active smokers. Hypertension 55:722–728

Colussi G, Bettinelli A, Tedeschi S, De Ferrari ME, Syren ML, Borsa N, Mattiello C, Casari G, Bianchetti MG (2007) A thiazide test for the diagnosis of renal tubular hypokalemic disorders. Clin J Am Soc Nephrol 2:454–460

Commare CE, Tappenden KA (2007) Development of the infant intestine: implications for nutrition support. Nutr Clin Pract 22:159–173

Cox ER, Halloran DR, Homan SM, Welliver S, Mager DE (2008) Trends in the prevalence of chronic medication use in children: 2002–2005. Pediatrics 122:e1053–e1061

Dalton R (2007) The development of sexual behavior. In: Kliegman RM, Behrman RE, Jenson HB, Stanton BF (eds) Nelson textbook of pediatrics, 18th edn. Saunders Elsevier, Philadelphia

Davis ID, Avner ED (2007) Acute poststreptococcal glomerulonephritis. In: Kliegman RM, Behrman RE, Jenson HB, Stanton BF (eds) Nelson textbook of pediatrics, 18th edn. Saunders Elsevier, Philadelphia

de Wildt SN, Kearns GL, Hop WC, Murry DJ, Bdel-Rahman SM, van den Anker JN (2002) Pharmacokinetics and metabolism of oral midazolam in preterm infants. Br J Clin Pharmacol 53:390–392

Donelli MG, Zucchetti M, Robatto A, Perlangeli V, D'Incalci M, Masera G, Rossi MR (1995) Pharmacokinetics of HD-MTX in infants, children, and adolescents with non-B acute lymphoblastic leukemia. Med Pediatr Oncol 24:154–159

Doyle LW, Ehrenkranz RA, Halliday HL (2010) Dexamethasone treatment in the first week of life for preventing bronchopulmonary dysplasia in preterm infants: a systematic review. Neonatology 98:217–224

Dubois J, Dehaene-Lambertz G, Perrin M, Mangin JF, Cointepas Y, Duchesnay E, Le BD, Hertz-Pannier L (2008) Asynchrony of the early maturation of white matter bundles in healthy infants: quantitative landmarks revealed noninvasively by diffusion tensor imaging. Hum Brain Mapp 29:14–27

Ducharme FM, Ni CM, Greenstone I, Lasserson TJ (2010) Addition of long-acting beta2-agonists to inhaled steroids versus higher dose inhaled steroids in adults and children with persistent asthma. Cochrane Database Syst Rev 4: CD005533

Dwyer JB, McQuown SC, Leslie FM (2009) The dynamic effects of nicotine on the developing brain. Pharmacol Ther 122:125–139

Ellis KJ (2000) Human body composition: in vivo methods. Physiol Rev 80:649–680

Evans N, Moorcraft J (1992) Effect of patency of the ductus arteriosus on blood pressure in very preterm infants. Arch Dis Child 67:1169–1173

Fawer CL, Torrado A, Guignard JP (1979) Maturation of renal function in full-term and premature neonates. Helv Paediatr Acta 34:11–21

Fettermann GH, Shuplock NA, Philipp FJ, Gregg HS (1965) The growth and maturation of human glomeruli and proximal convolutions from term to adulthood: studies by microdissection. Pediatrics 35:601–619

Finkelstein JW (1994) The effect of developmental changes in adolescence on drug disposition. J Adolesc Health 15:612–618

Fischl R (1902) Ueber Behandlung und Medikation bei Kindern im Allgemeinen. In: Biedert PH (ed) Lehrbuch der Kinderkrankheiten. Verlag von Ferdinand Enke, Stuttgart

FitzGerald GA, Patrono C (2001) The coxibs, selective inhibitors of cyclooxygenase-2. N Engl J Med 345:433–442

Fitzgerald M, Walker SM (2009) Infant pain management: a developmental neurobiological approach. Nat Clin Pract Neurol 5:35–50

Fleck C, Bräunlich H (1995) Renal handling of drugs and amino acids after impairment of kidney or liver function – influences of maturity and protective treatment. Pharmacol Ther 67:53–77

Fomon SJ, Nelson SE (2002) Body composition of the male and female reference infants. Annu Rev Nutr 22:1–17

Food and Drug Administration (2000) International Conference on Harmonisation; guidance on E11 clinical investigation of medicinal products in the pediatric population; availability. Notice. Fed Regist 65:78493–78494

Fraser J, Nadeau J, Robertson D, Wood AJ (1981) Regulation of human leukocyte beta receptors by endogenous catecholamines: relationship of leukocyte beta receptor density to the cardiac sensitivity to isoproterenol. J Clin Invest 67:1777–1784

Freye E (1996) Development of sensory information processing – the ontogenesis of opioid binding sites in nociceptive afferents and their significance in the clinical setting. Acta Anaesthesiol Scand Suppl 109:98–101

Frölich JC (1997) A classification of NSAIDs according to the relative inhibition of cyclooxygenase isoenzymes. Trends Pharmacol Sci 18:30–34

Gadomski AM, Bhasale AL (2006) Bronchodilators for bronchiolitis. Cochrane Database Syst Rev 3: CD001266

Gal P, Ransom JL, Davis SA (2006) Possible ibuprofen-induced kernicterus in a near-term infant with moderate hyperbilirubinemia. J Pediatr Pharmacol Ther 11:245–250

Glass HC, Wirrell E (2009) Controversies in neonatal seizure management. J Child Neurol 24:591–599

Goto S, Seo T, Murata T, Nakada N, Ueda N, Ishitsu T, Nakagawa K (2007) Population estimation of the effects of cytochrome P450 2C9 and 2C19 polymorphisms on phenobarbital clearance in Japanese. Ther Drug Monit 29:118–121

Green TP, Thompson TR, Johnson DE, Lock JE (1983) Diuresis and pulmonary function in premature infants with respiratory distress syndrome. J Pediatr 103:618–623

Guerrini R (2006) Epilepsy in children. Lancet 367:499–524

Guignard JP (2002) The adverse renal effects of prostaglandin-synthesis inhibitors in the newborn rabbit. Semin Perinatol 26:398–405

Hammerman C, Glaser J, Kaplan M, Schimmel MS, Ferber B, Eidelman AI (1998) Indomethacin tocolysis increases postnatal patent ductus arteriosus severity. Pediatrics 102:E56

Hammerman C, Shchors I, Jacobson S, Schimmel MS, Bromiker R, Kaplan M, Nir A (2008) Ibuprofen versus continuous indomethacin in premature neonates with patent ductus arteriosus: is the difference in the mode of administration? Pediatr Res 64:291–297

Hartley R, Green M, Quinn MW, Rushforth JA, Levene MI (1994) Development of morphine glucuronidation in premature neonates. Biol Neonate 66:1–9

Hausner E, Fiszman ML, Hanig J, Harlow P, Zornberg G, Sobel S (2008) Long-term consequences of drugs on the paediatric cardiovascular system. Drug Saf 31:1083–1096

Hellström A, Ley D, Hansen-Pupp I, Niklasson A, Smith L, Lofqvist C, Hard AL (2009) New insights into the development of retinopathy of prematurity – importance of early weight gain. Acta Paediatr 99:502–508

Hendeles L, Weinberger M (1983) Theophylline. A "state of the art" review. Pharmacotherapy 3:2–44

Hohmeister J, Kroll A, Wollgarten-Hadamek I, Zohsel K, Demirakca S, Hermann C (2010) Cerebral processing of pain in school-age children with neonatal nociceptive input: an exploratory fMRI study. Pain 150:257–267

Holmes GL (2009) The long-term effects of neonatal seizures. Clin Perinatol 36:901–914

Holmström G, van Wijngaarden P, Coster DJ, Williams KA (2007) Genetic susceptibility to retinopathy of prematurity: the evidence from clinical and experimental animal studies. Br J Ophthalmol 91:1704–1708

Holopainen IE (2008) Seizures in the developing brain: cellular and molecular mechanisms of neuronal damage, neurogenesis and cellular reorganization. Neurochem Int 52:935–947

Holt PG, Upham JW, Sly PD (2005) Contemporaneous maturation of immunologic and respiratory functions during early childhood: implications for development of asthma prevention strategies. J Allergy Clin Immunol 116:16–24

Honda A, Sugimoto Y, Namba T, Watabe A, Irie A, Negishi M, Narumiya S, Ichikawa A (1993) Cloning and expression of a cDNA for mouse prostaglandin E receptor EP2 subtype. J Biol Chem 268:7759–7762

Hunt CE (2006) Ontogeny of autonomic regulation in late preterm infants born at 34–37 weeks postmenstrual age. Semin Perinatol 30:73–76

Hunt CE, Hauck FR (2007) Sudden infant death syndrome. In: Kliegman RM, Behrman RE, Jenson HB, Stanton BF (eds) Nelson textbook of pediatrics, 18th edn. Saunders Elsevier, Philadelphia

Huss M, Hölling H, Kurth BM, Schlack R (2008) How often are German children and adolescents diagnosed with ADHD? Prevalence based on the judgment of health care professionals: results of the German health and examination survey (KiGGS). Eur Child Adolesc Psychiatry 17(Suppl 1):52–58

Hussain T, Greenhalgh K, McLeod KA (2009) Hypoglycaemic syncope in children secondary to beta-blockers. Arch Dis Child 94:968–969

Irwin CE Jr (2003) Somatic growth and development during adolescence. In: Rudolph CD, Rudolph AM, Hostetter MK, Lister G, Siegel NJ (eds) Rudolph's pediatrics, 21st edn. McGraw Hill Medical, New York

Jain A, Agarwal R, Sankar MJ, Deorari AK, Paul VK (2008a) Hypocalcemia in the newborn. Indian J Pediatr 75:165–169

Jain A, Aggarwal R, Jeevasanker M, Agarwal R, Deorari AK, Paul VK (2008b) Hypoglycemia in the newborn. Indian J Pediatr 75:63–67

Jeck N, Schlingmann KP, Reinalter SC, Komhoff M, Peters M, Waldegger S, Seyberth HW (2005) Salt handling in the distal nephron: lessons learned from inherited human disorders. Am J Physiol Regul Integr Comp Physiol 288:R782–R795

Johnson TN, Thomson M (2008) Intestinal metabolism and transport of drugs in children: the effects of age and disease. J Pediatr Gastroenterol Nutr 47:3–10

Johnson TN, Tanner MS, Taylor CJ, Tucker GT (2001) Enterocytic CYP3A4 in a paediatric population: developmental changes and the effect of coeliac disease and cystic fibrosis. Br J Clin Pharmacol 51:451–460

Kadan-Lottick NS (2007) Epidemiology of childhood and adolescent cancer. In: Kliegman RM, Behrman RE, Jenson HB, Stanton BF (eds) Nelson textbook of pediatrics, 18th edn. Saunders Elsevier, Philadelphia

Kanabar D, Dale S, Rawat M (2007) A review of ibuprofen and acetaminophen use in febrile children and the occurrence of asthma-related symptoms. Clin Ther 29:2716–2723

Kauffman RE (2005) Drug action and therapy in infants and children. In: Yaffe SJ, Aranda JV (eds) Neonatal and pediatric pharmacology – therapeutic principles in practice, 3rd edn. Lippincott Williams & Wilkins, Philadelphia

Kauffman RE, Lieh-Lai M (2004) Ibuprofen and increased morbidity in children with asthma: fact or fiction? Paediatr Drugs 6:267–272

Kauffman RE, Nelson MV (1992) Effect of age on ibuprofen pharmacokinetics and antipyretic response. J Pediatr 121:969–973

Kearns GL, Abdel-Rahman SM, Alander SW, Blowey DL, Leeder JS, Kauffman RE (2003) Developmental pharmacology – drug disposition, action, and therapy in infants and children. N Engl J Med 349:1157–1167

Kennedy M (2008) Hormonal regulation of hepatic drug-metabolizing enzyme activity during adolescence. Clin Pharmacol Ther 84:662–673

Kermorvant-Duchemin E, Sapieha P, Sirinyan M, Beauchamp M, Checchin D, Hardy P, Sennlaub F, Lachapelle P, Chemtob S (2010) Understanding ischemic retinopathies: emerging concepts from oxygen-induced retinopathy. Doc Ophthalmol 120:51–60

Kerschner JE (2007) Otitis media. In: Kliegman RM, Behrman RE, Jenson HB, Stanton BF (eds) Nelson textbook of pediatrics, 18th edn. Saunders Elsevier, Philadelphia

Kinney HC (2009) Brainstem mechanisms underlying the sudden infant death syndrome: evidence from human pathologic studies. Dev Psychobiol 51:223–233

Köckerling A, Reinalter SC, Seyberth HW (1996) Impaired response to furosemide in hyperprostaglandin E syndrome: evidence for a tubular defect in the loop of Henle. J Pediatr 129:519–528

Konduri GG, Kim UO (2009) Advances in the diagnosis and management of persistent pulmonary hypertension of the newborn. Pediatr Clin North Am 56:579–600

Koren G, Boucher N (2009) Adverse effects in neonates exposed to SSRIs and SNRI in late gestation – Motherisk update 2008. Can J Clin Pharmacol 16:e66–e67

Koukouritaki SB, Manro JR, Marsh SA, Stevens JC, Rettie AE, McCarver DG, Hines RN (2004) Developmental expression of human hepatic CYP2C9 and CYP2C19. J Pharmacol Exp Ther 308:965–974

Kuhle S, Male C, Mitchell L (2003) Developmental hemostasis: pro- and anticoagulant systems during childhood. Semin Thromb Hemost 29:329–338

Läer S, Elshoff JP, Meibohm B, Weil J, Mir TS, Zhang W, Hulpke-Wette M (2005) Development of a safe and effective pediatric dosing regimen for sotalol based on population pharmacokinetics and pharmacodynamics in children with supraventricular tachycardia. J Am Coll Cardiol 46:1322–1330

Lambert GH, Schoeller DA, Kotake AN, Flores C, Hay D (1986) The effect of age, gender, and sexual maturation on the caffeine breath test. Dev Pharmacol Ther 9:375–388

Latasch L, Freye E (2002) Pain and opioids in preterm and newborns. Anaesthesist 51:272–284

Lebenthal A, Lebenthal E (1999) The ontogeny of the small intestinal epithelium. JPEN J Parenter Enteral Nutr 23:S3–S6

Lenney W, Milner AD (1978) At what age do bronchodilator drugs work? Arch Dis Child 53:532–535

Leonhardt A, Seyberth HW (2003) Do we need another NSAID instead of indomethacin for treatment of ductus arteriosus in preterm infants? Acta Paediatr 92:996–999

Leonhardt A, Glaser A, Wegmann M, Schranz D, Seyberth H, Nusing R (2003) Expression of prostanoid receptors in human ductus arteriosus. Br J Pharmacol 138:655–659

Leonhardt A, Strehl R, Barth H, Seyberth HW (2004) High efficacy and minor renal effects of indomethacin treatment during individualized fluid intake in premature infants with patent ductus arteriosus. Acta Paediatr 93:233–240

Leung DYM (2007) Allergy and the immumologic basis of atopic disease. In: Kliegman RM, Behrman RE, Jenson HB, Stanton BF (eds) Nelson textbook of pediatrics, 18th edn. Saunders Elsevier, Philadelphia

Levene M (2007) Minimising neonatal brain injury: how research in the past five years has changed my clinical practice. Arch Dis Child 92:261–265

Linday LA, Engle MA, Reidenberg MM (1981) Maturation and renal digoxin clearance. Clin Pharmacol Ther 30:735–738

Linday LA, Drayer DE, Khan MA, Cicalese C, Reidenberg MM (1984) Pubertal changes in net renal tubular secretion of digoxin. Clin Pharmacol Ther 35:438–446

Litalien C, Theoret Y, Faure C (2005) Pharmacokinetics of proton pump inhibitors in children. Clin Pharmacokinet 44:441–466

Liu AH, Covar RA, Spahn JD, Leung DYM (2007) Childhood asthma. In: Kliegman RM, Behrman RE, Jenson HB, Stanton BF (eds) Nelson textbook of pediatrics, 18th edn. Saunders Elsevier, Philadelphia

Liu H, Manganiello V, Waleh N, Clyman RI (2008) Expression, activity, and function of phosphodiesterases in the mature and immature ductus arteriosus. Pediatr Res 64:477–481

Löscher W, Klotz U, Zimprich F, Schmidt D (2009) The clinical impact of pharmacogenetics on the treatment of epilepsy. Epilepsia 50:1–23

Lowry JA, Jarrett RV, Wasserman G, Pettett G, Kauffman RE (2001) Theophylline toxicokinetics in premature newborns. Arch Pediatr Adolesc Med 155:934–939

Lynn AM, Nespeca MK, Opheim KE, Slattery JT (1993) Respiratory effects of intravenous morphine infusions in neonates, infants, and children after cardiac surgery. Anesth Analg 77:695–701

Madadi P, Ross CJ, Hayden MR, Carleton BC, Gaedigk A, Leeder JS, Koren G (2009) Pharmacogenetics of neonatal opioid toxicity following maternal use of codeine during breastfeeding: a case-control study. Clin Pharmacol Ther 85:31–35

Mandelli M, Tognoni G, Garattini S (1978) Clinical pharmacokinetics of diazepam. Clin Pharmacokinet 3:72–91

Marcell AB, Irwin CE Jr (2003a) Risk-taking behaviors: substance use and abuse. In: Rudolph CD, Rudolph AM, Hostetter MK, Lister G, Siegel NJ (eds) Rudolph's pediatrics, 21st edn. McGraw Hill Medical, New York

Marcell AB, Irwin CE Jr (2003b) Risk-taking behaviors: unintentional injuries. In: Rudolph CD, Rudolph AM, Hostetter MK, Lister G, Siegel NJ (eds) Rudolph's pediatrics, 21st edn. McGraw Hill Medical, New York

Marcell AV, Irwin CE Jr (2003c) Risk-taking behaviors: sexual behavior. In: Rudolph CD, Rudolph AM, Hostetter MK, Lister G, Siegel NJ (eds) Rudolph's pediatrics, 21st edn. McGraw Hill Medical, New York

Marcell AV, Irwin, Jr CE (2003d) Risk-taking behaviors: covariation of risk behavoirs. In: Rudolph CD, Rudolph AM, Hostetter MK, Lister G, Siegel NJ (eds) Rudolph's Pediatrics, 21st edn. McGraw Hill Medical, New York

Marshall JD, Kearns GL (1999) Developmental pharmacodynamics of cyclosporine. Clin Pharmacol Ther 66:66–75

McCracken GH Jr (1986) Aminoglycoside toxicity in infants and children. Am J Med 80:172–178

McIlleron H, Willemse M, Werely CJ, Hussey GD, Schaaf HS, Smith PJ, Donald PR (2009) Isoniazid plasma concentrations in a cohort of South African children with tuberculosis: implications for international pediatric dosing guidelines. Clin Infect Dis 48:1547–1553

Miki Y, Suzuki T, Tazawa C, Blumberg B, Sasano H (2005) Steroid and xenobiotic receptor (SXR), cytochrome P450 3A4 and multidrug resistance gene 1 in human adult and fetal tissues. Mol Cell Endocrinol 231:75–85

Miller ML (2007) Evaluation of suspected rheumatic disease. In: Kliegman RM, Behrman RE, Jenson HB, Stanton BF (eds) Nelson textbook of pediatrics, 18th edn. Saunders Elsevier, Philadelphia

Mirochnick MH, Miceli JJ, Kramer PA, Chapron DJ, Raye JR (1988) Furosemide pharmacokinetics in very low birth weight infants. J Pediatr 112:653–657

Momma K, Toyoshima K, Takeuchi D, Imamura S, Nakanishi T (2005a) In vivo reopening of the neonatal ductus arteriosus by a prostanoid EP4-receptor agonist in the rat. Prostaglandins Other Lipid Mediat 78:117–128

Momma K, Toyoshima K, Takeuchi D, Imamura S, Nakanishi T (2005b) In vivo constriction of the fetal and neonatal ductus arteriosus by a prostanoid EP4-receptor antagonist in rats. Pediatr Res 58:971–975

Momma K, Toyoshima K, Ito K, Sugiyama K, Imamura S, Sun F, Nakanishi T (2009) Delayed neonatal closure of the ductus arteriosus following early in utero exposure to indomethacin in the rat. Neonatology 96:69–79

Moscicki AB (2003) Common menstrual problems. In: Rudolph CD, Rudolph AM, Hostetter MK, Lister G, Siegel NJ (eds) Rudolph's pediatrics, 21st edn. McGraw Hill Medical, New York

Mulrooney DA, Yeazel MW, Kawashima T, Mertens AC, Mitby P, Stovall M, Donaldson SS, Green DM, Sklar CA, Robison LL, Leisenring WM (2009) Cardiac outcomes in a cohort of adult survivors of childhood and adolescent cancer: retrospective analysis of the Childhood Cancer Survivor Study cohort. BMJ 339:b4606

Murry DJ, Crom WR, Reddick WE, Bhargava R, Evans WE (1995) Liver volume as a determinant of drug clearance in children and adolescents. Drug Metab Dispos 23:1110–1116

Nakanishi T, Gu H, Hagiwara N, Momma K (1993) Mechanisms of oxygen-induced contraction of ductus arteriosus isolated from the fetal rabbit. Circ Res 72:1218–1228

Narayanan M, Schlueter M, Clyman RI (1999) Incidence and outcome of a 10-fold indomethacin overdose in premature infants. J Pediatr 135:105–107

Natarajan G, Botica ML, Thomas R, Aranda JV (2007) Therapeutic drug monitoring for caffeine in preterm neonates: an unnecessary exercise? Pediatrics 119:936–940

Neu J (2007) Gastrointestinal development and meeting the nutritional needs of premature infants. Am J Clin Nutr 85:629S–634S

Nissen SE (2006) ADHD drugs and cardiovascular risk. N Engl J Med 354:1445–1448

No authors listed (2004) Morbidity and mortality among outborn neonates at 10 tertiary care institutions in India during the year 2000. J Trop Pediatr 50:170–174

Norton ME, Merrill J, Cooper BA, Kuller JA, Clyman RI (1993) Neonatal complications after the administration of indomethacin for preterm labor. N Engl J Med 329:1602–1607

Ohlsson A, Walia R, Shah S (2008) Ibuprofen for the treatment of patent ductus arteriosus in preterm and/or low birth weight infants. Cochrane Database Syst Rev: CD003481

Olkkola KT, Maunuksela EL, Korpela R, Rosenberg PH (1988) Kinetics and dynamics of postoperative intravenous morphine in children. Clin Pharmacol Ther 44:128–136

Pacifici GM (2009) Clinical pharmacokinetics of aminoglycosides in the neonate: a review. Eur J Clin Pharmacol 65:419–427

Paradisis M, Evans N, Kluckow M, Osborn D (2009) Randomized trial of milrinone versus placebo for prevention of low systemic blood flow in very preterm infants. J Pediatr 154:189–195

Paus T, Keshavan M, Giedd JN (2008) Why do many psychiatric disorders emerge during adolescence? Nat Rev Neurosci 9:947–957

Peters M, Jeck N, Reinalter S, Leonhardt A, Tonshoff B, Klaus GG, Konrad M, Seyberth HW (2002) Clinical presentation of genetically defined patients with hypokalemic salt-losing tubulopathies. Am J Med 112:183–190

Peterson RG, Simmons MA, Rumack BH, Levine RL, Brooks JG (1980) Pharmacology of furosemide in the premature newborn infant. J Pediatr 97:139–143

Pons G, Rey E, Carrier O, Richard MO, Moran C, Badoual J, Olive G (1989) Maturation of AFMU excretion in infants. Fundam Clin Pharmacol 3:589–595

Powers PS, Bruty H (2009) Pharmacotherapy for eating disorders and obesity. Child Adolesc Psychiatr Clin N Am 18:175–187

Prevot A, Mosig D, Guignard JP (2002) The effects of losartan on renal function in the newborn rabbit. Pediatr Res 51:728–732

Raishevich N, Jensen P (2007) Attention-deficit/hyperactivity disorder. In: Kliegman RM, Behrman RE, Jenson HB, Stanton BF (eds) Nelson textbook of pediatrics, 18th edn. Saunders Elsevier, Philadelphia

Raju TN, Higgins RD, Stark AR, Leveno KJ (2006) Optimizing care and outcome for late-preterm (near-term) infants: a summary of the workshop sponsored by the National Institute of Child Health and Human Development. Pediatrics 118:1207–1214

Ramachandrappa A, Jain L (2009) Health issues of the late preterm infant. Pediatr Clin North Am 56:565–577

Rane A (2005) Drug metabolism and disposition in infants and children. Neonatal and pediatric pharmacology – therapeutic principles in practice, 3rd edn. Lippincott Williams and Wilkins, Philadelphia

Redmond GP, Bell JJ, Perel JM (1978) Effect of human growth hormone on amobarbital metabolism in children. Clin Pharmacol Ther 24:213–218

Reed MD, Rodarte A, Blumer JL, Khoo KC, Akbari B, Pou S, Pharmd KGL (2001) The single-dose pharmacokinetics of midazolam and its primary metabolite in pediatric patients after oral and intravenous administration. J Clin Pharmacol 41:1359–1369

Reese J, Waleh N, Poole SD, Brown N, Roman C, Clyman RI (2009) Chronic in utero cyclooxygenase inhibition alters PGE2-regulated ductus arteriosus contractile pathways and prevents postnatal closure. Pediatr Res 66:155–161

Reinalter SC, Jeck N, Peters M, Seyberth HW (2004) Pharmacotyping of hypokalaemic salt-losing tubular disorders. Acta Physiol Scand 181:513–521

Roan Y, Galant SP (1982) Decreased neutrophil beta adrenergic receptors in the neonate. Pediatr Res 16:591–593

Rodrigues AD (2005) Impact of CYP2C9 genotype on pharmacokinetics: are all cyclooxygenase inhibitors the same? Drug Metab Dispos 33:1567–1575

Sankar R, Painter MJ (2005) Neonatal seizures: after all these years we still love what doesn't work. Neurology 64:776–777

Sans V, de la Dumas RE, Berge J, Grenier N, Boralevi F, Mazereeuw-Hautier J, Lipsker D, Dupuis E, Ezzedine K, Vergnes P, Taieb A, Leaute-Labreze C (2009) Propranolol for severe infantile hemangiomas: follow-up report. Pediatrics 124:e423–e431

Satwani P, Morris E, van de Ven C, Cairo MS (2005) Dysregulation of expression of immunoregulatory and cytokine genes and its association with the immaturity in neonatal phagocytic and cellular immunity. Biol Neonate 88:214–227

Schindler M (2002) Do bronchodilators have an effect on bronchiolitis? Crit Care 6:111–112

Schuster V, von Stockhausen HB, Seyberth HW (1990) Effects of highly overdosed indomethacin in a preterm infant with symptomatic patent ductus arteriosus. Eur J Pediatr 149:651–653

Seyberth HW (2008) An improved terminology and classification of Bartter-like syndromes. Nat Clin Pract Nephrol 4:560–567

Seyberth HW, Kühl PG (1988) The role of eicosanoids in paediatrics. Eur J Pediatr 147:341–349

Seyberth HW, Rascher W, Hackenthal R, Wille L (1983) Effect of prolonged indomethacin therapy on renal function and selected vasoactive hormones in very-low-birth-weight infants with symptomatic patent ductus arteriosus. J Pediatr 103:979–984

Seyberth HW, Müller H, Ulmer HE, Wille L (1984) Urinary excretion rates of 6-keto-PGF1 alpha in preterm infants recovering from respiratory distress with and without patent ductus arteriosus. Pediatr Res 18:520–524

Seyberth HW, Leonhardt A, Tönshoff B, Gordjani N (1991) Prostanoids in paediatric kidney diseases. Pediatr Nephrol 5:639–649

Shankaran S, Kauffman RE (1984) Use of chloramphenicol palmitate in neonates. J Pediatr 105:113–116

Shirkey HC (1975) Pediatric therapy, 5th edn. The C.V. Mosby Company, Saint Louis

Sjöqvist F, Garle M, Rane A (2008) Use of doping agents, particularly anabolic steroids, in sports and society. Lancet 371:1872–1882

Slotkin TA, Auman JT, Seidler FJ (2003) Ontogenesis of beta-adrenoceptor signaling: implications for perinatal physiology and for fetal effects of tocolytic drugs. J Pharmacol Exp Ther 306:1–7

Smith GC (1998) The pharmacology of the ductus arteriosus. Pharmacol Rev 50:35–58

Smith GC, McGrath JC (1994) Interactions between indomethacin, noradrenaline and vasodilators in the fetal rabbit ductus arteriosus. Br J Pharmacol 111:1245–1251

Smith GC, Wu WX, Nijland MJ, Koenen SV, Nathanielsz PW (2001) Effect of gestational age, corticosteroids, and birth on expression of prostanoid EP receptor genes in lamb and baboon ductus arteriosus. J Cardiovasc Pharmacol 37:697–704

Steer PA, Henderson-Smart DJ (2000) Caffeine versus theophylline for apnea in preterm infants. Cochrane Database Syst Rev: CD000273

Stevens TP, Harrington EW, Blennow M, Soll RF (2007) Early surfactant administration with brief ventilation vs. selective surfactant and continued mechanical ventilation for preterm infants with or at risk for respiratory distress syndrome. Cochrane Database Syst Rev: CD003063

Stewart CF, Hampton EM (1987) Effect of maturation on drug disposition in pediatric patients. Clin Pharm 6:548–564

Strolin BM, Whomsley R, Baltes EL (2005) Differences in absorption, distribution, metabolism and excretion of xenobiotics between the paediatric and adult populations. Expert Opin Drug Metab Toxicol 1:447–471

Subbarao P, Ratjen F (2006) Beta2-agonists for asthma: the pediatric perspective. Clin Rev Allergy Immunol 31:209–218

Szabó EZ, Luginbuehl I, Bissonnette B (2009) Impact of anesthetic agents on cerebrovascular physiology in children. Paediatr Anaesth 19:108–118

Taddio A, Katz J, Ilersich AL, Koren G (1997) Effect of neonatal circumcision on pain response during subsequent routine vaccination. Lancet 349:599–603

Takahashi H, Ishikawa S, Nomoto S, Nishigaki Y, Ando F, Kashima T, Kimura S, Kanamori M, Echizen H (2000) Developmental changes in pharmacokinetics and pharmacodynamics of warfarin enantiomers in Japanese children. Clin Pharmacol Ther 68:541–555

Tanner JM, Davies PS (1985) Clinical longitudinal standards for height and height velocity for North American children. J Pediatr 107:317–329

Thébaud B, Michelakis ED, Wu XC, Moudgil R, Kuzyk M, Dyck JR, Harry G, Hashimoto K, Haromy A, Rebeyka I, Archer SL (2004) Oxygen-sensitive Kv channel gene transfer confers oxygen responsiveness to preterm rabbit and remodeled human ductus arteriosus: implications for infants with patent ductus arteriosus. Circulation 110:1372–1379

Thompson AM, Bizzarro MJ (2008) Necrotizing enterocolitis in newborns: pathogenesis, prevention and management. Drugs 68:1227–1238

Tobin JR (2008) Paradoxical effects of midazolam in the very young. Anesthesiology 108:6–7

Toyoshima K, Momma K, Imamura S, Nakanishi T (2006) In vivo dilatation of the fetal and postnatal ductus arteriosus by inhibition of phosphodiesterase 3 in rats. Biol Neonate 89:251–256

Tubergen DG, Bleyer A (2007) The leukemias. In: Kliegman RM, Behrman RE, Jenson HB, Stanton BF (eds) Nelson textbook of pediatrics, 18th edn. Saunders Elsevier, Philadelphia

Vogelstein B, Kowarski A, Lietman PS (1977) The pharmacokinetics of amikacin in children. J Pediatr 91:333–339

Waleh N, Kajino H, Marrache AM, Ginzinger D, Roman C, Seidner SR, Moss TJ, Fouron JC, Vazquez-Tello A, Chemtob S, Clyman RI (2004) Prostaglandin E2 – mediated relaxation of the ductus arteriosus: effects of gestational age on g protein-coupled receptor expression, signaling, and vasomotor control. Circulation 110:2326–2332

Waleh N, Reese J, Kajino H, Roman C, Seidner S, McCurnin D, Clyman RI (2009) Oxygen-induced tension in the sheep ductus arteriosus: effects of gestation on potassium and calcium channel regulation. Pediatr Res 65:285–290

Walker SM, Franck LS, Fitzgerald M, Myles J, Stocks J, Marlow N (2009) Long-term impact of neonatal intensive care and surgery on somatosensory perception in children born extremely preterm. Pain 141:79–87

Wang L, Pozzato V, Turato G, Madamanchi A, Murphy TM, Chitano P (2008) Reduced spontaneous relaxation in immature guinea pig airway smooth muscle is associated with increased prostanoid release. Am J Physiol Lung Cell Mol Physiol 294:L964–L973

Wheatley CM, Dickinson JL, Mackey DA, Craig JE, Sale MM (2002) Retinopathy of prematurity: recent advances in our understanding. Br J Ophthalmol 86:696–700

Whitsett JA, Noguchi A, Moore JJ (1982) Developmental aspects of alpha- and beta-adrenergic receptors. Semin Perinatol 6:125–141

Witter FR, Zimmerman AW, Reichmann JP, Connors SL (2009) In utero beta 2 adrenergic agonist exposure and adverse neurophysiologic and behavioral outcomes. Am J Obstet Gynecol 201:553–559

Wright DH, Abran D, Bhattacharya M, Hou X, Bernier SG, Bouayad A, Fouron JC, Vazquez-Tello A, Beauchamp MH, Clyman RI, Peri K, Varma DR, Chemtob S (2001) Prostanoid receptors: ontogeny and implications in vascular physiology. Am J Physiol Regul Integr Comp Physiol 281:R1343–R1360

Yaffe SJ, Friedman WF, Rogers D, Lang P, Ragni M, Saccar C (1980) The disposition of indomethacin in preterm babies. J Pediatr 97:1001–1006

Yang D, Pearce RE, Wang X, Gaedigk R, Wan YJ, Yan B (2009) Human carboxylesterases HCE1 and HCE2: ontogenic expression, inter-individual variability and differential hydrolysis of oseltamivir, aspirin, deltamethrin and permethrin. Biochem Pharmacol 77:238–247

Developmental Pharmacokinetics

Johannes N. van den Anker, Matthias Schwab, and Gregory L. Kearns

Contents

J.N. van den Anker (✉)
Division of Pediatric Clinical Pharmacology, Department of Pediatrics, Children's National
Medical Center, 111 Michigan Avenue, NW, Washington, DC 20010, USA
e-mail: jvandena@cnmc.org

M. Schwab
Dr. Margarete Fischer-Bosch-Institute of Clinical Pharmacology, Auerbachstrasse 112,
70376 Stuttgart, Germany

Department of Clinical Pharmacology, Institute of Experimental and Clinical Pharmacology and
Toxicology, University Hospital, Tübingen, Germany

G.L. Kearns
Division of Pediatric Pharmacology and Medical Toxicology, Department of Medical Research,
Children's Mercy Hospital, Kansas City, MO, USA

H.W. Seyberth et al. (eds.), *Pediatric Clinical Pharmacology*,
Handbook of Experimental Pharmacology 205,
DOI 10.1007/978-3-642-20195-0_2, © Springer-Verlag Berlin Heidelberg 2011

Abstract The advances in developmental pharmacokinetics during the past decade reside with an enhanced understanding of the influence of growth and development on drug absorption, distribution, metabolism, and excretion (ADME). However, significant information gaps remain with respect to our ability to characterize the impact of ontogeny on the activity of important drug metabolizing enzymes, transporters, and other targets. The ultimate goal of rational drug therapy in neonates, infants, children, and adolescents resides with the ability to individualize it based on known developmental differences in drug disposition and action. The clinical challenge in achieving this is accounting for the variability in all of the contravening factors that influence pharmacokinetics and pharmacodynamics (e.g., genetic variants of ADME genes, different disease phenotypes, disease progression, and concomitant treatment). Application of novel technologies in the fields of pharmacometrics (e.g., in silico simulation of exposure–response relationships; disease progression modeling), pharmacogenomics and biomarker development (e.g., creation of pharmacodynamic surrogate endpoints suitable for pediatric use) are increasingly making integrated approaches for developmentally appropriate dose regimen selection possible.

Keywords Developmental   pharmacology   •   Pediatric   pharmacology   •   Neonatal pharmacology • Neonates • Pharmacokinetics • Pharmacogenomics • Pharmacodynamics • Drug metabolizing enzymes

1   Introduction

Human growth and development consists of a continuum of biologic events that includes somatic growth, neurobehavioral maturation, and eventual reproduction. The impact of these developmental changes in drug disposition is largely related to changes in body composition (e.g., body water content, plasma protein concentrations) and function of organs important in metabolism (e.g., the liver) and excretion (e.g., the kidney). During the first decade of life, these changes are dynamic and can be nonlinear and discordant making standardized dosing inadequate for effective drug dosing across the span of childhood. Consequently, "standard dosing" of many drugs during rapid phases of growth/development where both drug disposition and response may be altered is generally inadequate for the purpose of optimizing drug therapy. This goal can only be achieved through fundamental and integrative understanding of how ontogeny influences pharmacokinetics and pharmacodynamics.

Developmental pharmacokinetics must take into account normal growth and developmental pathways (Bartelink et al. 2006; Johnson et al. 2006). A better understanding of the various physiologic variables regulating and determining the fate of drugs in the body and their pharmacologic effects has dramatically improved both the safety and the efficacy of drug therapy for neonates, infants, children, and adolescents (Kearns et al. 2003a; Van Den Anker and Rakhmanina 2006). The impact of development on the pharmacokinetics of a given drug is dependent, to a great degree, upon age-related changes in the body composition and the acquisition of function of organs and organ systems that are important in determining drug metabolism as well as drug transport and excretion (Edginton et al. 2006; Anderson and Holford 2008). Although it is often convenient to classify pediatric patients on the basis of postnatal age for the study and provision of drug therapy (e.g., newborn infants aged 1 month or less, infants between 1 and 24 months of age, children between 2 and 12 years of age, and adolescents between 12 and 16–18 years of age), it is important to recognize that changes in physiology that characterize development may not correspond to these age-defined breakpoints and are also not linearly related to age. In fact, the most dramatic changes in drug disposition occur during the first 12–18 months of life, when the acquisition of organ function is most dynamic (Kearns et al. 2003a; Van Den Anker and Rakhmanina 2006). Additionally, independent from developmental aspects, it is important to mention that the pharmacokinetics of a given drug may be altered in pediatric patients also due to intrinsic (e.g., genotype, inherited diseases) and/or extrinsic (e.g., acquired diseases, diet, co-medication) factors that may occur during the first months and years of life (Blake et al. 2006; Van Den Anker et al. 1994; Allegaert et al. 2008; Leeder 2003; Krekels et al. 2007; Leeder et al. 2010). In principle, however, these factors are also important for nonpediatric populations such as adult geriatric patients. To study pediatric pharmacokinetics it is very useful to examine the impact of development on those physiologic variables that govern drug absorption, distribution, metabolism, and excretion (Bartelink et al. 2006; Johnson et al. 2006; Edginton et al. 2006) which is summarized by the commonly used term ADME.

2 Drug Absorption

For therapeutic agents administered by extravascular routes, the process of absorption is reflected by the ability of a drug to overcome chemical, physical, mechanical, and biological barriers. Developmental differences in the physiologic composition and function of these barriers can alter the rate and/or extent of drug absorption (Kearns et al. 2003a; Van Den Anker and Rakhmanina 2006). While factors influencing drug absorption are multifactorial in nature, developmental changes in the absorptive surfaces (e.g., gastrointestinal tract, skin) can be determinants of bioavailability (Kearns et al. 2003a; Van Den Anker and Rakhmanina 2006). The peroral route is the principal means for drug administration to infants, children, and adolescents but the skin represents an often overlooked, but important organ for systemic drug absorption as well. Therefore, the drug absorption part of this chapter will focus on drug absorption from the gastrointestinal tract and through the skin.

2.1   The Gastrointestinal Tract

The most important factors that influence drug absorption from the gastrointestinal tract are related to the physiology of the stomach, intestine, and biliary tract. The pH of the stomach is practically neutral at birth, decreases to around 3 within 48 h after birth, returns to neutral over the next 24 h, and remains that way for the next 10 days (Bartelink et al. 2006). Thereafter, it slowly declines again until it reaches adult values at about 2 years of age. These initial changes do not occur in premature infants, who seem to have little or no free acid during the first 14 days of life (Bartelink et al. 2006). The time of gastric emptying is delayed in the period immediately after birth for both full term and preterm neonates. It approaches adult values within the first 6–8 months of life (Strolin Benedetti and Baltes 2003). Intestinal transit time is prolonged in neonates because of reduced motility and peristalsis, but appears to be reduced in older infants as a result of increased intestinal motility (Strolin Benedetti and Baltes 2003; Kearns 2000). Other factors that may play a role in intestinal drug absorption are immaturity of the intestinal mucosa leading to increased permeability, immature biliary function, high levels of intestinal β-glucuronidase activity, reduced first-pass metabolism, maturation of carrier mechanisms, and variable microbial colonization (Kearns 2000). These developmental differences in the physiologic composition and function of these organs can alter the rate and/or extent of drug absorption. Changes in intraluminal pH can directly impact both drug stability and degree of ionization, thus influencing the relative amount of drug available for absorption. Acid labile drugs such as penicillin G and erythromycin are therefore more efficiently absorbed, whereas the same changes in gastric pH (developmentally or caused by the use of proton pump inhibitors) will result in clinically important decreases in the absorption of weak organic acids such as phenobarbital and phenytoin, necessitating adjustment of the amount of antiepileptic drug administered to the individual patient (Strolin Benedetti and Baltes 2003). Additionally, the ability to solubilize and subsequently absorb lipophilic drugs can be influenced by age-dependent changes in biliary function. Immature conjugation and/or transport of bile salts into the intestinal lumen results in low intraduodenal levels despite blood levels that exceed those seen in adults. Gastric emptying time is prolonged throughout infancy and child-hood consequent to reduced motility, which may retard drug passage into the intestine where the majority of absorption takes place (Kearns 2000). As a conse-quence, the rate of absorption of drugs with limited water solubility such as phenytoin and carbamazepine can be significantly altered resulting from these changes in gastrointestinal motility. Unfortunately, few studies have systematically evaluated the effect of developmental changes in gastric emptying and intestinal motility on drug absorption in infants and children. Anderson et al. showed that the oral acetaminophen (paracetamol) absorption rate was significantly lower in the first days of life before stabilizing 1 week after birth (Anderson et al. 2002). Another study showed that the time to reach the maximum concentration (t_{max}) of cisapride was significantly longer in preterm infants compared with term neonates (Kearns et al. 2003b). Generally, the rate at which most drugs are absorbed is generally slower and thus, the time to achieve maximum plasma concentrations is prolonged in neonates and young infants relative to older infants and children. Despite their incomplete characterization, developmental differences in the activity of intestinal drug metabolizing enzymes and efflux transporters have the potential to markedly alter drug bioavailability.

3   The Skin

The morphologic and functional development of the skin as well as the factors that influence penetration of drugs into and through the skin has been reviewed (Radde and McKercher 1985). Basically, the percutaneous absorption of a compound is directly related to the degree of skin hydration and relative absorptive surface area and inversely related to the thickness of the stratum corneum (Radde and McKercher 1985). The integument of the full-term neonate possesses an intact barrier function and is similar to that of an older child or adolescent. However, the ratio of surface area to body weight of the full-term neonate is much higher than that of an adult. Thus, the infant will be exposed to a relatively greater amount of drug topically than will older infants, children, or adolescents. In contrast, data of human skin from preterm infants indicates an inverse correlation between permeability and gestational age (Nachman and Esterly 1980). Permeability rates were 100- to 1,000-fold greater before 30 weeks gestation as compared with full-term neonates, with a three to fourfold greater permeation rate seen beyond 32 weeks (Ginsberg et al. 2004). In vivo studies suggest that this increased dermal permeability in preterm infants is a short-lived phenomenon with the permeability barrier of even the most premature neonates similar to that of full-term neonates by 2 weeks of postnatal life (Ginsberg et al. 2004). There are numerous reports in the literature underscoring the importance of skin absorption in neonates primarily showing toxicity after exposure to drugs or chemicals. These include pentachlorophenol-containing laundry detergents and hydrocortisone (Armstrong et al. 1969; Feinblatt et al. 1966). Therefore, extreme caution needs to be exercised in using topical therapy in neonates and young infants. In contrast, the possibility of turning enhanced skin absorption of drugs to the infant's advantage is an interesting idea and was explored exemplarily several years ago by using the percutaneous route to administer theophylline in preterm infants (Evans et al. 1985). A standard dose of theophylline gel was applied and serial theophylline levels were measured demonstrating that therapeutic theophylline levels were achieved in 11 of 13 infants and that the percutaneous route is a feasible method of administering theophylline in preterm infants.

4   Drug Distribution

Drug distribution is influenced by a variety of drug-specific physiochemical factors, including the role of drug transporters, blood/tissue protein binding, blood and tissue pH, and perfusion (Bartelink et al. 2006; Kearns et al. 2003a; Van Den Anker and Rakhmanina 2006). However, age-related changes in drug distribution are primarily related to developmental changes in body composition, the concentration of available binding proteins, and the capacity of plasma proteins to bind drugs. Age-dependent changes in body composition alter the physiologic "spaces" into which a drug may distribute (Friis-Hansen 1983). In very young infants, the total body water is high (80–90% of the bodyweight) while fat content is low (10–15% of the bodyweight). The amount of total body water decreases to 55–60% by adulthood. The extracellular water content is about 45% of the bodyweight in neonates, compared with 20% in adulthood (Friis-Hansen 1983). Larger extracellular and total body water spaces in neonates and young infants, coupled with adipose stores that have a higher water/lipid ratio than in adults, produce lower plasma concentrations for drugs that distribute into these respective compartments when administered in a weight-based fashion. Several hydrophilic drugs such as gentamicin and linezolid have a significantly larger volume of distribution in neonates than in infants or adults (Kearns et al. 2003c; De Hoog et al. 2005). The larger volume of distribution in neonates correlates with a larger extracellular water content. The pharmacokinetics of tramadol, a hydrophilic compound with a large volume of distribution in adults, could be described with a two-compartment model (Allegaert et al. 2005). The volume of distribution of the central compartment (a compartment more or less correlated to the extracellular water content) was increased in neonates compared to older children. The volume of distribution of the peripheral compartment (in which the drug is bound to tissue) was not affected by age (Allegaert et al. 2005). For lipophilic drugs that associate primarily with tissue, the influence of age on altering the apparent volume of distribution is not as readily apparent. The extent of drug binding to proteins in the plasma may influence the volume of distribution of drugs (Bartelink et al. 2006). Only free, unbound, drug can be distributed from the vascular space into other body fluids and, ultimately, to tissues where drug–receptor interaction occurs. Albumin, total protein, and total globulins such as $\alpha 1$ acid-glycoprotein are the most important circulating proteins responsible for this drug binding in plasma. The absolute concentration of these proteins is influenced by age, nutrition, and disease. Changes in the composition and amount of these circulating plasma proteins can also influence the distribution of highly bound drugs (Bartelink et al. 2006; Edginton et al. 2006). A reduction in both the quantity and binding affinity of circulating plasma proteins in the neonate and young infant often produces an increase in the free fraction of drug, thereby influencing the availability of the active moiety and potentially, its subsequent hepatic and/or renal clearance. Other factors associated with development and/or disease such as variability in regional blood flow, organ perfusion, permeability of cell membranes, changes in acid–base balance, and cardiac output can also influence drug binding and/or distribution. Finally, drug transporters such as the ABC efflux pump P-glycoprotein (MDR1/ABCB1), which show not only an ontogenic profile in the small intestine but also in the lung, can influence drug distribution because these transporters can markedly influence the extent to which drugs cross membranes in the body and whether drugs can penetrate or are secreted from the target sites (e.g., cerebrospinal fluid).

5 Drug Metabolism

Drug metabolism reflects the biotransformation of an endogenous or exogenous molecule by one or more enzymes to moieties, which are more hydrophilic and thus can be more easily excreted (Bartelink et al. 2006; Kearns et al. 2003a; Van Den Anker and Rakhmanina 2006). While metabolism of a drug generally reduces its ability to produce a pharmacologic action, it also can result in a metabolite that has significant potency, and thereby, contributes to the overall pharmacological effect of the drug. In the case of a prodrug such as codeine, biotransformation is required to produce the pharmacologically active metabolite morphine. Although drug metabolism takes place in several tissues (e.g., intestine, skin, lungs, liver), hepatic metabolism has been investigated most intensively and this metabolism has been divided conventionally into two phases (Bartelink et al. 2006; Kearns et al. 2003a; Van Den Anker and Rakhmanina 2006). Phase I hepatic metabolism usually results in modifying the therapeutic agent or xenobiotic (e.g., through oxidation) in order to make the molecule more polar. Phase II hepatic metabolism usually results in addition of a small molecule (e.g., glucuronide) to the therapeutic agent in order to make it more polar. While there are many enzymes that are capable of catalyzing the biotransformation of drugs, the quantitatively most important are represented by the cytochromes P450 (CYP450) (Nelson et al. 1996). The specific CYP450 isoforms responsible for the majority of human drug metabolism are represented by CYP3A4/5, CYP1A2, CYP2B6, CYP2D6, CYP2C9, CYP2C19, and CYP2E1 (Brown et al. 2008).

Development has a profound effect on the expression of CYP450. Distinct patterns of isoform-specific developmental CYP expression have been observed postnatally. As reflected by recent reviews, distinct patterns of isoform-specific developmental changes in drug biotransformation are apparent for many Phase I and Phase II drug metabolizing enzymes (Hines and McCarver 2002; McCarver and Hines 2002; De Wildt et al. 1999; Alcorn and McNamara 2002). Very recently, Hines (Hines 2008) has categorized the development of enzymes involved in human metabolism into three main categories: (1) those expressed during the whole or part of the fetal period, but silenced or expressed at low levels within 1–2 years after birth; (2) those expressed at relatively constant levels through-out fetal development, but increased to some extent postnatally; and (3) those whose onset of expression can occur in the third trimester, but substantial increase is noted in the first 1–2 years after birth. Based on literature data, CYP3A7,

Flavin-containing monooxygenase 1 (FMO1), sulfotransferase 1A3/4 (SULT1A3/4), SULT1E1, and maybe alcohol dehydrogenase 1A (ADH1A) belong to the first group. To the second group belong CYP2A6, 3A5, 2C9, 2C19, 2D6, 2E1, and SULT1A1. The third group includes ADH1C, ADH1B, CYP1A1, 1A2, 2A 6, 2A7, 2B6, 2B7, 2C8, 2C9, 2F1, 3A4, FMO3, SULT2A1, glucoronosyltransferases (UGT), and N-acetyltransferase 2 (Hines 2008; Balistreri et al. 1984; Card et al. 1989).

In addition to these in vitro data, there has been an explosion in the amount of information generated about metabolism of therapeutic agents in children during the last two decades. In vivo data have been generated largely through two means (Blake et al. 2005, 2007). One is through dedicated ontogeny studies in which a probe drug (e.g., dextromethorphan or acetaminophen/paracetamol) is given to children of various age groups or to the same children over a period of time (Blake et al. 2005, 2007). The other manner in which these in vivo data have been developed is serendipitously over the course of industry-sponsored or investigator-initiated pediatric clinical trials, which utilize the traditional age groups, and both anticipated as well as unexpected results reveal new data about the drug metabolizing enzymes involved. The most important examples of studies that have resulted in clinically important insight into the ontogeny of drug metabolism are summarized in the following paragraph.

Midazolam plasma clearance, which primarily reflects hepatic CYP3A4/5 activity after intravenous administration (De Wildt et al. 2001; Kinirons et al. 1999), increases approximately fivefold (1.2–9 ml/min/kg) over the first 3 months of life (Payne et al. 1989). Carbamazepine plasma clearance, also largely dependent upon CYP3A4 (Kerr et al. 1994), is greater in children relative to adults (Pynnönen et al. 1977; Riva et al. 1985; Rane et al. 1975), thereby necessitating higher weight-adjusted (i.e., mg/kg) doses of the drug to produce therapeutic plasma concentrations. CYP2C9 and to a lesser extent, CYP2C19, are primarily responsible for phenytoin biotransformation (Bajpai et al. 1996). Phenytoin apparent half life is prolonged (~75 h) in preterm infants but decreases to ~20 h in term infants less than 1 week postnatal age and to ~8 h after 2 weeks of age (Loughnan et al. 1977). Saturable phenytoin metabolism does not appear until approximately 10 days of postnatal age, demonstrating the developmental acquisition of CYP2C9 activity.

Caffeine and theophylline are the most common CYP1A2 substrates used in pediatrics. Caffeine elimination in vivo mirrors that observed in vitro with full 3-demethylation activity (mediated by CYP1A2) observed by approximately 4 months of age (Aranda et al. 1979). Formation of CYP1A2-dependent theophylline metabolites reaches adult levels by approximately 4–5 months of postnatal age (Kraus et al. 1993), and in older infants and young children, theophylline plasma clearance generally exceeds adult values (Milavetz et al. 1986). Furthermore, caffeine 3-demethylation in adolescent females appears to decline to adult levels at Tanner stage II relative to males where it occurs at stages IV/V, thus demonstrating an apparent sex difference in the ontogeny of CYP1A2.

The following sections of this chapter will focus on neonates and young infants because no other group defines such a period of rapid growth and development. It is well established that infants who are barely into their second trimester of gestational life born as small as a few hundred grams (400–500 g) can survive. On the other extreme, by the end of the first month of postnatal life, large for gestational age infants may weigh upwards of several kilograms. Indeed, the 95th weight percentile is approximately 5 kg. No other age groups can be defined in differences measured logarithmically. As one might expect, there are similar tremendous developmental changes in hepatic drug metabolizing enzymes during this time frame. Understanding these implications is important for individualized clinical development programs.

6 Phase I Enzymes

6.1 CYP3A

The CYP3A subfamily represents the majority of CYP total content in the liver (Brown et al. 2008). Indeed, it has been shown that over one-half of all drugs prescribed are metabolized by CYP3A (Zanger et al. 2008). The CYP3A subfamily consists of CYP3A4, 3A5, 3A7, and 3A43. CYP3A43 is not known to play a significant role in hepatic metabolism. It has been established that CYP3A4 is the predominant CYP3A enzyme in adults, whereas CYP3A7 is the predominant CYP3A enzyme in the fetus and infants. Moreover, there is a great deal of overlap of specificity of ability for CYP3A4 and CYP3A7 to metabolize therapeutic agents. In 2003, Stevens et al. published the results of examining the largest collection of fetal and pediatric liver samples to date. The study included 212 samples. Stevens and colleagues demonstrated that CYP3A7 is highest between 94 and 168 postconceptional days on a pmol/mg basis of total hepatic protein (Stevens et al. 2003). The level at birth is less than half that of the high prenatal value. However, it remains higher than that of even adult CYP3A4 levels. Furthermore, these hepatic samples demonstrated that there is minimal CYP3A4 activity prenatally that continues to increase after birth. Nevertheless, CYP3A7 content remains higher than CYP3A4 content until at least 6 months of age.

To date, two probe drugs have been researched extensively, which have demonstrated the lower activity of CYP3A4 at birth and in neonates. In 2001, De Wildt et al. published the results of midazolam metabolism given to 24 preterm infants. Only 19 of 24 preterm infants produced detectable levels of 1-OH-midazolam. Furthermore, these results firmly established that premature infants had lower CYP3A4 activity than full-term infants, than did children and adults historically. Oral cisapride has also been demonstrated to be a suitable substrate for CYP3A4 activity (Kearns et al. 2003b). Cisapride has demonstrated a similarly low activity for CYP3A4 in the neonatal period, as did midazolam (Kearns et al. 2003b; De Wildt et al. 2001).

In conclusion, CYP3A7 activity is very high before birth and continues to have high activity after birth and is even present into adulthood. CYP3A4 possesses very low activity at birth and very slowly increases in the neonatal period. Thus, when designing studies with substrates for CYP3A4 in young infants and children, great care needs to be taken to adjust for this low activity in order to achieve the goal of the FDA guidance that in children exposure and C_{max} are not higher than that in adults.

6.2 CYP1A2

One of the first CYP enzymes to be studied utilizing a probe drug in the first year of life is CYP1A2. Two methylxanthines (caffeine and theophylline) have been utilized extensively to evaluate CYP1A2 in vivo in young children (Evans et al. 1989; Erenberg et al. 2000; Lambert et al. 1986; Tateishi et al. 1999). Theophylline and caffeine are two commonly utilized medications in neonates for the treatment of apnea. These medications are frequently continued form the neonatal period during the first year of life. At birth, caffeine-3-demethylation, a measure of CYP1A2 activity, is very low. Consequently, Erenberg et al. published that the efficacious dose of caffeine is 10 mg/kg every day (Erenberg et al. 2000). The half-life of caffeine is 72–96 h in infants compared to approximately 5 h in older children and adults. Similarly, 8-hydroxylation of theophylline is reduced at birth. Nevertheless, longitudinal data indicate a rapid maturation process for CYP1A2, as it appears to reach adult levels within the first year of life, often within the first 6 months of life. Finally, it is important to note that caffeine activity is highly inducible by drugs, diet, and exogenous toxins such as cigarette smoke. In the adult literature, variability in CYP1A2 activity up to 100-fold has been reported. Moreover, Blake et al. reported that caffeine elimination half-life in neonates who are breast-fed is longer than that of formula-fed infants (Blake et al. 2006); information which suggests that the composition of infant diet (i.e., an environmental factor) can influence the pattern of ontogenic expression of a drug metabolizing enzyme.

In conclusion, it is evident that CYP1A2 activity is highly reduced in young infants. Additionally, activity of the enzyme is highly inducible. Finally, maturation of CYP1A2 activity is rapid in the first year of life. Therefore, when designing clinical studies, which include neonates, great care must be taken to assure that this variability in drug response is properly assessed, especially within the first 6–12 months of life.

6.3 CYP2D6

CYP2D6 is one of the most polymorphically expressed enzymes in humans (Zanger et al. 2004; Gaedigk et al. 2008). Some estimates indicate that fewer than 90% of individuals are homozygous for the wild-type allele. In 1991, Treluyer et al. published the results of liver samples from fetuses aged 17–40 weeks postconception. These results demonstrated that the concentration of hepatic CYP2D6 protein was very low or undetectable in these fetuses. This lack of CYP2D6 activity at birth led to the hypothesis that birth-related events may trigger maturation of the enzyme. In 2007, Blake et al. published in vivo results that provided further understanding of CYP2D6 activity in the first year of life. These results came from dosing infants with dextromethorphan at 0.5, 1, 2, 4, 6, and 12 months of age and measuring the metabolites in urine. These dextromethorphan results demonstrate indeed that there is low activity at birth, but that there is rapid acquisition of CYP2D6 activity in the first year of life. Already within the first 2 weeks of life there is measurable acquisition of CYP2D6 activity. Despite the discussion in the literature about the fact that the increase in renal function might conceal the enzyme development resulting in an apparent plateau of the metabolic ratio after 2 weeks (Johnson et al. 2008), very recent data show that an infant with a postmenstrual age of 52 weeks has already mature hepatic CYP2D6 activity (Allegaert et al. 2011).

Taken together, these results demonstrate the need for careful pharmacokinetic studies in infants and toddlers who are provided a pharmacologic agent, which is primarily metabolized by CYP2D6 (e.g., codeine, beta-blockers, propafenone). Not only does one need to be cognizant of potential infants who are predestined by their genome to be poor metabolizers, but potential studies need to realize the implications of low levels of CYP2D6 at birth and also the rapid maturation process that occurs within the first year of life (Stevens et al. 2008).

6.4   CYP2C9/CYP2C19

Lee et al. (2002) and Koukouritaki et al. (2004) have published the most extensive reviews to date on CYP2C activity in humans. They demonstrate that the two main representatives of the CYP2C subfamily of enzymes (CYP2C9 and CYP2C19) conveniently follow the CYP2C rule of 20%. Approximately 20% of hepatic CYP content of adult livers is CYP2C and these CYP2C enzymes metabolize 20% of pharmaceuticals developed to date.

Although not to the same extent as CYP2D6, the two main CYP2C representatives are polymorphically expressed. To date, over 30 alleles of CYP2C9 of CYP2C9 have been identified and more than 25 alleles of CYP2C19 of CYP2C19 have been reported in the literature (Lee et al. 2002; Koukouritaki et al. 2004). Just as with CYP2D6, some of these polymorphisms may result in poor metabolizer status, which may confound studies in infants and young children.

The ontogeny of CYP2C9 is much better established than CYP2C19. Indeed, hepatic liver samples have shown that CYP2C9 activity is functionally very low just prior to birth. However, much like CYP2D6, this activity increases quickly in the first year of life. The classic example of the effects of this very low level of CYP2C9 activity at birth can be seen with phenytoin (Suzuki et al. 1994). Indeed, the recommended daily dose for newborns is 5 mg/kg/day, but by 6 months to 3 years of age this increases to 8–10 mg/kg/day consequent to increased CYP2C9 activity.

Two major pharmaceutical classes of drugs (i.e., benzodiazepines and proton pump inhibitors) have major representative therapeutic agents that are metabolized by CYP2C19 (Kearns et al. 2003d). Indeed, characteristic representatives from these classes are used in the literature to indirectly ascertain the ontogeny of CYP2C19 activity. Hydroxylation of diazepam is attributed to CYP2C19 activity and is a classic example of the effects of the maturation process of CYP2C19 (Jung et al. 1997). In neonates, the half-life of diazepam is reported to be 50–90 h. Within the first year of life, that half-life of 40–50 h is much closer to the adult value, which is reported as 20–50 h (Klotz 2007).

More recently, the effects of the ontogeny on proton pump inhibitor metabolism have been reviewed. To date, all proton pump inhibitors other than rabeprazole are metabolized by CYP2C19. Of the drugs in this class, the biotransformation of pantoprazole is predominantly dependent upon CYP2C19 activity (Kearns and Winter 2003). When the weight-normalized apparent oral clearance of pantoprazole is examined in pediatric patients from 1 month to 16 years of age (Fig. 1), a developmental profile for the acquisition of CYP2C19 activity is apparent. As expected, exposures of the CYP2C19 metabolism-dependent proton pump inhibitors are universally increased in the youngest infants when genetic polymorphisms of CYP2C19 are fully accounted (Kearns and Winter 2003; Jung et al. 1997).

Taken together, these results demonstrate an important trend when designing pharmaceutical studies that depend on hepatic metabolism through the two major CYP2C enzyme pathways. It is extremely important to be cognizant of the limited activity of these enzymes in early childhood. Moreover, much like with CYP2D6, it is important to recognize the impact of genetic polymorphisms when studying individuals who take substrates of these enzymes (Brandolese et al. 2001). Finally, the first 3 months of life represents a dramatic maturation time for the activity of many drug metabolizing enzymes. When considered in the context of a similar dramatic, nonlinear increase in body size (i.e., both weight and length), individualization of drug dose based on pharmacokinetic data is often a real challenge, especially for agents where attainment of critical target plasma concentrations (or systemic exposures) is necessary. Therefore, one can assume that there will be great variability of exposure in studies with infants in this age group, especially when "standard doses" of a drug are given without adjustment during the first few months of life.

6.5 CYP2E1

CYP2E1 is being increasingly recognized for its importance in the oxidative metabolism of a wide variety of pharmaceuticals (e.g., acetaminophen, halothane,

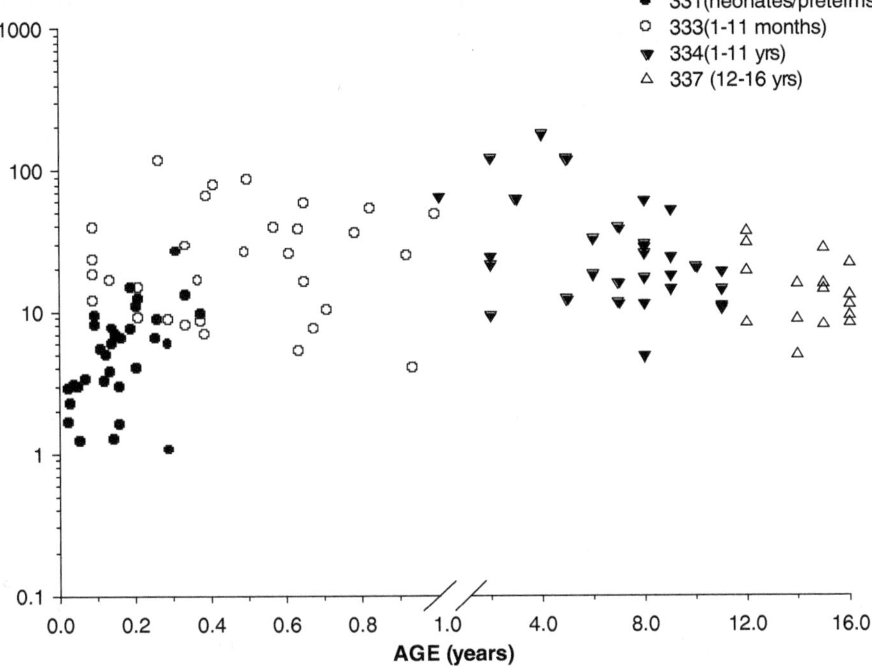

Fig. 1 Aggregate apparent oral clearance (CL/F) data for pantoprazole obtained from four pediatric clinical pharmacokinetic studies of the drug (study numbers 331, 333, 334, and 337) performed as part of pediatric labeling studies conducted under a written request from the U.S. Food and Drug Administration. All studies involved administration of a single oral dose of pantoprazole given as the proprietary drug formulation. To illustrate the association of development with pantoprazole pharmacokinetics, the value of CL/F has been normalized to a "standard" adult weight of 70 kg

and ethanol) (Jimenez-Lopez and Cederbaum 2005). However, only in the last 5 years has the developmental pattern of this important enzyme been well understood (Johnsrud et al. 2003). Nevertheless, human hepatic CYP2E1 developmental expression is difficult to appreciate due to the multiple levels of regulation in its activity. For example, CYP2E1 is known to be elevated in individuals who have high levels of ethanol consumption, in individuals who are obese, and finally in individuals who have type 2 diabetes (Caro and Cederbaum 2004). Finally, an increasing number of genetic polymorphisms, which lead to lower CYP2E1 protein concentration, have been demonstrated in the literature (Hanioka et al. 2003).

To date, Johnsrud et al. have published the largest study of the activity of fetal and pediatric liver samples to determine the ontogeny of CYP2E1 (Johnsrud et al. 2003). Measurable CYP2E1 activity was demonstrated in 18 of 49 second trimester livers and 12 of 15 third trimester samples. Moreover, measurements of mean concentrations of CYP2E1 protein as part of total milligrams of microsomal protein found that second trimester infants averaged 0.35 pmol/mg, third trimester infants 6.7 pmol/mg, newborns 8.8 pmol/mg and older infants aged 30–90 days 23.8 pmol/mg, and finally children aged 90 days to 18 years 41.4 pmol/mg. Thus, this implies a rapid maturation starting in late fetal life and continuing through early infancy in CYP2E1 activity. It would appear that these data demonstrate that careful attention would be required in studies of new CYP2E1 substrates in infants under the age of 90 days.

7   Drug Excretion

The kidney is the primary organ responsible for the excretion of drugs and their metabolites. Maturation of renal function is a dynamic process that begins early during fetal organogenesis and is complete by early childhood (Rhodin et al. 2009; Chen et al. 2006). The developmental increase in glomerular filtration rate (GFR) involves active nephrogenesis, a process that begins at 9 weeks and is complete by 36 weeks of gestation, followed by postnatal changes in renal and intrarenal blood flow. Following birth, the GFR is approximately 2–4 ml/min/kg in term neonates and as low as 0.6–0.8 ml/min/kg in preterm neonates (Van den Anker et al. 1995a). GFR increases rapidly during the first 2 weeks of life followed by a steady rise until adult values are reached by 8–12 months. This increase in GFR in the first weeks of life is mainly because of an increase in renal blood flow. Similarly, tubular secretory pathways are immature at birth and gain adult capacity during the first year of life.

There is a clear controversy regarding the use of serum creatinine to predict renal function in children (Filler and Lepage 2003). Serum creatinine depends on many factors and residual maternally derived creatinine interferes with the assay in the first days of life in neonates (Capparelli et al. 2001). In addition, factors that have a negative influence on the use of plasma creatinine to predict renal function are renal tubule integrity issues and GFR values of less than 20 mL/min/1.73 m^2. In these individuals, GFR is probably overestimated. If creatinine is measured with the Jaffé reaction ketoacids, serum bilirubin and cephalosporins interfere with the reaction and therefore the use of an enzymatic method should be advised because of less interference as compared to the Jaffé method (Van den Anker et al. 1995c). A more direct approach to estimate the GFR is to use a marker that is freely permeable across the glomerular capillary and neither secreted nor reabsorbed by the tubulus. Markers that have been mentioned to measure the GFR are inulin, polyfructosan S, cystatin C, ^{51}Cr-EDTA, ^{125}I-iothalamate, or mannitol (Filler and Lepage 2003; Hayton 2002). A marker to estimate the active tubular secretion in children is p-aminohippuric acid (Hayton 2002).

However, a comparison between serum creatinine with inulin clearance in preterm infants showed a good and clinical useful correlation and supported serum creatinine as an appropriate measure of GFR in preterm infants already on day 3 of life (Van Den Anker et al. 1995c).

Collectively, the aforementioned changes in GFR dramatically alter the plasma clearance of compounds with extensive renal elimination and thus provide a major determinant for age-appropriate dose regimen selection. Pharmacokinetic studies of drugs primarily excreted by glomerular filtration such as ceftazidime and famotidine have demonstrated significant correlations between plasma drug clearance and normal, expected maturational changes in renal function (Van den Anker et al. 1995a; James et al. 1998). For example, tobramycin is eliminated predominantly by glomerular filtration, necessitating dosing intervals of 36–48 h in preterm and 24 h in term newborns (De Hoog et al. 2002). Failure to account for the ontogeny of renal function and adjust aminoglycoside dosing regimens accordingly can result in exposure to potentially toxic serum concentrations. Also, concomitant medications (e.g., betamethasone, indomethacin) may alter the normal pattern of renal maturation in the neonate (Van Den Anker et al. 1994). Thus, for drugs with extensive renal elimination, both maturational and treatment associated changes in kidney function must be considered and used to individualize treatment regimens in an age-appropriate fashion.

8 Other Factors Influencing the Absorption, Distribution, Metabolism, and Excretion of Drugs in Neonates and Young Infants

In addition to growth and development, there are several other major variables that will influence the pharmacokinetic parameters of drugs such as inborn or acquired diseases, environmental influences such as body cooling, and pharmacogenomics. It is outside the scope of this chapter to provide extensive information on these important variables but a few will be highlighted here.

Hypoxic–ischemic events are encountered regularly in sick neonates and these events might result in a decrease in the rate and amount of drug absorption as well as impaired renal function. There are data to show that after perinatal asphyxia the GFR in neonates is 50% less as compared to neonates born without asphyxia, resulting in a decreased clearance of renally cleared drugs (Van den Anker et al. 1995b). The persistence and/or closure of a patent ductus arteriosus has a major impact on both the volume of distribution and elimination of frequently used drugs in the newborn (Van den Anker et al. 1995d). This has been shown for drugs such as ceftazidime where the existence of a patent ductus and or the exposure to indomethacin to close this ductus was associated with a decreased GFR and a larger volume of distribution of ceftazidime, a solely renally cleared drug. In another study investigating ibuprofen, there was a significant increase in the clearance of ibuprofen after closure of the ductus (Van Overmeire et al. 2001). Finally, total body cooling is a new treatment modality that is being used to improve the neurological outcome of neonates who suffered from perinatal asphyxia. In a study investigating the pharmacokinetics of morphine in neonates with and without body cooling, a clinically impressive decrease in morphine clearance was seen in neonates on body cooling (Roka et al. 2008).

9   Pharmacogenomics: Impact for Pediatric Populations

The contribution of genetic factors to explain heterogeneity of drug response in infants and children is another important issue with the ultimate goal for better treatment of children based on the individual genetic makeup. One of the major tasks is to optimally adapt the choice and amount of a drug to the individual need of a patient and, for instance, to prevent overdosing with the risk of adverse drug reactions. Genetic variability influences almost all ADME processes including drug absorption (e.g., via the intestinal drug transporter P-glycoprotein/ABCB1), drug metabolism (e.g., cytochrome P450 enzymes 2C9, 2C19, 2D6), and drug elimination, thereby resulting in alteration of pharmacokinetics and subsequently of pharmacodynamic processes.

There is an increasing body of evidence that genetic variants in drug metabolizing enzymes (e.g., CYP450 enzymes; http://www/cypalleles.ki.se/;) as well as in drug transporters (e.g., ABCB1/P-gp, SLCO1B1/OATP1B) (Schwab et al. 2003; Nies et al. 2008; Niemi et al. 2011) are functional relevant (e.g., loss of function variants or gain of function polymorphisms) with in part dramatic changes in mRNA and/or protein expression and function (Zanger et al. 2008). Genetic variants in drug targets such as receptor molecules or intracellular structures of signal transduction and gene regulation directly and/or indirectly may also influence drug response and tolerability in the neonate and young infant. Based on several novel and promising genomic technologies such as high-throughput genotyping (e.g., MaldiTof mass spectrometry), genome-wide association studies, and next generation sequencing, pharmacogenomic knowledge will improve our understanding of pharmacotherapy in children but will also stimulate the drug development process for innovative agents in the future (Russo et al. 2010).

To illustrate the impact of pediatric pharmacogenomics the link between development and genetics related to CYP2D6, one of the most studied enzymes, will be described. Genetic variation in CYP2D6 has been the subject of several comprehensive reviews in recent years (Zanger et al. 2004; Stevens et al. 2008). Poor (PM), intermediate (IM), extensive (EM), and ultrarapid (UM) metabolizer phenotypes are observed when a population is challenged with a probe substrate. Inheritance of two recessive loss-of-function alleles results in the "poor-metabolizer phenotype," which is found in about 5–10% of Caucasians and about 1–2% of Asian subjects (see earlier). At the other end of the spectrum, the presence of CYP2D6 gene duplication/multiplication events, which occurs at a frequency of 1–2% in Caucasians, most often is associated with enhanced clearance of CYP2D6 substrates although cases of increased toxicity due to increased formation of pharmacologically active metabolites have also been reported. Recently, this was even illustrated by a case of a breastfeeding woman with a UM phenotype, treated with codeine for pain after delivery, who formed so much morphine out of codeine that she intoxicated her newborn infant (Koren et al. 2006).

The ultimate utility of genomic information in the context of pharmacokinetics is when the genotype is shown to be predictive of the phenotype; specifically, when it can reliably predict the functional activity of a given enzyme and/or drug transporter. This is exemplified by use of the CYP2D6 activity score, which is derived based upon the functional impact (on CYP2D6 activity) of a given combination of *CYP2D6* alleles. A potential caveat with use of the CYP2D6 activity score resides with the fact that it has been validated in adults in whom the phenotypic CYP2D6 activity is fully developed (Zanger et al. 2001). In other words, the contribution of the genetic variation (e.g., CYP2D6 polymorphisms) to the phenotypic variability in drug disposition in adults has been explored. Very recently, Gaedigk et al. reported the use of this activity score also in infants (Gaedigk et al. 2008), but we still have to fit this genetic variation into the age-dependent maturation during infancy. At present we know that age and genetic determinants of CYP2D6 expression constitute significant determinants of inter-individual variability in CYP2D6-dependent metabolism during ontogeny. Very recently, it was documented that the in vivo phenotypic CYP2D6 activity was concordant with the genotype from 42 weeks postmenstrual age onwards (Allegaert et al. 2008; Blake et al. 2007). This indicates that for clinicians treating neonates, young infants, children, and adolescents the genetic variation in CYP2D6 is the major player to consider if prescribing CYP2D6 substrates.

In summary, both genetic and environmental factors contribute to inter-individual variability in the PK of medications metabolized by CYP2D6 (Leeder 2003; Krekels et al. 2007). In this context, a recent paper using a whole body physiology-based pharmacokinetic (PBPK) modeling approach to investigate the contribution of CYP2D6 genetics on codeine administration in breastfeeding mothers and their babies supports the evidence that pediatric pharmacogenomics comprises more than a single gene, and developmental aspects of physiological processes need to be considered (Willmann et al. 2009).

If CYP2D6 genotyping is becoming a standard laboratory test and the CYP2D6 activity score has been validated in infants, children, and adolescents, this will surely improve our capacity to predict the doses of CYP2D6 substrates required to treat the neonates, young infants, children, and adolescents in a more safe and effective way.

10 The Interface of Pharmacokinetics and Pharmacodynamics

Although, it is generally accepted that developmental differences in drug action exist, there is little scientific evidence of real age related pharmacodynamic variation among children of different age groups and adults. Age-related pharmacokinetic variation in drug clearance has the potential to alter the systemic

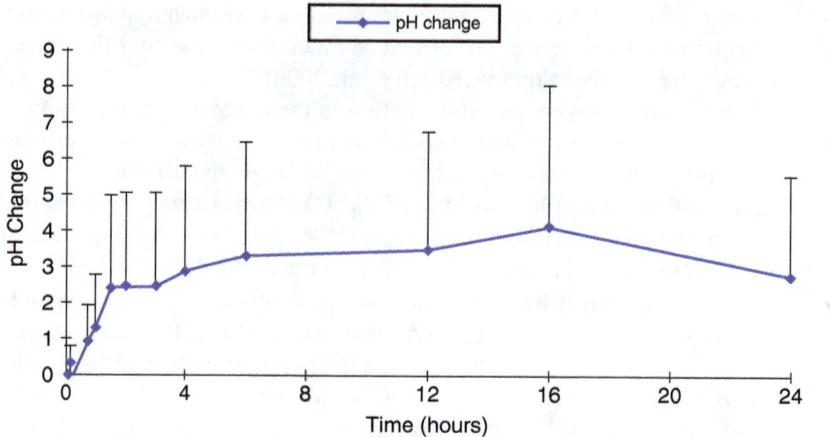

Fig. 2 Time dependent change in intragastric pH in a population of neonates administered a single intravenous dose of famotidine. Figure adapted from James et al. (1998)

exposure of drug from given dose with the consequence of producing less or more drug being available at the receptor(s) consequent to whether drug clearance is decreased or increased relative to values in adults. The resultant alteration in the dose–concentration profile may result in an attenuated (ineffective) or exaggerated (toxicity) pharmacodynamic response in an infant or child, a situation which is especially relevant for drugs with a narrow therapeutic index (e.g., aminoglycoside antibiotics, digoxin, antiarrhythmic agents). Thus, in some circumstances, apparent developmental differences in drug response/effect may be simply explained on pharmacokinetic basis. This is illustrated by the H_2 antagonist famotidine where consequent to a marked reduction in plasma clearance (i.e., renal elimination), a single intravenous dose produced a sustained increase in the intragastric pH in neonates for a 24-h postdose period (Fig. 2) (James et al. 1998).

11 Pediatric Dose Selection Based upon Pharmacokinetic Principles

Most current age-specific dosing requirements are based on the known influence of ontogeny on drug disposition. Current gaps in our knowledge (e.g., incomplete developmental profiles for hepatic and extrahepatic drug metabolizing enzymes, lack of knowledge with regard to expression of drug transporters that may influence drug clearance and/or bioavailability) prevent the use of simple formulas and/or allometric scaling for effective pediatric dose prediction; a fact especially true in very young infants where the relationship between body size and the maturation of pathways predominantly responsible for drug clearance are not linear (Holford 2010). Such approaches (e.g., allometric scaling) may have some potential clinical utility in children older than 3 years of age and adolescents whose organ function and body composition approximates that of young adults.

Age-specific dosing regimens for selected commonly used drugs where developmental differences in the dose–concentration profile have been well characterized serve to illustrate this point. For drugs whose plasma concentrations are routinely measured clinically (e.g., aminoglycosides, digoxin, caffeine, phenytoin, phenobarbital, carbamazepine, methotrexate, cyclosporine, tacrolimus, mycophenolate mofetil), or for whom pharmacokinetic characteristics were defined in pediatric patients during the drug development process, individualization of treatment based on patient-derived and in selected instances, population-estimated pharmacokinetic parameters is easily achieved. However, in the absence of such pharmacokinetic data and/or established pediatric dosing guidelines, alternate methods for dose selection must be used.

As discussed previously, the majority of age-adjusted pediatric drug dosing regimens utilize either body weight or surface area as surrogates to reflect the developmental determinants of drug disposition. Dose selection based on body weight or body surface areas will generally produce similar plasma concentration profiles except for those drugs whose apparent volume of distribution (V_d) corresponds to the extracellular fluid pool (i.e., $V_d < 0.3$ L/kg), where a body surface area based approach is preferable. In contrast, for drugs whose apparent V_d exceeds the extracellular fluid space (i.e., >0.3 L/kg), a body weight based approach for dose selection is preferable and as a result is the most frequently used approach for dosing in pediatrics.

When the pediatric dose for a given drug is not known these principles can be used to best approximate a proper dose for the initiation of treatment. Ritschel and Kearns (2009) have described an approach to determine dose in infants that is illustrated by the following equations:

$$\text{Infant dose (if } V_d < 0.3 \, \text{L/kg}) = (\text{infant BSA in m}^2 / 1.73 \, \text{m}^2) \times \text{adult dose},$$

$$\text{Infant dose (if } V_d \geq 0.3 \, \text{L/kg}) = (\text{infant BW in kg} / 70 \, \text{kg}) \times \text{adult dose}.$$

This approach is only useful for selection of dose size, and does not offer information regarding dosing interval since the equations contain no specific variable that describes potential age-associated differences in drug clearance. It is also important to note that this approach assumes that the body height and weight of a given child are appropriate (i.e., normal) for age and there are no abnormalities in body composition (e.g., edema, ascites) that can be produced by disease.

In neonates and young infants, the dosing interval for drugs with significant (i.e., $>50\%$) renal elimination by glomerular filtration can be approximated by estimation of the apparent elimination half-life ($t_{1/2}$) of the drug at a given point in development by using the following equations:

$$k_{el\ infant} = k_{el\ adult}\{[((GFR_{infant}/GFR_{adult}) - 1) \times F_{el}] + 1\},$$

$$T_{1/2\ infant} = 0.693/k_{el\ infant},$$

where k_{el} represents the average terminal apparent terminal elimination rate constant, GFR is an estimate of the glomerular filtration rate (which can be obtained from either a creatinine clearance determination or age-related normal values), and F_{el} is the fraction of drug excreted unchanged in the urine.

Alternatively, projection of pediatric dose requirement can be performed using in silico techniques (e.g., whole body physiologically based pharmacokinetic/pharmacodynamic models, population-based simulation, PK-Sim Packages, Simcyp Pediatric ADME Simulator) (Johnson and Rostami-Hodjegan 2011). The success of these approaches (i.e., prediction accuracy) is based upon the availability and reliability of parameter estimates (either pharmacokinetic, pharmacodynamic, or pharmacogenomic) and their prior knowledge in the specific subpopulation being used for dose projection (Espie et al. 2009). These caveats are especially important during early infancy where dynamic changes in drug disposition and action are likely consequent to ontogeny and developmental maturity in drug clearance pathways has not yet been attained.

12 Conclusions

The pediatric patient population consisting of neonates, infants, children, and adolescents shows unique differences in pharmacokinetic parameters as compared to adults and therefore requires specific dosage recommendations. While the paucity of pharmacokinetic and physiological data makes it difficult to precisely determine drug doses in pediatric patients, knowledge of the effects of growth, maturation, environmental influences, and pharmacogenetic background on absorption, distribution, metabolism, and elimination of frequently used medicines will allow more appropriate dosing recommendations for this patient population. Clearly, much more research is needed to fully understand the impact of development on the disposition of a drug. As described in this chapter, studies with substrates as markers for hepatic metabolic activity or renal function and in vitro data are very useful for a better understanding of this impact. Finally, there is an urgent need to better understand the metabolic activity, carrier mechanisms, and drug transporters related to the gastrointestinal tract.

Acknowledgements Johannes van den Anker is supported in part by FP7 grants TINN (223614), TINN2 (260908), and NEUROSIS (223060), and Matthias Schwab is supported in part by the FP7 grant NEUROSIS (223060).

References

Alcorn J, McNamara PJ (2002) Ontogeny of hepatic and renal systemic clearance pathways in infants: part I. Clin Pharmacokinet 41:959–998

Allegaert K, Anderson BJ, Verbesselt R, Debeer A, de Hoon J, Devlieger H et al (2005) Tramadol disposition in the very young: an attempt to assess in vivo cytochrome P-450 activity. Br J Anaesth 95:231–239

Allegaert K, van Schaik RH, Vermeersch S, Verbesselt R, Cossey V, Vanhole C et al (2008) Postmenstrual age and CYP2D6 polymorphisms determine tramadol O-demethylation in critically ill neonates and infants. Pediatr Res 63:674–679

Allegaert K, Rochette A, Veyckemans F (2011) Developmental pharmacology of tramadol during infancy: ontogeny, pharmacogenetics and elimination clearance. Paediatr Anaesth 21(3): 266–273

Anderson BJ, Holford NH (2008) Mechanism-based concepts of size and maturity in pharmacokinetics. Annu Rev Pharmacol Toxicol 48:303–332

Anderson BJ, van Lingen RA, Hansen TG, Lin YC, Holford NH (2002) Acetaminophen developmental pharmacokinetics in premature neonates and infants: a pooled population analysis. Anaesthesiology 96:1336–1345

Aranda JV, Collinge JM, Zinman R, Watters G (1979) Maturation of caffeine elimination in infancy. Arch Dis Child 54:946–949

Armstrong RW, Eichner ER, Klein DE, Barthel WF, Bennett JV, Jonsson V et al (1969) Pentachlorophenol poisoning in a nursery for newborn infants. II. Epidemiologic and toxicologic studies. J Pediatr 75:317–325

Bajpai M, Roskos LK, Shen DD, Levy RH (1996) Roles of cytochrome P4502C9 and cytochrome P4502C19 in the stereoselective metabolism of phenytoin to its major metabolite. Drug Metab Dispos 24:1401–1403

Balistreri W, Zimmer L, Suchy FJ, Bove KE (1984) Bile salt sulfotransferase: alterations during maturation and non-inducibility during substrate ingestion. J Lipid Res 25:228–235

Bartelink IH, Rademaker CM, Schobben AF, van den Anker JN (2006) Guidelines on paediatric dosing on the basis of developmental physiology and pharmacokinetic considerations. Clin Pharmacokinet 45:1077–1097

Blake MJ, Castro L, Leeder JS, Kearns GL (2005) Ontogeny of drug metabolizing enzymes in the neonate. Semin Fetal Neonatal Med 10:123–128

Blake MJ, Abdel-Rahman SM, Pearce RE, Leeder JS, Kearns GL (2006) Effect of diet on the development of drug metabolism by cytochrome P-450 enzymes in healthy infants. Pediatr Res 60:717–723

Blake MJ, Gaedigk A, Pearce RE, Bomgaars LR, Christensen ML, Stowe C et al (2007) Ontogeny of dextromethorphan O- and N-demethylation in the first year of life. Clin Pharmacol Ther 81:510–516

Brandolese R, Scordo MG, Spina E, Gusella M, Padrini R (2001) Severe phenytoin intoxication in a subject homozygous for CYP2C9*3. Clin Pharmacol Ther 70:391–394

Brown CM, Reisfeld B, Mayeno AN (2008) Cytochromes P450: a structure-based summary of biotransformations using representative substrates. Drug Metab Rev 40:169–184

Capparelli EV, Lane JR, Romanowski GL, McFeely EJ, Murray W, Sousa P et al (2001) The influences of renal function and maturation on vancomycin elimination in newborns and infants. J Clin Pharmacol 41:927–934

Card SE, Tompkins SF, Brien JF (1989) Ontogeny of the activity of alcohol dehydrogenase and aldehyde dehydrogenases in the liver and placenta of the guinea pig. Biochem Pharmacol 38:2535–2541

Caro AA, Cederbaum AI (2004) Oxidative stress, toxicology, and pharmacology of CYP2E1. Annu Rev Pharmacol Toxicol 44:27–42

Chen N, Aleksa K, Woodland C, Rieder M, Koren GL (2006) Ontogeny of drug elimination by the human kidney. Pediatr Nephrol 21:160–168

De Hoog M, Mouton JW, Schoemaker RC, Verduin CM, van den Anker JN (2002) Extended-interval dosing of tobramycin in neonates: implications for therapeutic drug monitoring. Clin Pharmacol Ther 71:349–358

De Hoog M, Mouton JW, van den Anker JN (2005) New dosing strategies for antibacterial agents in the neonate. Semin Fetal Neonatal Med 10:185–194

De Wildt SN, Kearns GL, Leeder JS, van den Anker JN (1999) Glucuronidation in humans: pharmacogenetic and developmental aspects. Clin Pharmacokinet 36:439–452

De Wildt SN, Kearns GL, Hop WC, Murry DJ, Abdel-Rahman SM, van den Anker JN (2001) Pharmacokinetics and metabolism of intravenous midazolam in preterm infants. Clin Pharmacol Ther 70:525–531

Edginton AN, Schmitt W, Voith B, Willmann S (2006) A mechanistic approach for the scaling of clearance in children. Clin Pharmacokinet 45:683–704

Erenberg A, Leff RD, Haack DG, Mosdell KW, Hicks GM, Wynne BA (2000) Caffeine citrate for the treatment of apnea of prematurity: a double-blind, placebo-controlled study. Pharmacotherapy 20:644–652

Espie P, Tytgat D, Sargentini-Maier ML, Poggesi I, Watelet JB (2009) Physiologically based pharmacokinetics (PBPK). Drug Metab Rev 41:391–407

Evans NJ, Rutter N, Hadgraft J, Parr G (1985) Percutaneous administration of theophylline in the preterm infant. J Pediatr 107:307–311

Evans WE, Relling MV, Petros WP, Meyer WH, Mirro J Jr, Crom WR (1989) Dextromethorphan and caffeine as probes for simultaneous determination of debrisoquin-oxidation and N-acetylation phenotypes in children. Clin Pharmacol Ther 45:568–573

Feinblatt BI, Aceto T, Beckhorn G, Bruck E (1966) Percutaneous absorption of hydrocortisone in children. Am J Dis Child 112:218–224

Filler G, Lepage N (2003) Should the Schwartz formula for estimation of GFR be replaced by cystatin C formula? Pediatr Nephrol 18:981–985

Friis-Hansen B (1983) Water distribution in the foetus and newborn infant. Acta Paediatr Scand 305:7–11

Gaedigk A, Simon D, Pearce RE, Bradford LD, Kennedy MJ, Leeder JS (2008) The CYP2D6 activity score: translating genotype information into a quantitative measure of phenotype. Clin Pharmacol Ther 83:234–242

Ginsberg G, Hattis D, Miller M, Sonawane B (2004) Pediatric pharmacokinetic data: implications for environmental risk assessment for children. Pediatrics 113:973–983

Hanioka N, Tanaka-Kagawa T, Miyata Y, Matsushima E, Makino Y, Ohno A et al (2003) Functional characterization of three human cytochrome P450 2E1 variants with amino acid substitutions. Xenobiotica 33:575–586

Hayton WL (2002) Maturation and growth of renal function: dosing renally cleared drugs in children. AAPS PharmSci 2:e3

Hines RN (2008) The ontogeny of drug metabolism enzymes and implications for adverse drug events. Pharmacol Ther 118:250–267

Hines RN, McCarver DG (2002) The ontogeny of human drug-metabolizing enzymes: phase I oxidative enzymes. J Pharmacol Exp Ther 300:355–360

Holford N (2010) Dosing in children. Clin Pharmacol Ther 87:367–370

James LP, Marotti T, Stowe C, Farrar HC, Taylor B, Kearns GL (1998) Pharmacokinetics and pharmacodynamics of famotidine in infants. J Clin Pharmacol 38:1089–1095

Jimenez-Lopez JM, Cederbaum AI (2005) CYP2E1-dependent oxidative stress and toxicity: role in ethanol-induced liver injury. Expert Opin Drug Metab Toxicol 1:671–685

Johnson TN, Rostami-Hodjegan A (2011) Resurgence in the use of physiologically based pharmacokinetic models in pediatric clinical pharmacology: parallel shift in incorporating the knowledge of biological elements and increased applicability to drug development and clinical practice. Paediatr Anaesth 21(3):291–301

Johnson TN, Rostami-Hodjegan A, Tucker GT (2006) Prediction of the clearance of eleven drugs and associated variability in neonates, infants and children. Clin Pharmacokinet 45:931–956

Johnson TN, Tucker GT, Rostami-Hodjegan A (2008) Development of CYP2D6 and CYP3A4 in the first year of life. Clin Pharmacol Ther 83:670–671

Johnsrud EK, Koukouritaki SB, Divakaran K, Brunengraber LL, Hines RN, McCarver DG (2003) Human hepatic CYP2E1 expression during development. J Pharmacol Exp Ther 307:402–407

Jung F, Richardson TH, Raucy JL, Johnson EF (1997) Diazepam metabolism by cDNA-expressed human 2C P450s: identification of P4502C18 and P4502C19 as low K(M) diazepam N-demethylases. Drug Metab Dispos 25:133–139

Kearns GL (2000) Impact of developmental pharmacology on pediatric study design: overcoming the challenges. J Allergy Clin Immunol 106:S128–S139

Kearns GL, Winter HS (2003) Proton pump inhibitors in pediatrics: relevant pharmacokinetics and pharmacodynamics. J Pediatr Gastroenterol Nutr 37(Suppl I)):S52–S59

Kearns GL, Abdel-Rahman SM, Alander SW, Blowey DL, Leeder JS, Kauffman RE (2003a) Developmental pharmacology – drug disposition, action, and therapy in infants and children. N Engl J Med 349:1157–1167

Kearns GL, Robinson PK, Wilson JT, Wilson-Costello D, Knight GR, Ward RM et al (2003b) Cisapride disposition in neonates and infants: in vivo reflection of cytochrome P450 3A4 ontogeny. Clin Pharmacol Ther 4:312–325

Kearns GL, Jungbluth GL, Abdel-Rahman SM, Hopkins NK, Welshman IR, Grzebyk RP et al (2003c) Impact of ontogeny on linezolid disposition in neonates and infants. Clin Pharmacol Ther 74:413–422

Kearns GL, Anderson T, James LP, Gaedigk A, Kraynak RA, Abdel-Rahman SM et al (2003d) Omeprazole disposition in children following single dose administration. J Clin Pharmacol 43:840–848

Kerr BM, Thummel KE, Wurden CJ, Klein SM, Kroetz DL, Gonzalez FJ et al (1994) Human liver carbamazepine metabolism. Role of CYP3A4 and CYP2C8 in 10,11-epoxide formation. Biochem Pharmacol 47:1969–1979

Kinirons MT, O'Shea D, Kim RB, Groopman JD, Thummel KE, Wood AJ et al (1999) Failure of erythromycin breath test to correlate with midazolam clearance as a probe of cytochrome P4503A. Clin Pharmacol Ther 66:224–231

Klotz U (2007) The role of pharmacogenetics in the metabolism of antiepileptic drugs: pharmacokinetics and therapeutic implications. Clin Pharmacokinet 46:271–279

Koren G, Cairns J, Chitayat D, Gaedigk A, Leeder JS (2006) Pharmacogenetics of morphine poisoning in a breastfed neonate of a codeine-prescribed mother. Lancet 368:704

Koukouritaki SB, Manro JR, Marsh SA, Stevens JC, Rettie AE, McCarver DG et al (2004) Developmental expression of human hepatic CYP2C9 and CYP2C19. J Pharmacol Exp Ther 308:965–974

Kraus DM, Fischer JH, Reitz SJ, Kecskes SA, Yeh TF, McCulloch KM et al (1993) Alterations in theophylline metabolism during the first year of life. Clin Pharmacol Ther 54:351–359

Krekels EH, van den Anker JN, Baiardi P, Cella M, Cheng KY, Gibb DM et al (2007) Pharmacogenetics and paediatric drug development: issues and consequences to labelling and dosing recommendations. Expert Opin Pharmacother 8:1787–1799

Lambert GH, Schoeller DA, Kotake AN, Flores C, Hay D (1986) The effect of age, gender, and sexual maturation on the caffeine breath test. Dev Pharmacol Ther 9:375–388

Lee CR, Goldstein JA, Pieper JA (2002) Cytochrome P450 2C9 polymorphisms: a comprehensive review of the in vitro and human data. Pharmacogenetics 12:251–263

Leeder JS (2003) Developmental and pediatric pharmacogenomics. Pharmacogenomics 4:331–341

Leeder JS, Kearns GL, Spielberg SP, van den Anker JN (2010) Understanding the relative roles of pharmacogenetics and ontogeny in pediatric drug development and regulatory science. J Clin Pharmacol 50(12):1377–1387

Loughnan PM, Greenwald A, Purton WW, Aranda JV, Watters G, Neims AH (1977) Pharmacokinetic observations of phenytoin disposition in the newborn and young infant. Arch Dis Child 52:302–309

McCarver DG, Hines RN (2002) The ontogeny of human drug metabolizing enzymes: phase II conjugation enzymes and regulatory mechanisms. J Pharmacol Exp Ther 300:361–366

Milavetz G, Vaughan LM, Weinberger MM, Hendeles L (1986) Evaluation of a scheme for establishing and maintaining dosage of theophylline in ambulatory patients with chronic asthma. J Pediatr 109:351–354

Nachman RL, Esterly NB (1980) Increased skin permeability in preterm infants. J Pediatr 96:99–103

Nelson DR, Koymans L, Kamataki T, Stegeman JJ, Feyereisen R, Waxman DJ et al (1996) P450 superfamily: update on new sequences, gene mapping, accession numbers and nomenclature. Pharmacogenetics 6:1–42

Niemi M, Pasanen MK, Neuvonen PJ (2011) Organic anion transporting polypeptide1B1: a genetically polymorphic transporter of major importance for hepatic drug uptake. Pharmacol Rev 63(1):157–181

Nies AT, Schwab M, Keppler D (2008) Interplay of conjugating enzymes with OATP uptake transporters and ABCC/MRP efflux pumps in the elimination of drugs. Expert Opin Drug Metab Toxicol 4:545–568

Payne K, Mattheyse FJ, Liedenberg D, Dawes T (1989) The pharmacokinetics of midazolam in paediatric patients. Eur J Clin Pharmacol 37:267–272

Pynnönen S, Sillanpää M, Frey H, Iisalo E (1977) Carbamazepine and its 10,11-epoxide in children and adults with epilepsy. Eur J Clin Pharmacol 11:129–133

Radde IC, McKercher HG (1985) Transport through membranes and development of membrane transport. In: MacLeod SM, Radde IC (eds) Textbook of pediatric clinical pharmacology. PSG, Littleton, MA, pp 1–16

Rane A, Bertilsson L, Palmer L (1975) Disposition of placentally transferred carbamazepine (Tegretol) in the newborn. Eur J Clin Pharmacol 8:283–284

Rhodin MM, Anderson BJ, Peters AM, Coulthard MG, Wilkins B, Cole M et al (2009) Human renal function maturation: a quantitative description using weight and postmenstrual age. Pediatr Nephrol 24:67–76

Ritschel WA, Kearns GL (eds) (2009) Handbook of basic pharmacokinetics, 7th edn. American Pharmacists Association, Washington, DC, pp 274–276

Riva R, Contin M, Albani F, Perucca E, Procaccianti G, Baruzzi A (1985) Free concentration of carbamazepine and carbamazepine-10,11-epoxide in children and adults. Influence of age and phenobarbitone co-medication. Clin Pharmacokinet 10:524–531

Roka A, Melinda KT, Vasarhelyi B, Machay T, Azzopardi D, Szabo M (2008) Elevated morphine concentrations in neonates treated with morphine and prolonged hypothermia for hypoxic ischemic encephalopathy. Pediatrics 121:e844–e849

Russo R, Capasso M, Paolucci P, Iolascon A, TEDDY European Network of Excellence (2010) Pediatric pharmacogenetic and pharmacogenomic studies: the current state and future perspectives. Eur J Clin Pharmacol ePub 2011;67 suppl 1:17–27 Epub 2010 Nov 11

Schwab M, Eichelbaum M, Fromm MF (2003) Genetic polymorphisms of the human MDR1 drug transporter. Annu Rev Pharmacol Toxicol 43:285–307

Stevens JC, Hines RN, Gu C, Koukouritaki SB, Manro JR, Tandler PJ et al (2003) Developmental expression of the major human hepatic CYP3A enzymes. J Pharmacol Exp Ther 307:573–582

Stevens JC, Marsh SA, Zaya MJ, Regina KJ, Divakaran K, Le M et al (2008) Developmental changes in human liver CYP2D6 expression. Drug Metab Dispos 36:1587–1593

Strolin Benedetti M, Baltes EL (2003) Drug metabolism and disposition in children. Fundam Clin Pharmacol 17:281–299

Suzuki Y, Mimaki T, Cox S, Koepke J, Hayes J, Walson PD (1994) Phenytoin age-dose-concentration relationship in children. Ther Drug Monitor 16(2):145–150

Tateishi T, Asoh M, Yamaguchi A, Yoda T, Okano YJ, Koitabashi Y (1999) Developmental changes in urinary elimination of theophylline and its metabolites in pediatric patients. Pediatr Res 45:66–70

Treluyer JM, Jacqz-Aigrain E, Alvarez F, Cresteil T (1991) Expression of CYP2D6 in developing human liver. Eur J Biochem 202:583–588

Van den Anker JN, Rakhmanina NY (2006) Pharmacological research in pediatrics: from neonates to adolescents. Adv Drug Deliv Rev 58:4–14

Van den Anker JN, Hop W, de Groot R, van der Heijden AJ, Broerse HM, Lindemans J et al (1994) Effects of prenatal exposure to betamethasone and indomethacin on the glomerular filtration rate in the preterm infant. Pediatr Res 36:578–581

Van den Anker JN, Schoemaker R, Hop W, van der Heijden BJ, Weber A, Sauer PJ et al (1995a) Ceftazidime pharmacokinetics in preterm infants: effects of renal function and gestational age. Clin Pharmacol Ther 58:650–659

Van den Anker JN, Van der Heijden AJ, Hop WCJ, Schoemaker RC, Broerse HM, Neijens HJ et al (1995b) The effect of asphyxia on the pharmacokinetics of ceftazidime in the term newborn. Pediatr Res 38:808–811

Van den Anker JN, de Groot R, Broerse HM, Sauer PJ, van der Heijden BJ, Neijens HJ et al (1995c) Assessment of glomerular filtration rate in preterm infants by serum creatinine: comparison with inulin clearance. Pediatrics 96:1156–1158

Van den Anker JN, Hop WCJ, Schoemaker RC, Van der Heijden AJ, Neijens HJ, De Groot R (1995d) Ceftazidime pharmacokinetics in preterm infants: effects of postnatal age and postnatal exposure to indomethacin. Br J Clin Pharmacol 40:439–443

Van Overmeire B, Touw D, Schepens PJC, Kearns GL, van den Anker JN (2001) Ibuprofen pharmacokinetics in preterm infants with patent ductus arteriosus. Clin Pharmacol Ther 70:336–343

Willmann S, Edgington AN, Coboeken K, Ahr G, Lippert J (2009) Risk to the breast-fed neonate from codeine treatment to the mother: a quantitative mechanistic modelling study. Clin Pharmacol Ther 86:634–643

Zanger UM, Fischer J, Raimundo S, Stuven T, Evert BO, Schwab M, Eichelbaum M (2001) Comprehensive analysis of the genetic factors determining expression and function of hepatic CYP2D6. Pharmacogenetics 11:573–585

Zanger UM, Raimundo S, Eichelbaum M (2004) Cytochrome P450 2D6: overview and update on pharmacology, genetics and biochemistry. Naunyn-Schmiedebergs Arch Pharmacol 369:23–37

Zanger UM, Turpeinen M, Klein K, Schwab M (2008) Functional pharmacogenetics/genomics of human cytochromes P450 involved in drug biotransformation. Anal Bioanal Chem 392:1093–1108

Principles of Therapeutic Drug Monitoring

Wei Zhao and Evelyne Jacqz-Aigrain

Contents

Abstract Therapeutic drug monitoring (TDM) is central to optimize drug efficacy in children, because the pharmacokinetics and pharmacodynamics of most drugs differ greatly between children and adults. Many factors should be analyzed to implement TDM in the pediatric population, including a validated pharmacological parameter and an analytical method adapted to children as limited sampling volumes and high sensitivity are required. The use of population approaches, new analytical methods such as saliva and dried blood spots, and pharmacodynamic monitoring give attractive options to improve TDM, individualize therapy in order to optimize efficacy and reduce adverse drug reactions.

Keywords Monitoring • Concentration • Therapeutic index • Pharmacokinetics • Pharmacodynamics • Bayesian estimation

W. Zhao • E. Jacqz-Aigrain (✉)
Department of Pediatric Pharmacology and Pharmacogenetics, Clinical Investigation Center, CIC Inserm 9202, French network of Pediatric Investigation Centers (CICPaed), Hôpital Robert Debré, 48 Boulevard Sérurier, 75935 Paris, France
e-mail: evelyne.jacqz-aigrain@rdb.aphp.fr

H.W. Seyberth et al. (eds.), *Pediatric Clinical Pharmacology*,
Handbook of Experimental Pharmacology 205,
DOI 10.1007/978-3-642-20195-0_3, © Springer-Verlag Berlin Heidelberg 2011

1 Therapeutic Drug Monitoring: Definition, Which Drug to Measure?

TDM is used, in combination with parameters of the patient's clinical condition to help guide decisions regarding drug dosing in individual patients (Walson 1998) in order to optimize therapeutic efficacy and minimize adverse events. The general requirements for a drug to be considered for TDM are presented in Table 1.

2 Pharmacological Differences Between Adults and Children

Although criteria for TDM pertain to both adults and children, children are more likely to benefit from TDM, as in contrast to the adult situation, validated dosage recommendations are limited for many drugs prescribed in children. Indeed, approximately 70% of drugs prescribed to children, and more than 93% to critically ill neonates, are unlicensed or used in an off-label manner ('t Jong et al. 2000, 2002; Conroy et al. 2000). As growth and development are a continuum, with continuous changes in physiological parameters during childhood, marked differences in the pharmacokinetic and pharmacodynamic behavior of many drugs are reported between children and adults. All pharmacokinetic phases are involved (Kearns et al. 2003): in such situations, pediatric dosage is empirical. As a result, therapeutic failures, adverse events, and even fatalities may occur (Ince et al. 2009).

Oral absorption may be altered by changes in gastroenterological physiology with age. During the neonatal period, intragastric pH is relatively high (greater than 4), as both basal acid output and the total volume of gastric secretions are limited. As a consequence, the bioavailability of acid labile compounds is increased

Table 1 Requirements to set up TDM for a given drug (Touw et al. 2005; Soldin and Soldin 2002)

- A relationship exists between drug plasma (blood) concentration and effect and is stronger than between drug dosage and effect
- The drug has a narrow therapeutic index, i.e., small difference between the therapeutic and toxic concentrations, between the low concentration, without effect and the high concentration, associated with toxicity
- The concentrations resulting from a given dose are unpredictable as a result of inter- and intra-individual variability
- The clinical effects are not easily measurable
- A rapid and reliable analytical method is validated to determine drug and metabolites concentrations

In addition, TDM can also be useful:

- If toxicity is suspected
- In the absence of drug response when subtherapeutic concentrations are suspected or compliance is questionable
- When dose adjustment is required as a result of drug interactions or changes in clinical state

compared to older children (Agunod et al. 1969; Rodbro et al. 1967). Furthermore, in infants younger than 6 months, gastric emptying is much slower, which probably prolongs the time required to achieve maximal plasma levels. Most of these physiological variables affecting oral absorption are immature, reaching adult values, between 5 and 10 years of age. *Percutaneous absorption* is enhanced in infants, which may be partly accounted by the presence of a thinner stratum corneum in the preterm neonate (Rutter 1987) and by the relatively greater extent of cutaneous perfusion and hydration of the epidermis throughout childhood (Okah et al. 1995; Fluhr et al. 2000). Rectal absorption may also be enhanced in neonates and infants (Kearns et al. 2003). *Intramuscular absorption* depends on several physiological factors: reduced skeletal-muscle blood flow and inefficient muscular contractions may reduce the rate of intramuscular drug absorption. On the other hand, the relatively higher density of skeletal-muscle capillaries in infants may increase absorption (Greenblatt and Koch-Weser 1976; Carry et al. 1986).

Distribution may be altered by the differences in body composition. In neonates and infants, the relatively larger total body water (70–75% in neonates versus 50–55% in adults) and extracellular water component (40% in neonates versus 20% in adults) and lower fat tissue (15% in infants versus 20% in adults) affect the distribution of drugs which are mainly distributed in body water and to a lesser extent of lipophilic drugs (Koren 1997). In addition, the lower protein binding in neonates and infant increases the free fraction of drugs highly bound in older children and adults.

Metabolism is influenced by numerous factors and primarily by age. In the neonate, the hepatic microsomal enzyme system is immature. Drug-metabolizing activities by cytochrome P450 oxidases (CYP, phase I enzymes) and conjugating enzymes (phase II enzymes) are substantially lower and vary extensively between patients (See Chapter: Pharmacokinetics and maturation/development). This explains why the variability of pharmacokinetic parameters such as clearance or elimination half-life is much higher in children than in adults. TDM is therefore very useful during this period, because of the lack of validated dosage regimens and the rapid change of enzyme activities.

Renal elimination. The glomerular filtration rate (GFR) is much lower in neonates than in older infants, children, or adults. GFR matures during infancy and approaches an adult rate by 6–12 months postnatal age. The maturation process of renal structure and function includes prolongation and maturation of renal tubules, increase in renal blood flow, and improvement of filtration efficiency. In addition, blood flow is shifted from the deeper to the more superficial nephrons (Koren 1997).

Pharmacodynamic differences also exist between the pediatric and adult populations. Indeed, children do not always respond to drug treatment similarly to adults. One of the examples is warfarin. Developmental changes in the pharmacokinetics and pharmacodynamics of warfarin enantiomers were studied in prepubertal, pubertal, and adult patients given long-term warfarin therapy. The results showed that the patients from these three age groups had comparable mean plasma concentrations of unbound warfarin enantiomers. However, the prepubertal patients showed significantly lower plasma concentrations of protein C and prothrombin fragments 1 + 2 and greater international normalized ratio (INR ratio between the coagulation time of a sample of blood and the normal coagulation time, when coagulation takes place in certain standardized conditions) and dose normalized INR than the adults. This increased response to warfarin should be taken into account when starting treating children with warfarin (Takahashi et al. 2000).

3　TDM in Practice

3.1　Timing of Sampling for TDM in Children (Table 2)

Drugs are usually administered at repeated doses with a constant dosage interval, either orally or intravenously. Blood or plasma concentrations rise and fall in each inter-dose interval, from peak to trough. For drugs with linear elimination given at a fixed dosage regimen, drug concentrations reach steady-state conditions after 4–5 half-lives. Approximated steady-state concentrations may be reached earlier if a loading dose is given. This estimation does not apply to drugs with saturable elimination when given at the usual dose, i.e., phenytoin and theophylline. In such cases of dose dependant kinetics, the drug concentrations increase disproportionately. During continuous infusion, no fluctuations are expected in blood/plasma concentrations at steady state. In some situations, drugs should be monitored before steady-state levels are reached to ensure the efficacy and avoid toxicity (1) when the half-live is long, in order to detect overdosing before steady state; (2) in individuals with impaired metabolism or renal clearance; and (3) in case of potential drug interactions. In all cases, detailed information on patient's disease and clinical conditions, biological parameters of interest, drug, dosage regimen and associated therapies, and time of sampling relative to the time of drug administration are essential to interpret the results (Gross 2001).

Table 2 Technical aspects of TDM; sample collection, analytical methods

Delay between start of treatment and time of sampling
Sampling time (peak or trough?)
Number of samples
Conditions of sampling
Type of sample (blood, plasma, saliva, dried spot, etc.)
Volume of each sample
Appropriate collecting tube
Validated analytical method

3.2 Technical Aspects of TDM: Sample Collection, Analytical Methods

The influence of the blood collecting tube on the concentrations measured should be taken into consideration. Indeed, several studies have reported that inappropriate tubes containing serum separator gels can significantly affect the determination of phenytoin (Dasgupta et al. 1994; Quattrocchi et al. 1983) or ribavirin, the latter being more stable in gel-containing tubes than in dry or ethylenediaminetetra-acetic acid tubes (Marquet et al. 2010). Therefore, it is strongly recommended to evaluate the matrix effect of blood collecting tubes when validating a new analytic method for TDM. Another important issue in pediatric TDM is for techniques validated for very small sample volumes, especially in neonates, with low total blood volume (40 mL for a preterm infant of 500 g). Moreover, as hematocrit is higher in young infants, more blood has to be drawn to obtain a similar volume of plasma. To optimize TDM, a TDM laboratory has to develop analytical methods adapted to the age of the patients, particularly for neonates. In addition, all laboratories should make analytical procedures available to clinicians that include for each drug the optimal sampling time and sampling volume required, the type of blood collecting tubes, clinical and biological parameters required to interpret the measured concentration (Koren 1997). Differences between analytical methods may have a major impact on the results. Monitoring of immunosuppressants is taken here as an example. Because of their high inter- and intra-individual variability and narrow therapeutic index, TDM of immunosuppressants is mandatory both in children and in adults whatever the indication, but primarily to prevent transplant rejection and toxicity in organ transplanted children. Immunoassay techniques are widely used for TDM as they are easy to perform and are less time consuming than chromatographic methods. However, although often regarded as "specific" for the parent drug, the antibody may cross-react with other compounds, including metabolites of the drug. Therefore, the concentrations are often overestimated as compared with chromatographic assays. Due to the cross reactivity of mycophenolic acid (MPA) with its acyl-glucuronide metabolite (AcMPAG) in enzyme-multiplied immunoassay technique (EMIT), the concentrations of MPA determined by EMIT were systematically higher than by high-performance liquid chromatography with ultraviolet (HPLC-UV) method, with an average positive bias of 15% in pediatric transplant recipients (Irtan et al. 2008). In general, these differences do not affect significantly the clinical value of TDM, although they have an impact on the target concentration and contribute to the variability of drug concentrations reported in the literature. However, in defined clinical conditions where the concentrations of metabolites contribute significantly to the measured drug concentration, the differences between analytical assays should be taken into account to interpret the results. This is the case, for example, in liver transplanted patients immediately posttransplant receiving mycophenolate mofetil (MMF) the prodrug of MPA, where overestimation of MPA concentration may occur and be misleading (Schütz et al. 1998).

3.3 Which Samples to Analyze: Blood or Saliva, Dried Blood Spot?

TDM is usually performed in blood/plasma after venous sampling. Children, and primarily younger ones, usually fear needles and injections and alternative sampling techniques will satisfy both children and their parents.

Saliva sampling is an alternative procedure both noninvasive and painless. When compared to venous blood sampling, saliva sampling has the following advantages: (1) Sample collection with minimal patient discomfort. (2) Repeated samples easier to obtain and very useful in patients receiving chronic treatments. Saliva sampling has shown great interest for the TDM of anticonvulsant drugs as numerous studies have shown a good correlation between saliva and blood concentrations of carbamazepine, phenytoin, primidone, and ethosuximide (Herkes and Eadie 1990; Gorodischer et al. 1997; Liu and Delgado 1999). However, although saliva sampling has gained adequate acceptance in pharmacokinetic and pharmacodynamic research studies, its use in clinical practice remains limited (Drobitch and Svensson 1992). Limiting factors are linked to saliva collection and sample analysis and include salivary flow rate and pH, sampling conditions, contamination and protein binding have been shown to influence drug measurements. This is the case for valproic acid and some controversy exists for phenobarbital. Therefore, a standardized and well-controlled sampling procedure should be developed and validated to standardize the drug TDM in saliva (Liu and Delgado 1999; Mullangi et al. 2009)

The dried blood spot (DBS) sampling is another option for TDM in children. In DBS sampling, blood is obtained via a finger or heel prick with an automatic lancet and the drop of blood is collected on a sampling paper, then dried and easily kept and/or sent for analysis. DBS offers a number of advantages over conventional venous blood sampling, as (1) it is less invasive, avoiding classical venous puncture or canula, (2) it requires smaller blood volume (less than 100 μL), (3) storage is simpler and transfer is easier at room temperature, (4) DBS can be easily collected by the patient itself or his guardian with minimum training and sent by mail to the assigned laboratory, so that TDM results are available when patients visit the physician (Li and Tse 2010; Edelbroek et al. 2009). DBS is increasingly used for the TDM of a wide spectrum of drugs such as antiretroviral drugs (Koal et al. 2005; ter Heine et al. 2009a, b), immunosuppressants (Cheung et al. 2008; Hoogtanders et al. 2007; Wilhelm et al. 2009; van der Heijden et al. 2009), and antiepileptics (la Marca et al. 2008, 2009). The most important physiological factor that affects DBS results is hematocrit. Hematocrit affects blood viscosity and flux and impacts diffusion properties of blood applied on the filter paper. When hematocrit is high, diffusion in the paper is poor, a higher volume per punch is required for analysis and a higher concentration will be measured than when the hematocrit is low (Adam et al. 2000; Mei et al. 2001). This should be taken into account in pediatric patients as the hematocrit value varies with age, e.g., 0.28–0.67 in patients from birth to 1 year and 0.35–0.42 for children (2–12 years old) (Li and Tse 2010). In addition, assay sensitivity and specificity remain a challenge as blood volume is lower and analytical interferences may occur. Indeed HPLC coupled with either UV or fluorescence detection may not be suitable, the reference method being HPLC coupled with tandem mass spectrometry (MS/MS) used in most publications on DBS analysis.

The interpretation of drug concentrations measured during monitoring should take into account all the aspect and conditions of monitoring (including dose and dosage schedule, the type of biological sample, analytical technique used, start of treatment, potential drug interactions, etc.) and use reference concentrations to draw recommendations for dosage adaptation (Table 3).

Table 3 Therapeutic concentrations for different classes of drug

Class	Medication	Sampling time	Therapeutic range in children	Reference
Antiepileptic drugs	Carbamazepine	Predose	4–12 µg/mL	Scheyer and Cramer (1990)
	Phenobarbital	Any time during dosage interval after steady state	20–60 µg/mL	Warner et al. (1998)
	Phenytoin	Predose (oral dose); 1–4 h post-IV loading dose. At least 2 h post-IV dose	Infant: 6–11 µg/mL; Free drug: 1–2 µg/mL	Warner et al. (1998)
	Primidone	Predose	5–12 µg/mL	Warner et al. (1998)
	Valproic acid	Predose	50–120 µg/mL	Warner et al. (1998)
Aminoglycosides	Gentamicin	Predose	0.5–1 µg/mL	Touw et al. (2009)
		Peak	10–12 µg/mL	
	Tobramycin	Predose	0.5–1 µg/mL	Touw et al. (2009)
		Peak	10–12 µg/mL	
	Amikacin	Peak	24–35 µg/mL	Sherwin et al. (2009)
		AUC_{24h}	130–590 µg h/mL	
Glycopeptides	Vancomycin	Predose	5–10 µg/mL	de Hoog et al. (2004)
		Peak	20–40 µg/mL	
Immunosuppressants	Cyclosporine	Predose	Initial posttransplantation period: 150–250 µg/L (kidney, liver) Maintenance period: 100–150 µg/L (kidney); 130–200 µg/L (liver)	Brodehl (1994)
		2-h post oral dose	Initial posttransplantation period: 1,300–1,800 µg/L (kidney); 800–1,200 µg/L (liver)	
	Tacrolimus	Predose	Initial posttransplantation period: 10–20 ng/mL Maintenance period: 5–15 ng/mL	del Mar Fernández De Gatta et al. (2002)
	MPA (after administration of mycophenolate mofetil – MMF)	AUC_{12h}	30–60 mg h/L	del Mar Fernández De Gatta et al. (2002)
Miscellaneous	Theophylline	Predose	5–15 mg/L	Self et al. (1993)
	Digoxin	At least 6-h post dose	0.8–2 ng/mL	Steinberg and Notterman (1994)

4 New Approaches for TDM: Population Pharmacokinetics and Bayesian Estimator

Monitoring aims at measuring individual drug exposure based on validated pharmacokinetic parameters that better reflect drug effect than drug dosage. Drug monitoring may be based on different parameters: trough concentration (just before the following administration), peak concentration, or area under the curve (AUC) measured at steady state. Optimal interpretation of the result requires a validated therapeutic range: the lowest limit is the concentration that produces half of the maximum possible therapeutic effect while the upper limit is determined by toxicity and is the concentration at which toxicity will develop but only in a limited number of patients. A major limitation of TDM in children is that for many medications, target concentrations are not defined in children but only based on data obtained in adults.

"Population pharmacokinetic approaches" opened new ways for TDM. For population pharmacokinetic modeling, numerous drug concentrations, so-called observations, are obtained from a large number of patients, representing the entire population. The "nonlinear mixed effects modeling is based on the simultaneous analysis of all data obtained and Parametric method" means that the distribution of the pharmacokinetic parameters is assumed to be normal or log-normal. Both the interindividual and intraindividual pharmacokinetic variabilities are estimated separately. Covariate analysis is then performed, in which demographic and pathophysiologic (e.g., weight, age, liver and kidney function, disease severity and genetics, etc.) predictors of variability are identified. If these predictors are associated with clinically significant shifts in the therapeutic index, they may serve for the design of individualized dosage regimens. The population approach allows the analysis of either sparse and rich data, but also unbalanced data or a combination of data from experimental settings and clinical practice (Ince et al. 2009; Zhao et al. 2009, 2010).

4.1 Bayesian Estimation

The most useful TDM application of population pharmacokinetics is dose individualization using a posteriori method – Bayesian estimation (also called "maximum a posteriori Bayesian estimation"). It relies upon the following formula:

$$\mathrm{p}(P/C) = K \bullet \mathrm{p}(C/P) \bullet \mathrm{p}(P)$$

stating that the posterior probability density $\mathrm{p}(P/C)$ of the pharmacokinetic parameter P, given the measured concentration C in a given patient, is proportional to the product of the likelihood of the data $\mathrm{p}(C/P)$ with the prior probability density of the parameters $\mathrm{p}(P)$ in the population to which the patient belongs. The likelihood depends on the pharmacokinetic model that describes the expected concentration for a given set of parameters and covariate values, and on the residual error model, which describes the deviation between the expected concentrations and the measured concentrations (Tod et al. 2001).

Bayesian estimation offers more flexibility in blood sampling times, owing to its precision and to the amount of information provided. Unlike the other a posteriori methods, Bayesian estimation is based on population pharmacokinetic studies and takes into account the pharmacokinetic characteristics of a typical population, individual patient's data including drug concentrations and covariates, but also takes into account the variability of the pharmacokinetics parameters in the population. In practice, the population pharmacokinetic parameters can be obtained from the index dataset, which is used a priori to determine the distribution of pharmacokinetic parameters in a given population or from the literature. In the last case, the external validation is mandatory, as numerous factors, such as age, weight, clinical condition, genetics, etc., can modify the population pharmacokinetic parameters. It should be demonstrated that the published model could correctly predict the concentrations in validation dataset.

An important issue is the validation of Bayesian estimation, either internal or external. When the number of patients receiving the drug is limited, internal validation using a circular permutation method can be considered. The full dataset is randomly divided into four subsets, each one containing 25% of data and the building group includes only part of the total data. The population parameters obtained in each combination of three subsets using 75% of data each time, corresponding to the building group are used to calculate the individual pharmacokinetic parameters of the remaining 25% of data defined as the internal validation group. This procedure is repeated four times (as there are four different combinations of 75 and 25% datasets). Predicted concentrations or AUCs using Bayesian estimation from four times of circular permutation are then compared with the corresponding observed values.

The methodology of external validation is used when a large number of patients are available, allowing the validation group to be different from the building group and not used to define the pharmacokinetic parameters. In this situation, the patients are randomly divided prior to any analysis, into the building vs. validation group. The population parameters obtained in the building group are used to calculate the individual data in the validation group, where individual predicted concentrations or AUCs using Bayesian estimation will be compared with the observed, measured values.

Whatever the processes of validation, according to the method described by Sheiner and Beal (1981), the criteria for evaluating the predictive performance of Bayesian estimation include the prediction bias prediction error (PE) and absolute prediction error (APE). They are calculated by using the following equations:

$$PE = (\text{predicted value} - \text{reference value})/\text{reference value and}$$

$$APE = ABS\,(\text{predicted value} - \text{reference value})/\text{reference value.}$$

PE and APE are expressed in the results as a percentage.

The lower the PE and APE, the more accurate and precise the prediction of Bayesian estimation are (Sheiner and Beal 1981).

Bayesian estimation have been increasingly employed in AUC-guided TDM (e.g., cyclosporine, Mycophenolate Mofetil, carboplatin) (Irtan et al. 2007; Payen et al. 2005; Peng et al. 1995) as well as in routine monitoring of drugs characterized by a very high interindividual pharmacokinetic variability such as methotrexate, tobramycin, gentamicin, etc. (Tod et al. 2001; Plard et al. 2007).

5 Pharmacodynamic Monitoring

The current TDM approach determines drug concentrations (or other pharmacokinetic parameters) in extracellular or whole blood fractions. It is used as a surrogate marker of effect, but in some cases it may be hampered by the absence of correlation between exposure and effect. In recent years, it was shown that the assessment of pharmacodynamic effects provides a mean to improve and individualize drug therapy. Numerous attempts have been made to develop biomarkers that would complete TDM, e.g., pharmacodynamic monitoring of immunosuppressive therapy, which is considered as a new strategy to tailor immunosuppressive therapy (Oellerich et al. 2006; Sommerer et al. 2009).

However, immunosuppressive effect is complex and involves drug-independent mediators, such as immunophilins for activity of cyclosporine and tacrolimus (calcineurin inhibitors, CNI). Concentrations based TDM is limited in its ability to measure drug effectiveness at its immunosuppressive site of action. As a result, measured concentrations within the therapeutic range do not guarantee absence of rejection or avoidance of toxicity in all patients and at all times. Pharmacodynamic approaches are designed to address this issue (van Rossum et al. 2010). Numerous tools have been developed for pharmacodynamic monitoring of CNI therapy, such as calcineurin inhibition, IL-2 production, expression of genes encoding cytokines, intra-lymphocyte ATP concentrations in $CD4^+$ cells, and T-cell cytometric and functional assays as markers of the degree of CNI-induced immunosuppression (de Jonge et al. 2009). Preliminary reports also show associations between the different pharmacodynamic markers and outcome as well as CNI pharmacokinetics (Fukudo et al. 2005; Sanquer et al. 2004; Brunet et al. 2007). However, the routinely clinical use of these pharmacodynamic markets remains to be validated in order to be implemented in clinical practice. Studies in larger patient populations are needed to evaluate the clinical value of these promising approaches.

Pharmacodynamic monitoring is not supposed to replace current concentrations based TDM rather a complementary combination of TDM and pharmacodynamic monitoring, which could help to improve pharmacotherapy for more effective and safe results in individual patients.

References

Adam BW, Alexander JR, Smith SJ, Chace DH, Loeber JG, Elvers LH, Hannon WH (2000) Recoveries of phenylalanine from two sets of dried blood spot reference materials: prediction from hematocrit, spot volume, and paper matrix. Clin Chem 46:126–128

Agunod M, Yamaguchi N, Lopez R, Luhby AL, Glass GB (1969) Correlative study of hydrochloric acid, pepsin, and intrinsic factor secretion in newborns and infants. Am J Dig Dis 14:400–414

Brodehl J (1994) Consensus statements on the optimal use of cyclosporine in pediatric patients. Transplant Proc 26:2759–2762

Brunet M, Crespo M, Millan O et al (2007) Pharmacokinetics and pharmacodynamics in renal transplant recipients under treatment with cyclosporine and myfortic. Transplant Proc 39:2160–2162

Carry MR, Ringel SP, Starcevich JM (1986) Distribution of capillaries in normal and diseased human skeletal muscle. Muscle Nerve 9:445–454

Cheung CY, van der Heijden J, Hoogtanders K, Christiaans M, Liu YL, Chan YH, Choi KS, van de Plas A, Shek CC, Chau KF, Li CS, van Hooff J, Stolk L (2008) Dried blood spot measurement: application in tacrolimus monitoring using limited sampling strategy and abbreviated AUC estimation. Transpl Int 21:140–145

Conroy S et al (2000) Survey of unlicensed and off label drug use in paediatric wards in European countries. European Network for Drug Investigation in Children. BMJ 320:79–82

Dasgupta A, Dean R, Saldana S, Konnaman G, McLawhon RW (1994) Absorption of therapeutic drugs by barrier gels in serum separator blood collection tubes. Am J Clin Pathol 101:456–461

de Hoog M, Mouton JW, van den Anker JN (2004) Vancomycin: pharmacokinetics and administration regimens in neonates. Clin Pharmacokinet 43:417–440

de Jonge H, Naesens M, Kuypers DR (2009) New insights into the pharmacokinetics and pharmacodynamics of the calcineurin inhibitors and mycophenolic acid: possible consequences for therapeutic drug monitoring in solid organ transplantation. Ther Drug Monit 31:416–435

del Mar Fernández De Gatta M, Santos-Buelga D, Domínguez-Gil A et al (2002) Immunosuppressive therapy for paediatric transplant patients: pharmacokinetic considerations. Clin Pharmacokinet 41:115–135

Drobitch RK, Svensson CK (1992) Therapeutic drug monitoring in saliva: an update. Clin Pharmacokinet 23:365–379

Edelbroek PM, van der Heijden J, Stolk LM (2009) Dried blood spot methods in therapeutic drug monitoring: methods, assays, and pitfalls. Ther Drug Monit 31:327–336

Fluhr JW, Pfisterer S, Gloor M (2000) Direct comparison of skin physiology in children and adults with bioengineering methods. Pediatr Dermatol 17:436–439

Fukudo M, Yano I, Masuda S et al (2005) Pharmacodynamic analysis of tacrolimus and cyclosporine in living-donor liver transplant patients. Clin Pharmacol Ther 78:168–181

Gorodischer R, Burtin P, Verjee Z, Hwang P, Koren G (1997) Is saliva suitable for therapeutic monitoring of anticonvulsants in children: an evaluation in the routine clinical setting. Ther Drug Monit 19:637–642

Greenblatt DJ, Koch-Weser J (1976) Intramuscular injection of drugs. N Engl J Med 295:542–546

Gross AS (2001) Best practice in therapeutic drug monitoring. Br J Clin Pharmacol 52(Suppl 1):5S–10S

Herkes GK, Eadie MJ (1990) Possible roles for frequent salivary antiepileptic drug monitoring in the management of epilepsy. Epilepsy Res 6:146–154

Hoogtanders K, van der Heijden J, Christiaans M, Edelbroek P, van Hooff JP, Stolk LM (2007) Therapeutic drug monitoring of tacrolimus with the dried blood spot method. J Pharm Biomed Anal 44:658–664

Ince I, de Wildt SN, Tibboel D, Danhof M, Knibbe CA (2009) Tailor-made drug treatment for children: creation of an infrastructure for data-sharing and population PK-PD modelling. Drug Discov Today 14:316–320

Irtan S, Azougagh S, Monchaud C, Popon M, Baudouin V, Jacqz-Aigrain E (2008) Comparison of high-performance liquid chromatography and enzyme-multiplied immunoassay technique to monitor mycophenolic acid in paediatric renal recipients. Pediatr Nephrol 23:1859–1865

Irtan S, Saint-Marcoux F, Rousseau A, Zhang D, Leroy V, Marquet P, Jacqz-Aigrain E (2007) Population pharmacokinetics and bayesian estimator of cyclosporine in pediatric renal transplant patients. Ther Drug Monit 29:96–102

Kearns GL, Abdel-Rahman SM, Alander SW, Blowey DL, Leeder JS, Kauffman RE (2003) Developmental pharmacology–drug disposition, action, and therapy in infants and children. N Engl J Med 18(349):1157–1167

Koal T, Burhenne H, Römling R, Svoboda M, Resch K, Kaever V (2005) Quantification of antiretroviral drugs in dried blood spot samples by means of liquid chromatography/tandem mass spectrometry. Rapid Commun Mass Spectrom 19:2995–3001

Koren G (1997) Therapeutic drug monitoring principles in the neonate. National Academy of Clinical Biochemistry. Clin Chem 43:222–227

la Marca G, Malvagia S, Filippi L, Fiorini P, Innocenti M, Luceri F, Pieraccini G, Moneti G, Francese S, Dani FR, Guerrini R (2008) Rapid assay of topiramate in dried blood spots by a new liquid chromatography–tandem mass spectrometric method. J Pharm Biomed Anal 48:1392–1396

la Marca G, Malvagia S, Filippi L, Luceri F, Moneti G, Guerrini R (2009) A new rapid micromethod for the assay of phenobarbital from dried blood spots by LC-tandem mass spectrometry. Epilepsia 50:2658–2662

Li W, Tse FL (2010) Dried blood spot sampling in combination with LC-MS/MS for quantitative analysis of small molecules. Biomed Chromatogr 24:49–65

Liu H, Delgado MR (1999) Therapeutic drug concentration monitoring using saliva samples. Focus on anticonvulsants. Clin Pharmacokinet 36:453–470

Marquet P, Sauvage FL, Loustaud-Ratti V, Babany G, Rousseau A, Lachâtre G (2010) Stability of ribavirin concentrations depending on the type of blood collection tube and preanalytical conditions. Ther Drug Monit 32:237–241

Mei JV, Alexander JR, Adam BW, Hannon WH (2001) Use of filter paper for the collection and analysis of human whole blood specimens. J Nutr 131:1631S–1636S

Mullangi R, Agrawal S, Srinivas NR (2009) Measurement of xenobiotics in saliva: is saliva an attractive alternative matrix? Case studies and analytical perspectives. Biomed Chromatogr 23:3–25

Oellerich M, Barten MJ, Armstrong VW (2006) Biomarkers: the link between therapeutic drug monitoring and pharmacodynamics. Ther Drug Monit 28:35–38

Okah FA, Wickett RR, Pickens WL, Hoath SB (1995) Surface electrical capacitance as a noninvasive bedside measure of epidermal barrier maturation in the newborn infant. Pediatrics 96:688–692

Payen S, Zhang D, Maisin A, Popon M, Bensman A, Bouissou F, Loirat C, Gomeni R, Bressolle F, Jacqz-Aigrain E (2005) Population pharmacokinetics of mycophenolic acid in kidney transplant pediatric and adolescent patients. Ther Drug Monit 27:378–388

Peng B, Boddy AV, Cole M, Pearson AD, Chatelut E, Rubie H, Newell DR (1995) Comparison of methods for the estimation of carboplatin pharmacokinetics in paediatric cancer patients. Eur J Cancer 31A:1804–1810

Plard C, Bressolle F, Fakhoury M, Zhang D, Yacouben K, Rieutord A, Jacqz-Aigrain E (2007) A limited sampling strategy to estimate individual pharmacokinetic parameters of methotrexate in children with acute lymphoblastic leukemia. Cancer Chemother Pharmacol 60:609–620

Quattrocchi F, Karnes HT, Robinson JD, Hendeles L (1983) Effect of serum separator blood collection tubes on drug concentrations. Ther Drug Monit 5:359–362

Rodbro P, Krasilnikoff PA, Christiansen PM (1967) Parietal cell secretory function in early childhood. Scand J Gastroenterol 2:209–213

Rutter N (1987) Percutaneous drug absorption in the newborn: hazards and uses. Clin Perinatol 14:911–930

Sanquer S, Schwarzinger M, Maury S et al (2004) Calcineurin activity as a functional index of immunosuppression after allogeneic stem-cell transplantation. Transplantation 77:854–858

Scheyer RD, Cramer JA (1990) Pharmacokinetics of antiepileptic drugs. Semin Neurol 10:414–420

Schütz E, Svinarov D, Shipkova M, Niedmann PD, Armstrong VW, Wieland E, Oellerich M (1998) Cyclosporin whole blood immunoassays (AxSYM, CEDIA, and Emit): a critical overview of performance characteristics and comparison with HPLC. Clin Chem 44:2158–2164

Self TH, Heilker GM, Alloway RR, Kelso TM, Abou-Shala N (1993) Reassessing the therapeutic range for theophylline on laboratory report forms: the importance of 5–15 micrograms/ml. Pharmacotherapy 13:590–594

Sheiner LB, Beal SL (1981) Some suggestions for measuring predictive performance. J Pharmacokinet Biopharm 9:503–512

Sherwin CM, Svahn S, Van der Linden A, Broadbent RS, Medlicott NJ, Reith DM (2009) Individualised dosing of amikacin in neonates: a pharmacokinetic/pharmacodynamic analysis. Eur J Clin Pharmacol 65:705–713

Soldin OP, Soldin SJ (2002) Review: therapeutic drug monitoring in pediatrics. Ther Drug Monit 24:1–8

Sommerer C, Giese T, Meuer S, Zeier M (2009) Pharmacodynamic monitoring of calcineurin inhibitor therapy: is there a clinical benefit? Nephrol Dial Transplant 24:21–27

Steinberg C, Notterman DA (1994) Pharmacokinetics of cardiovascular drugs in children. Inotropes and vasopressors. Clin Pharmacokinet 27:345–367

't Jong GW et al (2000) Unapproved and off-label use of drugs in a children's hospital. N Engl J Med 343:1125

't Jong GW et al (2002) Unlicensed and off-label drug use in a paediatric ward of a general hospital in the Netherlands. Eur J Clin Pharmacol 58:293–297

Takahashi H, Ishikawa S, Nomoto S, Nishigaki Y, Ando F, Kashima T, Kimura S, Kanamori M, Echizen H (2000) Developmental changes in pharmacokinetics and pharmacodynamics of warfarin enantiomers in Japanese children. Clin Pharmacol Ther 68:541–555

ter Heine R, Hillebrand MJ, Rosing H, van Gorp EC, Mulder JW, Beijnen JH, Huitema AD (2009a) Quantification of the HIV-integrase inhibitor raltegravir and detection of its main metabolite in human plasma, dried blood spots and peripheral blood mononuclear cell lysate by means of high-performance liquid chromatography tandem mass spectrometry. J Pharm Biomed Anal 49:451–458

ter Heine R, Rosing H, van Gorp EC, Mulder JW, Beijnen JH, Huitema AD (2009b) Quantification of etravirine (TMC125) in plasma, dried blood spots and peripheral blood mononuclear cell lysate by liquid chromatography tandem mass spectrometry. J Pharm Biomed Anal 49:393–400

ter Heine R, Rosing H, van Gorp EC, Mulder JW, van der Steeg WA, Beijnen JH, Huitema AD (2008) Quantification of protease inhibitors and nonnucleoside reverse transcriptase inhibitors in dried blood spots by liquid chromatography–triple quadrupole mass spectrometry. J Chromatogr B Anal Technol Biomed Life Sci 867:205–212

Tod MM, Padoin C, Petitjean O (2001) Individualising aminoglycoside dosage regimens after therapeutic drug monitoring: simple or complex pharmacokinetic methods? Clin Pharmacokinet 40:803–814

Touw DJ, Neef C, Thomson AH, Cost-effectiveness of Therapeutic Drug Monitoring Committee of the International Association for Therapeutic Drug Monitoring and Clinical Toxicology (2005) Cost-effectiveness of therapeutic drug monitoring: a systematic review. Ther Drug Monit 27:10–17

Touw DJ, Westerman EM, Sprij AJ (2009) Therapeutic drug monitoring of aminoglycosides in neonates. Clin Pharmacokinet 48:71–88

van der Heijden J, de Beer Y, Hoogtanders K, Christiaans M, de Jong GJ, Neef C, Stolk L (2009) Therapeutic drug monitoring of everolimus using the dried blood spot method in combination with liquid chromatography–mass spectrometry. J Pharm Biomed Anal 50:664–670 van Rossum HH, de Fijter JW, van Pelt J (2010) Pharmacodynamic monitoring of calcineurin inhibition therapy: principles, performance, and perspectives. Ther Drug Monit 32:3–10

Walson PD (1998) Therapeutic drug monitoring in special populations. Clin Chem 44:415–419

Warner A, Privitera M, Bates D (1998) Standards of laboratory practice: antiepileptic drug monitoring. National Academy of Clinical Biochemistry. Clin Chem 44:1085–1095

Wilhelm AJ, den Burger JC, Vos RM, Chahbouni A, Sinjewel A (2009) Analysis of cyclosporin A in dried blood spots using liquid chromatography tandem mass spectrometry. J Chromatogr B Anal Technol Biomed Life Sci 877:1595–1598

Zhao W, Elie V, Baudouin V, Bensman A, André JL, Brochard K, Broux F, Cailliez M, Loirat C, Jacqz-Aigrain E (2010) Population pharmacokinetics and Bayesian estimator of mycophenolic acid in children with idiopathic nephrotic syndrome. Br J Clin Pharmacol 69:358–366

Zhao W, Baudouin V, Zhang D, Deschênes G, Le Guellec C, Jacqz-Aigrain E (2009) Population pharmacokinetics of ganciclovir following administration of valganciclovir in paediatric renal transplant patients. Clin Pharmacokinet 48:321–328

Drug Delivery and Formulations

Jörg Breitkreutz and Joachim Boos

Contents

Abstract Paediatric drug delivery is a major challenge in drug development. Because of the heterogeneous nature of the patient group, ranging from newborns to adolescents, there is a need to use appropriate excipients, drug dosage forms and delivery devices for different age groups. So far, there is a lack of suitable and safe drug formulations for children, especially for the very young and seriously ill patients. The new EU legislation will enforce paediatric clinical trials and drug development. Current advances in paediatric drug delivery include interesting new concepts such as fast-dissolving drug formulations, including orodispersible tablets

J. Breitkreutz (✉)
Institut für Pharmazeutische Technologie und Biopharmazie, Heinrich-Heine-Universität Düsseldorf, Universitätsstraße 1, 40225 Düsseldorf, Germany
e-mail: joerg.breitkreutz@uni-duesseldorf.de

J. Boos
Klinik und Poliklinik für Kinder- und Jugendmedizin, Westfälische Wilhems-Universität, 48149 Münster, Germany

H.W. Seyberth et al. (eds.), *Pediatric Clinical Pharmacology*,
Handbook of Experimental Pharmacology 205,
DOI 10.1007/978-3-642-20195-0_4, © Springer-Verlag Berlin Heidelberg 2011

and oral thin strips (buccal wafers), and multiparticulate dosage forms based on mini-tabletting or pelletization technologies. Parenteral administration is likely to remain the first choice for children in the neonatal period and for emergency cases. Alternative routes of administration include transdermal, pulmonary and nasal drug delivery systems. A few products are already available on the market, but others still need further investigations and clinical proof of concept.

Keywords Paediatric drug formulations • Child-appropriate dosage forms • Excipients toxicity • Drug delivery devices • Compliance

Abbreviations

ADI	Acceptable daily intake
API	Active pharmaceutical ingredient
DPI	Dry powder inhaler
EMA	European Medicines Agency
FAO	Food and Agriculture Organization
GINA	Global Initiative on Asthma
JECFA	Joint Expert Committee on Food Additives
ODT	Orally disintegrating tablet
PDE	Permitted daily exposure
PIP	Paediatric Investigation Plan
pMDI	Pressured metered-dose inhaler
TSE	Transmissible spongiform encephalitis
UK	United Kingdom
WHO	World Health Organization

1 Administration Routes and Drug Dosage Forms

Limited evidence-based information around acceptability and preference of dosage forms in children are available, despite the fact that the therapeutic outcomes are closely linked to it. An ideal formulation should be beneficial for all subsets of the paediatric population, provide sufficient bioavailability of the active pharmaceutical ingredient (API), be palatable or at least acceptable, contain non-toxic, safe excipients, enable a safe and easy administration, own socio-cultural acceptance and provide precise advice in the product information (Table 1) (Breitkreutz and Boos 2007). However, it is unlikely in most cases that a "one-fits-all" solution will be available (Krause and Breitkreutz 2008). A variety of drug application routes and appropriate dosage forms have to be considered. Due to economical reasons, pharmaceutical companies and regulatory bodies have to elaborate compromises between an ideal and a realistic approach. In the reflection paper *Formulations of*

Table 1 List of basic criteria for paediatric drug formulations

Sufficient bioavailability
Safe excipients
Palatable and/or acceptable properties
Acceptable dose uniformity
Easy and safe administration
Socio-cultural acceptability
Precise and clear product information
Parent/caregiver friendly

Choice for the Paediatric Population released by the European Medicines Agency (EMA), the central regulatory office for medicinal products in the European Union, a matrix on the acceptability of administration routes and dosage forms in relation to age is provided (EMA 2006). The table is extremely helpful to elaborate a rough idea on the opportunities and challenges of drug administration, but is not legally binding. The source data of the matrix were expert opinions only and not scientifically derived results. However, when submitting the Paediatric Investigational Plan (PIP) to the EMA, which is now general requirement in the drug license procedure in Europe (Breitkreutz 2008), the provided table might be of additional benefit for preparing the regulatory discussions. However, recent advances in pharmaceutical technologies such as new drug dosage forms and novel functional excipients urgently require a general revision of the present reflection paper (Krause and Breitkreutz 2008).

1.1 Peroral Drug Delivery

Peroral drug administration is the preferred route of administration both in the paediatric and the adult population. In general, peroral dosage forms can be distinguished in solid or liquid forms. Semi-solid formulations, emulsions and suspensions are generally sub-summarized under "liquid" dosage forms. Liquid formulations offer the advantage of easy administration and a wide range for dose adaptation, but they also display major disadvantages (Breitkreutz et al. 1999). There are a limited number of safe excipients available for liquid formulations in contrast to solid dosage forms (see section "Excipients"). In aqueous formulations, there is a need for preservatives or antimicrobial devices to ensure the microbiological stability over storage and in-use conditions. Another major issue with liquid formulations is taste (see section "Compliance Issues"). Masking unpleasant taste of an API is much harder to achieve than with solid formulations where introducing barriers like polymer coatings is an often used option. Dose accuracy in using oral liquid preparations is another challenge. In a recently published survey on antibiotic suspensions in marketed German products it became evident that the accomplished dosing devices like dosing spoons and cups are inappropriate to measure correct doses (Fig. 1), at least if lower doses than the standard doses are

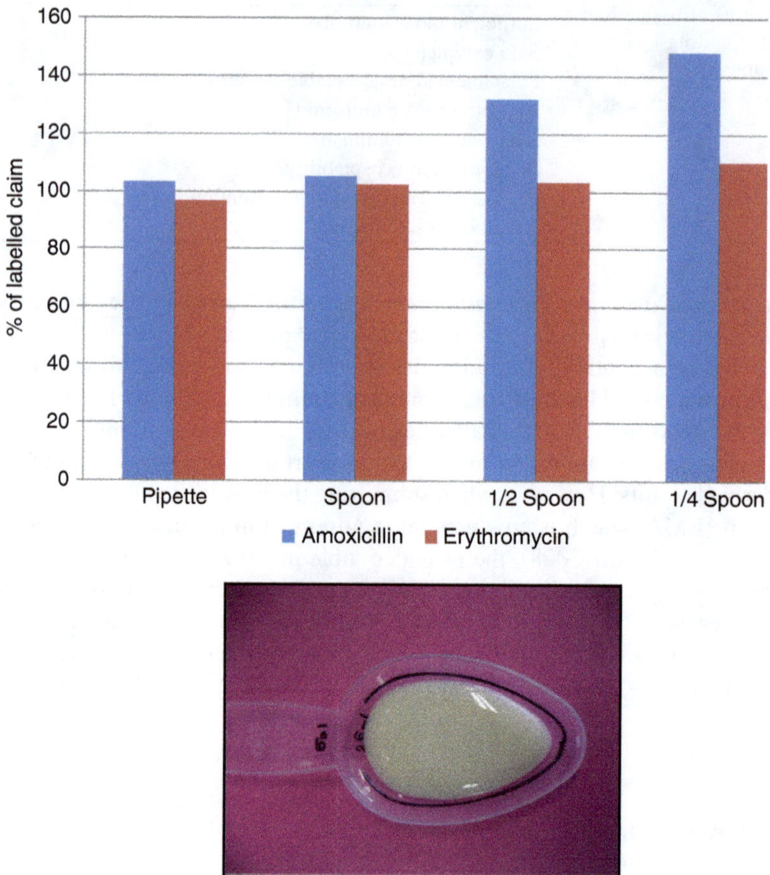

Fig. 1 Dosing errors when using measuring spoons in medicinal products (modified from Breitkreutz et al. 1999). Percentage shows the actually measured dose in relation to the labelled claim in all amoxicillin and erythromycin products available on the German market (*top*). The deviating volumes are due to the inadequate calibration of the spoons provided in the package (*bottom*: precisely measured 2.5 ml liquid, but graduation is still visible and hence, causes overdosing)

required (Griessmann et al. 2007). Parents make numerous administration errors especially when dosing the oral medication by dosing cups. Only 30% of the parents can accurately ($\pm$20% of the labelled dose) administer the correct dose by a cup with printed graduations and 50% by a cup with etched marks. Significant dosing errors (more than 40% deviation) were made by a quarter of all parents enrolled in the study (Yin et al. 2010). Oral syringes are much more precise, but also more expensive. Dose volumes may be critical, and it is considered that pre-school children should not receive more than 5 mL and school-children should not be dosed with more than 10 mL. It is evident that the less palatable the drug is, the smaller the overall volume should be.

To overcome the disadvantages in liquid formulations, dispersible tablets and effervescent dosage forms provide an alternative but are not without inherent issues. The large volume of required diluent causes a burden of liquid to be swallowed. The ingestion of bicarbonate in case of effervescent formulations may lead to gastrointestinal malfunctions. Often the resulting sodium and/or potassium content are rather high and particularly not suitable for renally impaired patients.

The general consensus on the acceptability of solid dosage forms provided in the EMA reflection paper (EMA 2006) is that children younger than 6 years (newborns, infants and pre-school children) have great difficulty with, or are even unable to swallow solid oral dosage forms. The threshold of 6 years is mainly based on a Dutch study on the consumption of dosage forms over age where a remarkable shift from liquid to solid formulations was detected (Schirm et al. 2003). The swallowing of monolithic dosage forms such as tablets or capsules can be trained, but some children will not be capable to learn it at all (Czyzewski et al. 2000). However, recent data from South Africa suggest that there is no significant difference in refusal rates of children receiving liquid and solid formulations (Polaha et al. 2008). There is ongoing research how the dimensions and geometries of monolithic dosage forms may affect the acceptability and swallowing. Mini-tablets with 3-mm diameter could be swallowed by a majority of 4-year-old children (Thomson et al. 2009). Multifunctional tablets which can be splitted into pieces and then dissolved prior to administration, but also swallowed may be another interesting option.

Swallowing issues are frequently overcome by crushing tablets or opening capsules and adding the resulting powder to beverages or soft food despite proof of accurate dosing, stability and bioequivalence. Sometimes the resulting powder is further diluted with powdered excipients and repackaged in sachets or capsules for extemporaneous dispensing with few, if any, compatibility and stability consideration. It is often neglected that food may have variable quality and composition and that food ingredients may reduce the API content. 6-Mercaptopurine for instance is completely degraded within minutes by xanthinoxidase which is still active in milk or milk products (Wessel et al. 2001). The validation of the prepared extemporaneous formulation is often poorly performed. In case of hydrochlorothiazide, it could be demonstrated that neither the magistral capsules nor some in literature proposed liquid formulations offer sufficient dose uniformity (Barnscheid 2008).

When tablets are not scored but yet split or cut to obtain the appropriate dose or to facilitate swallowing, dose accuracy cannot always be ensured: the weight of a split tablet can range from 50 to 150% of the actual half-tablet weight (van Santen et al. 2002). However, when using improved tablet geometries accurate dose adaptation can be performed for even one-eighth of the total dose (Kayitare et al. 2009). Only few products with scored tablets contain explicit information on divisibility and procedures for splitting (Quinzler et al. 2006). Splitting tablets into segments is not recommended with narrow therapeutic index drugs, potent or cytotoxic APIs. Some solid dosage forms (e.g. saliva-resistant, enteric-coated, sustained-release coated tablets, osmotically driven drug delivery systems) cannot be manipulated without affecting taste, release properties, and possible therapeutic effects, unless especially stated in the product information provided by the

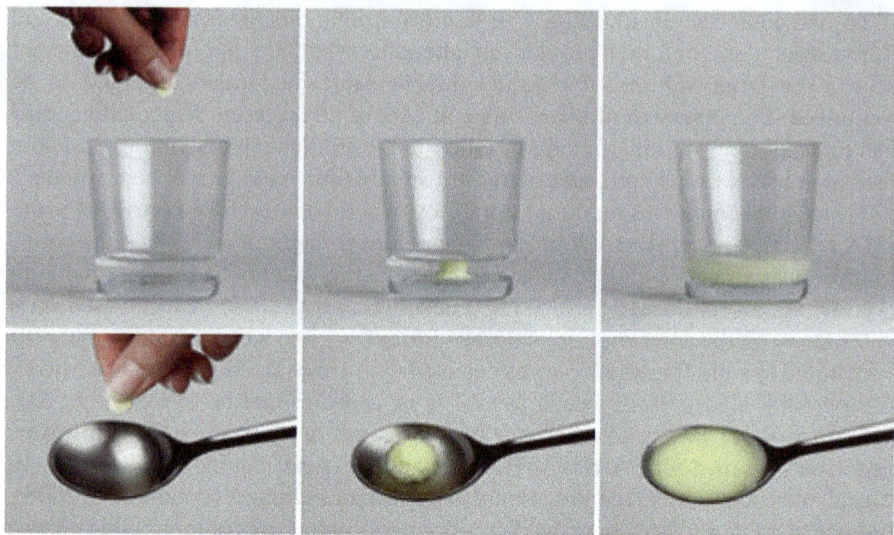

Fig. 2 Multifunctional tablet for paediatric use: Coartem® (Novartis). The tablet can be dissolved in glass or a small volume of liquid on a spoon prior to administration. The formulation is specifically designed for malaria treatment of children in developing countries with high temperatures and humidity

manufacturer in agreement with the regulatory authority (Breitkreutz et al. 1999). The use of splitting devices does usually not improve the dose uniformity of the obtained segments, and therefore, may also not replace the development of appropriate formulations.

A potentially very fruitful area for future research and development are so-called "enabling formulations" verified by the pharmaceutical companies to provide a defined diluent or dispersion vehicle which is mixed with the marketed solid dosage forms, preferably multiparticulates such as granules (sprinkles), pellets or mini-tablets. The resulting liquid or semi-solid formulation can be dosed intra-orally or using devices the child likes. The recently introduced products Co-Artem®, a fixed-dose antimalarial combination (Fig. 2), and Tracleer® for children, containing bosentan for pulmonary arterial hypertension, have been designed as tablets with breaking notches for splitting, but they can also be dissolved in water or at least dispersed forming a suspension for facilitating the oral uptake.

1.2 Oromucosal Drug Delivery

Solid preparations which spontaneously disperse in the oral cavity (e.g. orodispersible tablets, thin film strips, oral lyophilisates) stand also on the periphery of solids and liquids. There are exciting new opportunities and recent advances in this area. Oral lyophilisates, e.g. based on the Zydis® technology, have been introduced some years ago offering fast-disintegrating wafers instantaneously forming a drug solution within a few seconds (Seager 1998). As the production of the lyophilisates is quite energy and cost-consuming their use was limited to niche markets, e.g. for antiemetic drugs in high-dose cancer therapy. By introducing new functional excipients, such as ready-to-use powder mixtures for direct tabletting, new opportunities arise. By these excipients, mostly composed of co-processed mannitol, binders and super-disintegrants, orally disintegrating tablets (ODTs) can be developed offering almost the same disintegration profiles as oral lyophilisates, but produced on conventional tabletting equipment (Brown 2003). An interesting new approach has been recently introduced by combining the mini-tablet and the ODT concept (Fig. 3). These orodispersible mini-tablets dissolve within a few seconds in the mouth releasing the drug substance. In the best case only 2.5 mg drug can be loaded into a 2-mm mini-tablet, so that multiple dosing might be necessary. An unpleasant taste of the API may be another issue and could require taste-masking measures which would further reduce the dose loading. Oral film strips are another alternative in paediatrics and the first medicinal products, e.g. with antiemetic drugs or cough medication, have been introduced (Garsuch and Breitkreutz 2010). Depending on drug substance, the film area and height up to 70 mg, but usually only 15–25 mg API can be included in an oral film piece. The limitation of the orodispersible formulations in general is the poor drug load when maintaining the fast-dissolving properties. However, in paediatric medicines numerous drug molecules are used at low doses and are therefore potential candidates for oromucosal drug preparations. Another challenge is that only few excipients are available to improve medication's palatability and that using these excipients might cause a reduction of the maximum drug load. Moreover, it is to be noted that few studies have been performed to assess appropriate age, stage of development, and dosage form of choice regarding applicability, acceptability, and preference. Further it has to be considered that the absorption profile may be complicated as some molecules may be absorbed directly through the oral mucosa, but an uncertain ration of the dose is absorbed after swallowing.

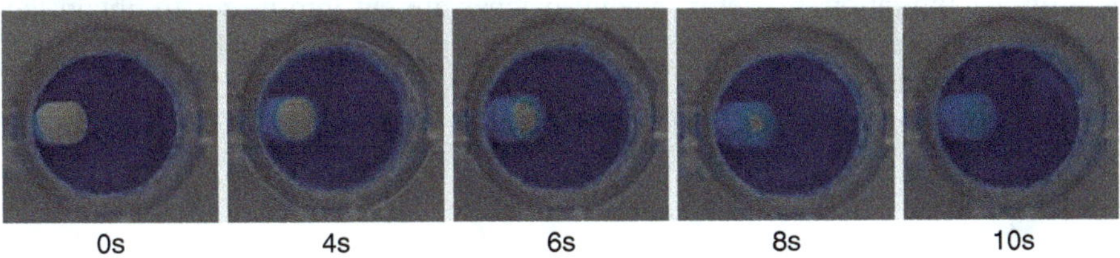

Fig. 3 Orally disintegrating mini-tablet (diameter: 2 mm) rapidly losing shape and partly dissolving in artificial saliva

1.3   Rectal Drug Delivery

The rectal administration route can be used for local (e.g. laxative or anti-inflammatory) or systemic (e.g. antipyretic or anticonvulsive) treatment. The administration of drugs by rectal formulations (e.g. suppositories, solution, soft capsules or ointments) can result in a wide variability in the rate and extent of absorption in children. The rectal administration of suppositories or enemas for systemic effects may nevertheless be chosen because the patient cannot take medication orally, because the oral dosage form is rejected as a result of palatability issues or because immediate absorption is required in emergency cases such as grand-mal seizures. However, the use of rectal preparations has major drawbacks. When administering rectal preparations, there is always the danger of premature expulsion. The rectal bioavailability is limited for a broad range of drug molecules (e.g. levodopa, phenytoin and penicillins), compared with oral or intestinal absorption (Krause and Breitkreutz 2008). Last but not least, the rectal route is poorly accepted by a number of patients and caregivers in certain countries and cultures.

1.4   Topical/Transdermal Drug Delivery

The development of the stratum corneum, the most prominent absorption barrier of human skin, is complete at birth but is more perfused and hydrated than in older children or adults. Therefore, neonates and infants have an underdeveloped epidermal barrier and are subject to excessive absorption of potentially toxic ingredients from topically applied products. Only few transdermal products (e.g. contraceptive drugs, caffeine, fentanyl, scopolamine, nicotine and methylphenidate) have been tested or marketed for use in the paediatric population and predominantly have targeted the elder children. Scopolamine is licensed only for children aged 14 years or more because accidental overdoses in younger patients resulted in hallucinogenic reactions. But still, the development of transdermal products in paediatric doses could be beneficial for children who are unable to tolerate or accept oral medications. The need for several sizes of patches to cover different doses might be a further limitation. Sometimes adult patches are cut into pieces to obtain the required size and dose. It is important to note that this is only possible with matrix-type patches and, even then, the release kinetic may be modified and may cause accidental overdosing.

1.5   Parenteral Drug Delivery

Parenteral administration routes enable drug administration to unconscious and uncooperative patients. In the neonatal period and in emergency cases, the intravenous administration of drugs is the most important therapeutic option. Preterm and term neonates often receive all their medications by permanent venous cannula. The drug delivery is often controlled by infusion pumps, such as the Perfusor® technology, which allows an individual dose regimen.

Few drug products are available specifically designed for the subcutaneous or intramuscular administration to children, whereas vaccines are provided with adequate doses and design. Other parenteral routes of administration (e.g. intrathecal, epidural, intraosseous, intraarterial or intracardiac) are used mostly in emergency cases, for anaesthesia or in palliative care.

Drug solutions for infusion are often prepared extemporaneously by the hospital pharmacy or by mixing products for parental use with marketed vehicles like Ringer's solution or isotonic sodium chloride solution. It is important to avoid any drug–drug or drug–excipient interactions when mixing two or more medicinal products. Ionic compounds may form ion pairs causing agglomeration and sedimentation. Excipients such as detergents or bile acids may complex the drug substance and thereby, change pharmacokinetics. By changing the pH value or the ionic strength of the original products during the mixing process particles may form that must be absent in intravenous, intraarterial or intracardiac preparations to avoid embolism. Many active substances for injection, but also some for infusion, are presented as lyophilized powders to be reconstituted before administration. A number of products require withdrawal of a single dose or at least a particular amount of the total dose if the product is intended for use in newborns, infants and toddlers.

The facility to accurately measure the required small volumes is of particular importance. There is a clinical need to limit the fluid uptake, especially in very young children. On the other hand the volumes and surfaces of tubes, pumps and cannulas have to considered when adjusting the flow rate and determining the total volume. If not, it might be possible that not a single drug molecule may enter the body of the child treated with a low dose and low volume of the drug. Hyperosmolar injections or extreme pH values may irritate peripheral veins and produce thrombophlebitis, extravasation and pain. In many studies, various errors in preparing and administering parenteral preparations have been reported. On paediatric wards in Germany and UK, a huge rate of 34–48% of falsely prepared or administered solutions have been estimated (Wirtz et al. 2003; Taxis and Barber 2004). The errors include inappropriate choice of solvents, incorrect calculation of doses, too fast infusion rates (especially for the bolus), omitting prescribed co-medication, wrong or incomplete labelling of the prepared bottles, and various incompatibilities between the ingredients of the mixture. In some cases, there was a fatal outcome from the iatrogenic medication errors. Specially developed parenteral medications for paediatric use are obviously advantageous. In a comparative study, significant differences in bioavailability and other pharmacokinetic parameters could be demonstrated for a specifically developed paediatric vial in comparison to an extemporaneously prepared solution used for the treatment of newborns (Allegaert et al. 2006).

Another critical issue is the migration of compounds of the applied medical devices such as catheters, pumps, valves and also containers into the liquid preparation. The migration of plasticizers such as phthalates from polyvinylchloride bags and tubes was determined as up to 400 mg/L diethylhexyl phthalate in fat emulsions for parenteral nutrition (Wurdack et al. 2006). Other potential contaminants from packaging materials and feeding tubes are monomers from the polymer synthesis, leaching aluminium ions, antioxidants and colouring agents.

1.6   Intranasal Drug Delivery

This drug delivery into the nose provides fast and direct access to systemic circulation without first-pass metabolism. Administration is not easy especially with uncooperative children, but small volumes involved, rapidity of execution, feasibility at home has made it more attractive, particularly for no-needle approach to acute illnesses. Aerosols with an appropriate device can avoid swallowing and is more precise in terms of dose. APIs such as benzodiazepines, fentanyl, diamorphine, midazolame and ketamine have been used successfully via this route. The key issue is to guarantee the released dose from a single actuation from the device, especially for children as the dose is low and small deviations from the intended dose may critically harm the patients.

1.7   Pulmonary Drug Delivery

Inhalative therapy is a major problem in paediatric drug delivery that comprises different aspects such as drug formulation, inhaled particle size and shape, device design and also physiological and psychological issues (Krause and Breitkreutz 2008). Still, the amount of drug deposited in the lung after using an inhalation device is often small in adults, but even less in children. Today, paediatric inhalative formulations are restricted to treat pulmonary disease like asthma locally and are not intended for a systemic treatment.

Compared to adults, children have lower tidal volumes, smaller functional residual capacity and shorter respiratory cycles. The distances and volumes of children's airways and the throat differ from the adult form and therefore influence drug deposition in the lungs. As a result the pulmonary deposition is mainly hampered by lower breathing volumes, short residence times in the airways and insufficient cooperation of the child.

Very young children are obligate nose breathers which can result in the total loss of drug particles before entering the lungs.

Several studies suggest that drug particle sizes should be adapted for use in children (Schüepp et al. 2005; Janssens et al. 2003). This is not only a problem of crystal engineering, but also of drug formulation and device development. Smaller particles deposit more peripherically and less in the upper airways whereas large particles mostly stay in the mouth or throat by impaction to the endothelial cells. In the case of dry powder inhalers (DPI) with interactive powder mixtures the outer deposition of large particles made from carriers like lactose is intended, but the smaller drug particles should enter the lung. In this particular case drug deposition in the lung is a function of breathing abilities (to release the total dose, to separate drug and excipients and to enable the direct flow of micronized drug particles into the lung), of the formulation (which excipients, which drug crystals) and of the device (breathing resistance, actuation, mouth adapter). It might be possible that various devices and formulations would be needed for the same drug to suit the requirements and properties of different age groups.

Pressured metered-dose inhalers (pMDI) have been sometimes successfully employed in the paediatric population. These products are designed to deliver a unit dose at high velocity with small particle size. However, self-administration is difficult for younger patients with reduced coordination abilities and less compliance consciousness.

To decrease oropharyngeal impaction and optimize utilization, various spacers can be used. Face masks enable the use of pMDI for very young infants whereas DPIs are only suitable for children with enough inspiratory flow to trigger particles' release and transport the particles deep in the lung. Nebulizers are applicable for all ages but very few are portable yet. Guidance for use of different inhaler types (i.e. nebulizers, pMDI and DPI) has been established by the Global Initiative on Asthma (GINA), a panel of clinical experts who look at the various inhaler types, their features, and patient experience. Their guidance has been incorporated in national regulatory guidance throughout the world. The most appropriate device should be selected for each child. Children younger than 4 years should use a pMDI plus a spacer with face mask or a nebulizer with face mask. Children aged 4–6 years should use a pMDI plus a spacer with mouthpiece, a DPI, or, if necessary, a nebulizer with face mask. For children using spacers, the spacer must fit the inhaler, and particular attention should be paid to ensure that the spacer fits the child's face. Children of any age older than 6 years who have difficulty using pMDIs should use a pMDI with a spacer, breath-actuated inhaler, DPI, or nebulizer. Particularly among children younger than 5 years, inhaler techniques may be poor and should be monitored closely. In order to improve devices and formulations, the development of in-vitro models fully reflecting the physiological conditions at different age groups of children are under development in our working group. The aim is to improve today's deposition rates by taking the differences in airways and capabilities into account.

2 Excipients

Pharmaceutical excipients are falsely regarded as "inactive ingredients" or "inert substances" (McIntyre and Choonara 2004). Excipients show similar pharmacokinetic profiles like APIs, with absorption, distribution into organs, metabolization

Table 2 Some excipients with elevated toxicological risk and severe outcome in children reported in the literature

Excipient	Patients at risk	Administration	Adverse reactions
Benzyl alcohol	<6 months	Oral, parenteral	Neurotoxicity, metabolic acidosis, >100 deaths
Polyethylene glycol (Macrogol)	<6 months	Parenteral	Metabolic acidosis
Aluminium salts	<6 months	Oral, parenteral	Encephalopathy, microcytic anaemia, osteodystrophy
Propylene glycol	<12 months	Oral, parenteral	Neurotoxicity, seizures, hyperosmolarity, death
Menthol	<12 months	Oral, nasal, dermal application to face or breast	Bronchoconstriction, death
Diethylene glycol	<18 years, all ages	Oral	Metabolic acidosis, hyperosmolarity, >500 deaths
Benzalkonium chloride	Hypersensitive patients, all ages	Oral, nasal, ocular	Bronchoconstriction in hypersensitive patients, loss of microvili function
Parabens	<18 years, all ages	Oral, parenteral, ocular, topical	Allergies, contact dermatitis, carcinogenic potential
Sulfites, bisulfites	Hypersensitive patients, all ages	Oral, parenteral	Anaphylactic reactions

with drug interaction capacity and elimination. To evaluate pharmaceutical excipients some predictive methods and agreed limits have been adapted from the risk assessment of food additives such as the Acceptable Daily Intake (ADI), established by the Joint Expert Committee on Food Additives (JECFA) of the World Health Organisation (WHO) and world's Food and Agriculture Organisation (FAO). However, it is questionable whether these limits can be used for the paediatric population (see Table 2). The toxicity is mainly attributed to children's insufficient or varying metabolic capacity in the first years of life. Mixing up of excipients in formulations, accidentally used high amounts of excipients, errors in correct labelling of ingredients and unforeseen toxic effects of excipients have been reported (McIntyre and Choonara 2004). Plenty of these unwanted events have been linked to diethylene glycol which was used as co-solvent in pharmaceutical preparations (84 deaths in Nigeria 2009), in tooth-paste (China 2009) or as an impurity in other excipients such as glycerol or propylene glycol (at least 21 deaths in Panama 2006 and 28 in Bangladesh 2009). Between 1995 and today at least 500 children died from iatrogenic intoxication with diethylene glycol.

2.1 Exposure and Risk

The risk of children exposed to pharmaceutical excipients is linked to their age and thereby, the maturation of organs and functions of the metabolic systems. The excipients may maintain for longer period in the juvenile body due to reduced metabolic capacity or minor renal elimination. They can easily enter the brain as the blood–brain barrier is more permeable than in adults. They can activate the immune system of the maturing organism and may induce allergies or anaphylactic reactions.

Excipients with an elevated risk in paediatrics linked to the pharmacokinetic properties are benzyl alcohol, ethanol, propylene glycol, polyethylene glycol and aluminium salts (such as aluminium stearate or aluminium hydroxides). Benzyl alcohol caused the "gasping syndrome" first described in 1981 by the accumulation of metabolites such as benzaldehyde and benzoic acid in blood (metabolic acidosis) and brain (neurotoxicity) causing more than 100 deaths worldwide (Gershanik et al. 1981). Metabolic acidosis is also a problem associated with high intake of polyethylene glycol and propylene glycol. Propylene glycol is regarded as very safe in the adult population. There is no limit to be considered when using propylene glycol in adulthood. In syrups for oral use it is often used as solvent, co-solvent or as a replacement for a preservative at very high concentrations. There have never been any reports on neurotoxic effects in adolescents and school-children. But in neonates, especially in low-weight newborns and pre-term babies, numerous deaths, severe brain damage and life-long handicaps have been reported (American Academy of Pediatrics 1997; MacDonald et al. 1987). Propylene glycol and its metabolites may enter the brain and may cause seizure and other neurotoxicological effect.

The neurotoxic potency of ethanol is well known, but the long-term effects of low ethanol doses are still under discussion. Ethanol levels in pre-term neonates or neonates with low birth weight have been recently investigated and raise concerns (Whittacker et al. 2009). In some paediatric patients, even lower limits must be considered, e.g. in children with liver and kidney malfunctions. In paediatric dialysis patients the use of propylene glycol, polyethylene glycols and aluminium salts should be completely prohibited. Hypersensitive patients may adversely react on allergen presented in the formulation such as parabens, benzalkonium chloride, colourants (azo dyes), sulfites, starches (glutens) or wool wax (Breitkreutz and Boos 2007). For parabens agonistic activity at hormone receptors is discussed and propyl paraben has been recently deleted from the list of permitted food additives in the EU. In some cases, the immune system will cause anaphylactic reaction which may be severe and live-threatening (dextran, sodium bisulfite, macrogolglycerol-ricinoleate). Moreover, it has to be considered that some children may suffer from rare diseases such as phenylketonuria, hereditary fructose intolerance and lactose intolerance. In phenylketonuria, the use of aspartame must be prohibited as it is a phenylalanine source. In fructose intolerance, the intake of the excipients fructose, sucrose and sorbitol should be avoided.

2.2 Impurities in Medicinal Products

The fatal intoxications with diethylene glycol as an impurity lead to a discussion about the quality of pharmaceutical excipients. Despite chemical impurities some more potential contaminants have been identified in materials derived from mammalian species with transmissible spongiform encephalitis (TSE), excipients with potential viral load, and substances with potential endotoxin and pyrogen load.

Some excipients in medicinal products are not labelled as they are only present in traces. Residual solvents, for instance, are used in the manufacturing process to solve a drug substance, a film former or a granulation binder. Residuals of catalysts from the synthesis of the compounds and salts from heavy metals from synthesis or packaging materials may be contained. Plasticizers from plastic containers may migrate into the liquid phase (see section "Parenteral Drug Delivery"). The residual burden of solvents is a good example, how difficult a risk assessment in paediatric is: The amount of residuals of organic solutes in a finished product is limited by the Permitted Daily Exposure (PDE). The organic solvents are categorized into three classes by the toxic potency. Solvents with highest toxicity are listed in class I, the less problematic solvents in class III. However, both the categorization and the fixed limits have been derived from risk assessment for adults, namely a woman with 50 kg body weight. It is not probable that these limits match the paediatric situation. Therefore, for the PIP procedure and for the market licensing procedure it is recommended to reduce the burden of potential contaminants as far as possible. Alternative manufacturing technologies such as aqueous film coating, dry powder coating, lipid coating and aqueous or solvent-free granulation methods are highly demanded and should be applied for paediatric medicines whenever possible.

3 Compliance Issues

Compliance and concordance issues have multivariate complex origins but an unacceptable taste is one major compliance issue (Cram et al. 2009). Two factors make taste preference and palatability critical in paediatric adherence. The dosage forms most commonly employed for paediatric formulations are liquids and orodispersible tablets. A perceived unpleasant taste is much more evident with these dosage forms than when a drug is administered as a conventional solid oral dosage form. Taste-masking of the unpleasant taste can be better achieved by coating the drug crystals or the complete dosage form by polymers (film-coated tablets) or sugars (dragees). It is widely believed that children younger than 6 years have more distinguished taste perception than older children and adults. Therefore, development of oral formulations for this age group is rather challenging. Taste buds and olfactory receptors are fully developed in early infancy and a profound aversion to bitter tasting substances is pronounced in all children of this age group. Bitter taste perception is obviously a safety and protection measure to prohibit the intake of toxic plant materials by the neonates and toddlers. By the recent introduction of analytical instruments, so called electronic tongues, the development of child-appropriate medicines is facilitated. Although these instruments are not reliable for absolute taste prediction, they offer the opportunity to rationalize the development by testing the taste-relevant molecules (APIs or excipients) and evaluating the effectiveness of taste-masking strategies (Woertz et al. 2010). In addition to taste formulation's smell, texture and visual appearance are important factors in the development of paediatric dosage forms for oral use.

Beside the taste perception children's adherence to therapy is affected by their cognitive skills, their acceptability or ability to swallow, their socio-cultural environment and personal strengths, affected or not by their disease. Recently, some new medicinal products have entered the market in order to avoid the stigmatization of the juvenile patient. Examples are improved injection devices with fancy design, e.g. with insulin or growth hormone, transdermal patches with fentanyl and pulsatile drug formulations with methylphenidate. In order to prevent school-children with attention deficiencies disorders from stigmatization, capsule formulations with mixed uncoated and coated pellets with delayed drug-release (e.g. Medikinet® retard) and oral osmotically releasing pulsed system (Concerta®) have been introduced to save the dosing during school-time.

The adherence to the therapy regimen is also related to the capabilities of the caregivers, which are the parents of the children in most cases. The education of parents and children plays a major role in dosing errors. Although it is even alerting that the use of dosing cups results in about 25% of dosing procedures to major dosing errors in general, the incidence of dosing errors almost doubles with limited literacy (Yin et al. 2010). But even with clear instructions it seems to be difficult to administer liquid preparations correctly. In another study only 66% of the volunteers measure the correct volume with a syringe and even less, 14.6% using a dosing cup although the majority of people strongly believed it would be correct (Sobhani et al. 2008). It can be concluded that clear advice and instructions, better visually than in words, must be provided with the medicinal products.

4 Conclusions

Drug delivery to children is still a major challenge. Key issues are age-appropriate formulations, safety of excipients, suitability of drug delivery devices and therapy compliance. Some improvements have been made recently. The most promising in oral drug delivery are orodispersible mini-tablets and thin film strips. In parenteral drug delivery age-adapted devices and profound knowledge on the preparation of extemporaneous or enabling formulations are of major importance. In pulmonary drug delivery new in vitro deposition models, adapted to physiological properties of children, may lead to better formulations and delivery devices. The new EU formulation will stimulate the research and development in paediatric medicines. Hopefully we will be able to match the unmet needs of paediatric patients soon.

References

Allegaert K, Anderson BJ, Vrancken M (2006) Impact of a paediatric vial on the magnitude of systematic medication errors in neonates. Paediatr Perinat Drug Ther 7:59–63

American Academy of Pediatrics (1997) "Inactive" ingredients in pharmaceutical products – a review. Pediatrics 99:268–278

Barnscheid L (2008) Kindgerechte Arzneizubereitungen mit diuretischen Wirkstoffen, Dissertation HHU Düsseldorf

Breitkreutz J (2008) European perspectives on pediatric formulations. Clin Ther 30:2146–2154

Breitkreutz J, Boos J (2007) Paediatric and geriatric drug delivery. Expert Opin Drug Deliv 4:37–45

Breitkreutz J, Wessel T, Boos J (1999) Dosage forms for peroral administration to children. Paediatr Perinat Drug Ther 3:25–33

Brown D (2003) Orally disintegrating tablets: taste over speed. Drug Deliv Technol 5:34–37

Cram A, Breitkreutz J, Desset-Brèthes S et al (2009) Challenges of developing palatable oral paediatric formulations. Int J Pharm 365:1–3

Czyzewski DI, Runyan D, Lopez MA (2000) Teaching and maintaining pill swallowing in HIV-infected children. AIDS Read 10:88–94

European Medicines Agency (EMA) (2006) Committee for Medicinal Products for Human Use. Reflection paper: formulations of choice for the paediatric population. EMEA/CHMP/PEG/194810/2005

Garsuch V, Breitkreutz J (2010) Comparative investigations on different polymers for the manufacturing of fast-dissolving oral films. J Pharm Pharmacol 62:539–545

Gershanik JJ, Boecler B, George W et al (1981) The gasping syndrome – benzyl alcohol (BA) poisoning? Clin Res 29:895A

Griessmann K, Breitkreutz J, Schubert-Zsilavecz M et al (2007) Dosing accuracy of measuring devices provided with antibiotic suspensions. Paediatr Perinat Drug Ther 8:61–70

Janssens H, De Jongste J, Hop W et al (2003) Extra-fine particles improve lung delivery of inhaled steroids in infants. Chest 123:2083–2088

Kayitare E, Vervaet C, Ntawukulilyayo JD et al (2009) Development of fixed dose combination tablets containing zidovudine and lamivudine for paediatric applications. Int J Pharm 370:41–46

Krause J, Breitkreutz J (2008) Improving drug delivery in paediatric medicine. Pharm Med 22:41–50

MacDonald MG, Getson PR, Glasgow AM et al (1987) Propylene glycol: increased incidence of seizures in low birth weight infants. Pediatrics 79:622–625

McIntyre J, Choonara I (2004) Drug toxicity in the neonate. Biol Neonate 86:218–221

Polaha J, Dalton WT, Lancaster BM (2008) Parenteral report of medication acceptance among youth: implications for everyday practice. South Med J 101:1106–1112

Quinzler R, Gasse C, Schneider A et al (2006) The frequency of inappropriate tablet splitting in primary care. Eur J Clin Pharmacol 62:1065–1073

Schirm E, Tobi H, de Vries TW et al (2003) Lack of appropriate formulations of medicines for children in the community. Acta Paediatr 92:1486–1489

Schüepp K, Jauernig J, Janssens H et al (2005) In vitro determination oft he optimal particle size for nebulized aerosol delivery to infants. J Aerosol Med 18:225–235

Seager H (1998) Drug-delivery products and the Zydis fast-dissolving dosage form. J Pharm Pharmacol 50:375–382

Sobhani P, Christopherson J, Ambrose PJ et al (2008) Accuracy of oral liquid measuring devices: comparison of dosing cup and oral dosing syringe. Ann Pharmacother 42:46–52

Taxis K, Barber N (2004) Incidence and severity of intravenous drug errors in a German hospital. Eur J Clin Pharmacol 59:815–817

Thomson SA, Tuleu C, Wong ICK et al (2009) Minitablets: a new modality to deliver medicines to preschool-age children. Pediatrics 123:e235–e238

Van Santen E, Barends DM, Frijlink HW (2002) Breaking of scored tablets: a review. Eur J Pharm Biopharm 53:139–145

Wessel T, Breitkreutz J, Ahlke E et al (2001) Problems in the maintenance therapy with mercuptopurine tablets [in German]. Krankenhauspharmazie 22:325–329

Whittacker A, Currie AE, Turner MA et al (2009) Toxic additives in medication for preterm infants. Arch Dis Child Fetal Neonatal Ed 94:F236–F240

Wirtz V, Taxis K, Barber N (2003) An observational study of intravenous medication errors in the United Kingdom and in Germany. Pharm World Sci 25:104–111

Woertz K, Tissen C, Breitkreutz J et al (2010) Performance qualification of an electronic tongue according to the ICH guideline Q2. J Pharm Biomed Anal 51:497–506

Wurdack W, Kittlaus A, Pecar R et al (2006) Release of components from primary package materials and their migration into drug and nutrition solutions [in German]. Krankenhauspharmazie 27:334–339

Yin HS, Mendelsohn AL, Wolf MS et al (2010) Parents' medication administration errors. Arch Pediatr Adolesc Med 164:181–186

Part II
Development of Pediatric Medicines

Development of Paediatric Medicines: Concepts and Principles

Klaus Rose and Oscar Della Pasqua

Contents

Abstract The term "off-label use of drugs in children" is common to current medical practice. A look into the historical context helps to elucidate the framework for the use of medicines in children. Proper drug labels are relatively new in history. They emerged half a century ago when U.S. legislation forced manufacturers to prove the safety and efficacy of drugs by adequate clinical

K. Rose (✉)
klausrose Consulting, Pediatric Drug Development & More, Birsstrasse 16, 4052 Basel, Switzerland
e-mail: rose@granzer.biz

O. Della Pasqua
Division of Pharmacology, Amsterdam Center for Drug Research, Leiden University, Einsteinweg 55, P.O. Box 9503, 2300 RA Leiden, The Netherlands

Clinical Pharmacology & Discovery Medicine, GlaxoSmithKline R&D, Stockley Park, Uxbridge UB11 1BT, United Kingdom
e-mail: odp72514@gsk.com

H.W. Seyberth et al. (eds.), *Pediatric Clinical Pharmacology*,
Handbook of Experimental Pharmacology 205,
DOI 10.1007/978-3-642-20195-0_5, © Springer-Verlag Berlin Heidelberg 2011

trials. Today pharmaceutical progress is so obvious and well established that the discrepancy between its benefit for adults as compared to children started to be perceived by champions in different institutions. There is an increased understanding of the child's physiology during developmental growth, of the maturation of enzyme systems, of the pharmacokinetics and pharmacodynamics and of the differences in disease processes. The involved institutions include legislators, government, regulatory authorities, academic scientists, pharmaceutical companies, the WHO, to name just the most prominent ones, but there are many more. Driving forces for the improvement of medicines for children include societal priorities, the involvement of science, the mission of regulatory authorities the role of clinical pharmacologists, paediatricians, and the characteristics of our market-driven economy with its chaotic, contradictory and lively elements. We do not live in an ideal world, but there is progress, and children are likely to benefit from it.

Keywords Paediatric drug development • Medicines for children • Neglected diseases • Incentives for paediatric clinical research • Public health • Regulatory authorities • Priorities in paediatric drug development • Historical context of paediatric drug development

1   Evolution of Paediatric Drug Development

Since its earliest origins, mankind, adults and children were challenged by accidents, diseases and hazards that required medical treatment. Until less than a century ago, women used to get pregnant at a very young age and usually gave birth to several children. The death rate of these children was horrific by today's standards, as was the frequency of mothers dying at childbirth. This situation occurred despite health care providers being available during all these millennia and centuries. Based on current medical knowledge little of what they could deliver was helpful, albeit state-of-the-art at the time. And these professionals had an amazingly high social reputation, with a status between priests and physicians. In parallel to the evolvement of modern medicines, the principles of professional health care practice and the criteria for the recognition of effective treatments also changed dramatically over the last centuries, with an ever accelerating speed of change. To a great extent, scientific principles have replaced common belief, tradition and superstition, all of which pervaded therapeutics over the centuries. The reputation of a member of the medical community has today something to do with his or her actual knowledge and therapeutic skills.

On the other hand, there is today an increasingly complex layer between the patient receiving treatment and the health care professional dispensing it. Therapeutics is based on an intricate process that we will define here as evidence synthesis. To assess the efficacy of a new drug, clinical trials are performed in hundreds or thousands of patients. The implementation and execution of these trials may involve multiple clinical research centres, which can be thousands of miles away, in another country, in another continent, or spread worldwide. To ensure that such trials adhere to the state-of-the art standards and procedures, a network of regulation exists that is recognised by national authorities and professionals worldwide (ICH 2010). In addition, regulatory authorities have established a comprehensive mechanism of monitoring and auditing. A clinical trial performed in China, India and Latin America may be audited by the FDA (2010), the EMA (2010), or even jointly by these two agencies. All the information gathered in a trial will at the end be processed, analysed and reported. The submission of such evidence to regulatory authorities triggers an evaluation process that may lead to approval or rejection of the proposed treatment or therapy. If the evaluation is positive, the evidence from clinical trial results becomes part of the label or summary of product characteristics (SPC) and of the patient information leaflet. In contrast to long gone times, none of the information regarding the indication, efficacy and safety of a treatment originates from the medical doctor who prescribes it. Instead, it is the result of pharmaceutical physicians, clinical scientists and other professionals who contribute to drug development. In this chapter, we try to grasp how this layer between patient and caregiver is being adapted to the specific needs of children.

The advent of industrialisation in combination with the awakening of medical sciences towards the end of the nineteenth century resulted in the identification and subsequent availability of new, efficacious medicines. This process has since then yielded powerful medications (e.g. antibiotics or steroids) for the treatment of adults. These drugs have been subsequently brought into paediatrics based on empiricism, an approach which has prevailed until recently.

Despite the development of pharmacology and clinical pharmacology as disciplines with increasing understanding of the mode of action of available drugs, including the requirements to demonstrate their efficacy, the formal assessment of treatment effects in children has remained limited due to cultural, practical and ethical reasons. In addition, the tools for the evaluation of efficacy and safety in children have been historically questionable by current standards in clinical research. Drugs developed early in the last century showed strong efficacy, but had also the potential for serious side-effects and adverse events. The first major tragedies (Taussig 1962; Wax 1995), leading to multiple deaths and malformations resulted in the mandate for manufacturers in the USA to yield proof of safety (1936) and efficacy (1960s, Kefauver-Harris amendments) (Hilts 2003; Rose and van den Anker 2010; Stoetter 2007). Since then, therapeutic claims have to be demonstrated by properly designed clinical trials and other measures. The requirement for data supporting product claims represented the beginning of the modern drug labelling system. The initial deep, nearly blind confidence in modern medications was in this way replaced by the need to impose control. In the United States, the Food and Drug Administration (FDA) became responsible for the assessment of the scientific and quality aspects of drug development. Comparable legislation followed in Europe, with some variations in the implementation in different individual countries.

The cultural and historical differences in medical practice in Europe have prevented consensus and created discrepancies in the level of evidence deemed appropriate for many adult indications and for most paediatric labels. The main consequence of such discrepancies includes the lack of clear dosing recommendations (i.e., dosing regimen) and formal proof of efficacy (i.e., therapeutic indication) for the majority of approved drugs. The acceptance of this practice by paediatricians, regulatory agencies, clinical researchers and parents has evolved into extensive off-label use of medicines in children from the beginning of the existence of modern labels. As a consequence of this practice, most companies in the United States and in Europe introduced paediatric disclaimers to avoid litigation.

Cultural perspectives about childhood have also influenced the way scientific evidence was generated. Until recently children have been regarded and treated as small adults, with dosing recommendations varying between rough estimates (children get half a tablet, babies a quarter) and empirical formulas, which varied by country and sometimes across regions or hospitals within the same country. Protagonism in research has enforced empiricism in therapeutic utilisation of drugs in children. From a prescriber's perspective, such practice has been justified by the need for easy rules and prevention of prescription errors. Furthermore, personal convictions often dominated the choice of eminent scientists. Still today, the question regarding what is the right dose for children remains often unanswered (Cella et al. 2010).

The awareness about the need for a dedicated programme for paediatric medicines exemplifies the slow shift in paradigm we are currently experiencing in drug development. In contrast to the perception of the 1960s, which considered evidence for safety and efficacy of a drug in adults sufficient to establish its use in children, today's society has become more sceptical and more demanding. In addition to a specific ICH guideline on paediatric drug development (ICH E11 2010), which has been in force since 2000, the United States and European Union paediatric regulations have introduced clear requirements for drug approval and label claims that demand more than just scattered scientific evidence from drug use in children. Safety and efficacy need to be proven based on a well-thought development plan adapted to the specific therapeutic needs of children. The regulatory authorities in the United States and Europe have had and still have a key role in driving forward this change.

Since the dawning of modern medicine development, our understanding of the differences between adults and children in terms of (patho)physiology and in pharmacokinetics (i.e., what the body does with the drug) and pharmacodynamics (i.e., what the drug does with the body) has expanded considerably. In parallel, advances in the assessment of exposure–response relationships have provided tools for exploring experimental designs and optimising the evaluation of pharmacokinetics, efficacy and safety in children. Clinical pharmacology has also supported the development of increasingly sophisticated knowledge on formulations and on the optimisation of drug delivery. Academic paediatric clinical pharmacology research has so far focused on drugs that were on the market and then systematically explored whether they could and should be used in children or not.

2 Challenges in the Transition from Retrospective to Prospective Assessment of Medicines for Children

It has not become yet evident to the international community that the current European legislation has introduced an unprecedented revolution. It forces pharmaceutical industry and researchers across all therapeutic areas to consider the future paediatric use of new chemical or biological entities, which are neither on the market, nor available to the adult population yet. This poses another important challenge: informal benchmarking from prior therapeutic utilisation in adults will not be available at the time a new drug or biological is first administered to children. The long-lasting arguments that in the past supported the empiricism used by paediatricians and paediatric pharmacologists will have less and less space in the years to come. Off-label use will not be supported by evidence of safety and efficacy in adults at the same extent post-launch data have provided in the past.

In contrast to the retrospective evaluation of a drug's pharmacokinetics, pharmacodynamics or clinical profile, which has been driven by academic research, considerations about the clinical development of new medicines and future use of a new compound in children will require direct involvement of the pharmaceutical industry and potentially other sponsors. The need to establish partnerships, to foster critical mass in academia and to enable effective public–private partnerships or other collaborative efforts has, however, not been defined by the law. This represents the single most important challenge to the success of this new era in paediatric drug development.

In summary, the evidence supporting paediatric drug utilisation is evolving from a rather simple research activity within the realms of academic expert groups to a global multidisciplinary effort where relevant stakeholders must work together. However, modern society is complex and cooperation cannot be taken for granted, particularly when different interests are at stake. Collaboration is not the result of logical thinking nor is it based on effective use of resources and expertise towards a common goal. It is imposed by a framework created by the paediatric legislation, the results of which are just beginning to become visible.

3 Priorities and Unmet Needs in Paediatric Diseases

Priorities and unmet medical needs vary across geographic regions not only because of biological, clinical and demographic reasons, but also due to political, economical and social differences in the perception of the implications of disease on child health and well-being. Let's take as example two diseases which are currently the focus of various research efforts: attention-deficit hyperactivity disorder (ADHD) and malaria. In the United States, ADHD is perceived as a developmental disorder that requires pharmaceutical treatment to facilitate school advancement of children, reducing the burden of parents and teachers. The same disorder is perceived differently in Europe. On the other hand, malaria pervades the lives of millions of children in Africa. Which of these two diseases should be prioritised in terms of R&D efforts and health care policies? Many voices may advocate malaria, but the answer to this question is complex and remains a social and ethical dilemma as long as the priorities of the major players depend primarily upon return-of-investment (RoI).

The majority of organisations in a market economy will have to consider direct or indirect return of investment to fulfil their social and economic role. Serious non-profit organisations and private–public partnerships, such as Drugs for Neglected Diseases Initiative (DNDi 2010) and Medicines against Malaria Venture (MMV 2010) have a research agenda and predefined targets to meet. Many more stake-holders can be found by web search engines, including charities, African govern-ments, the United Nations, the World Health Organisation (WHO 2010) and the Bill and Melinda Gates foundation (Gates Foundation 2010), all of which have their own agenda.

The aforementioned issues are not addressed by the legislation on medicines for children. In market-driven drug development, it is the management of individual companies that decides which therapeutic targets will be included into the R&D portfolio. A company has to aim for long-term survival, irrespective of the ethos and social responsibilities it may endorse. To survive in a global economy, enterprises must be able to maintain revenue. However, it is also true that there are millions of children on this planet that have diseases that could be treated with medications that are already available, but not accessible to the patients in need. There is no single solution to this and many other dilemmas. A different, joint public–private partnership model might be considered which would be recognised beyond the regulatory and geographical borders of single countries. Without an integrated, long-term action plan, it is unlikely that the needs of vulnerable popu-lations, whether ADHD patients in the United States or malaria-infected children in Africa, will be duly addressed.

3.1 Essentials in Paediatric Clinical Research

There are key elements where most scientists will agree are necessary in drug development if children are to be considered as integral part of it. Among other things, an assessment must be performed for each disease which delineates unmet medical needs and ongoing efforts in basic and applied research (e.g. understand-ing of disease processes, target identification). Another critical factor under-pinning a more effective approach to paediatric drug research is the ability to access and share data on disease, safety and treatment outcome across organi-sations. Currently, regulatory authorities are the only stakeholders who have the privilege to access, to review and to mine preclinical and clinical research data across a wide range of diseases. It could be argued that such valuable data should not remain obscure to the wider scientific community, that the benefits from sharing disease and treatment-related information represent an opportunity to every stakeholder, and that mechanisms could be implemented to protect commercial and patent interests without dismissing the impact that further integration of information can have on therapeutics. This discussion will go on for a long time.

Concerted efforts are also required to ensure optimal implementation of clinical development plans for each drug that reaches development stage. Unfortunately, little attention has been paid so far to the implementation of paediatric trials. The ethical, practical and financial burden associated with gathering evidence from pharmacokinetics, efficacy and safety in children remains irrespective of the therapeutic indication. In addition, lack of consensus exists in areas such as (1) accepted age-matched normal range for laboratory measurements (e.g., for haematology, biochemistry, urinanalysis), (2) requirements for the validation of clinical endpoints for the assessment of efficacy and safety, and (3) standards for long-term safety monitoring and pharmacovigilance. Moreover, guidelines and policies for paediatric drug development are still highly regulated on a regional base, despite the availability of a worldwide framework by ICH. Considerable differences remain between regions and personal views seem to dictate implementation policies. In contrast, the decision regarding which therapeutic area to invest is entirely up to local decision-makers usually from private companies. Investment choices from non-profit organisations such as the Bill Gates foundation (USA) or governmental institutes such as Institute Pasteur (France) and Fiocruz Institute (Brazil) are minority examples of a different modus operandi in R&D. Despite evidence for effective results, they have not had the impact on market drivers which individual companies have had so far. Channelling the debate on unmet medical needs and on the requirements for the level of evidence through non-profit organisations may represent an opportunity to further find common ground between private interests (patient advocacy groups, pharmaceutical companies) and public health policies.

The future of paediatric development will ultimately depend on decision-makers. However, fundamental modifications are required in the way decisions are made about medicines for children. One thinkable scenario would be a joint international governmental programme to reimburse new drugs with proven clinical benefit based on health outcome, comparable to the approach that has evolved over the last decades for vaccination and immunisation programmes across the world. Various rare diseases and therapeutic niches exist which would benefit from a similar framework. Entrepreneurial efforts could lead to start-up companies which can rely on return of investment. This mechanism would trigger opportunities for identifying investors and clinical development venture capital. New charities and research organisations with clear focus might evolve. In this public–private partnership paradigm, profit margins can be defined by consensus of all relevant stakeholders, rather than by shareholders.

4 Incentives and Rewards

Irrespective of a shift in the paradigm for sponsorship and prioritisation of diseases, the need for incentives and rewards in paediatric drug development will remain. The use of incentives has been the primary mechanism in the United States and more recently in the European Union. This type of reward, based on extension of patent protection, has triggered numerous paediatric development programmes for drugs which are still under protection. Through these programmes, children are now already more exposed to clinical research than they have ever been in the past. The key mechanism is the offer to pharmaceutical companies to prolong the duration of patent protection against generic competition for a limited time. In return, the originating company negotiates a paediatric development plan with the authorities. It is important to realise that patent protection is prolonged for the all marketed indications, i.e. adults and children. One could argue that adults have to pay for paediatric research – but what is wrong about that? Children cannot pay for themselves.

Incentivising paediatric research through patent extension or market exclusivity can only work under several conditions. Firstly, there must be competition with generic drugs and a third-party payer system. This first set of requirements exists in the United States and Europe, but much less in Japan and other markets. Therefore, the road to a comparable approach in other areas of the world is blocked. Other strategies must be contemplated there. Secondly, the respective market for which a patent extension is granted needs to have a critical mass that makes the added value of a patent extension large enough to trigger investments in paediatric research. Despite the population size of emerging market countries such as India, China and Brazil, at present these markets are not sufficiently large to offer serious incentives for paediatric research. Thirdly, the mechanisms underlying patent protection must be strong and sufficiently robust to prevent infringements. Again, the quoted countries are examples of emerging economies where patent protection mechanisms are still weak. In addition, current public health policies are aimed at providing the population with those drugs that cover the medical needs of the majority. As a result, few R&D companies based in these countries have been able to develop innovative medicines.

Incentivising paediatric research for innovative drugs has so far produced very limited incentives for older, off-patent drugs, most of which continue to be used in an empirically, off-licence manner. The U.S. government had promised to promote clinical investigations on off-patent drugs but for years did not provide the necessary funds. This situation has now started to change, and impressive NIH-guided development programme are under way now to scrutinise the use of many off-patent drugs in the paediatric population. A similar initiative has been implemented in the EU under the auspices of the Research Directorate, which allocates research grants on therapeutic areas, which have been identified as unmet medical needs.

5   A New Role for Regulatory Authorities

A few decades ago, it was unthinkable to envisage Western governments enforcing choices to pharmaceutical industry regarding which drugs should be developed for children. This has however evolved: the incentives of the paediatric legislation have to some degree influenced the directions industry pursues. The requirement for a paediatric investigational plan (PIP) to be submitted to the European Medicines Agency at an early stage of development is enforcing disclosure of key information, including planned therapeutic targets and indications for compounds in development. Even though at an early stage a company may not be certain whether the compound will ever become a marketed drug, this process enables regulators to scrutinise how efforts and resources are being allocated to drug targets and diseases. It is also prompting a dialogue on the contents of the paediatric programme, with direct impact on the level of evidence required for approval and consequently to the rewards. Indirectly, regulators have also got the opportunity to impose waivers on areas deemed unnecessary or low priority.

Nevertheless, as indicated previously, the majority of the off-patent drugs licensed for an adult indication continue to be used without scientific evidence for the dose rationale, benefits and risks in children. A different funding model is required to prioritise evaluation of these drugs. In this context, it is clear that regulation can play an important role in shaping the future of paediatric drug development. One should not, however, consider regulatory mechanisms as the only means to promote the advancements in the field. Incentives and regulatory requirements have to be seen in a much wider context. And there will always remain national and geographical borders.

6   Strategy for a Paediatric Development Plan

One of the main changes in the way drugs have been approved for paediatric use is the requirement for formal evidence of efficacy and safety as needed for adult indications. Historically, the implementation of paediatric legislation in the United States from 1997 to 2007 [FDA Modernization Act (FDAMA), Pediatric Research Equity Act (PREA), Best Pharmaceuticals for Children Act (BPCA), FDA Amendment Acts (FDAAA)] (2010) has driven paediatric product development without explicit timing for the generation of such evidence. The absence of a milestone for the implementation of paediatric plans has caused a major gap in R&D. Given that most clinical studies were phase IV commitments, poor integration of the clinical plans has become common practice for indications which include adults and children. Despite the controversy, this system has improved the off-label use of most licensed medicines.

The introduction of the paediatric legislation in the EU has added an important element to paediatric research. It defines the timing at which a paediatric plan should be in place. The regulation has changed the R&D landscape by introducing a milestone for the implementation of a proposal, the paediatric investigational plan, which could even occur in parallel to the development of the adult indication, where applicable.

A detailed description of the requirements for a paediatric development plan is out of the scope of this chapter, but the new EU legislation is triggering a profound review of strategy and key processes in adult and paediatric drug development. There are various challenges from a clinical and scientific perspective, including establishing the rationale for dose selection in clinical trials in children, identification and validation of primary endpoints for paediatric diseases and the assessment of long-term safety in paediatric trials. From a theoretical perspective, one important challenge is how to distinguish the influence of developmental growth and other external factors from drug-related effects. Of particular interest is the role of co-morbidities specific to childhood which may become important confounders of drug response in children. On the other hand, the shift in paradigm also poses a challenge to clinical practice, which will have to abandon informal, off-label prescription as the basis of therapeutic innovation. Paediatricians and clinical researchers have to face the requirements for the generation of formal evidence. This is and may remain a major cultural hurdle throughout the next generation. Paediatric prescription has been dominated by empiricism and myths about how to best treat children. This problem is compounded by the lack of scientific and technical training in paediatric clinical pharmacology, which would provide paediatricians with the appropriate set of skills to design better trials and accurately interpret findings from randomised clinical trials.

As indicated above, for the first time in the history of paediatric medicine, the assessment of risk–benefit ratio is becoming a prospective exercise. The dialogue between industry, academia, professional networks, regulators and patient organisations will be critical to ensure paediatric needs are prioritised and complexities understood accordingly.

Conceptually, the development of a paediatric strategy must account for a number of aspects, which can be categorised as follows:

1. *Level of evidence*. Arguments to support the need to generate efficacy data vs. using indirect inferences from extrapolation and bridging studies.
2. *Disease*. Understanding of differences or similarities in aetiology, epidemiology, symptoms and signs across populations. This includes the availability of common endpoints for the assessment of efficacy and safety in children of different ages vs. adults.
3. *Dosing rationale*. Understanding of the requirements for the dosing rationale which should be based on exposure–response relationships, rather than empirically defined by differences in body size. These considerations apply equally to efficacy and safety.
4. *Drug delivery*. Understanding of the implications of changes in dosage form and route of administration, taking into account the need for age-suitable formulations.

5. *Study implementation*. Major differences exist in terms of population size, patient stratification, sampling frequency, statistical design, which are required to generate evidence in children. Innovative designs can be used in conjunction with pharmacostatistical methods that enable assessment of pharmacokinetics, efficacy and safety. The use of placebo-controlled parallel group designs is by far the most used method and the least desirable design in children.
6. *Risk management*. Long-term safety and risk management of paediatric products can differ considerably from adult indications. The ability to distinguish the influence from developmental growth and other age-related factors from intrinsic drug effects is critical for establishing preventive actions and assessing drug-relatedness.

These points represent a pragmatic view of the principles defined by the ICH E11 and should form the basis for a global strategy. Clinical researchers, paediatricians and regulators have been aware of these needs for a long time, but very few experts are knowledgeable about how to properly evaluate drug use in the intended population.

It is worth mentioning that the data to support the use of a paediatric formulation and the information required to define the dosing rationale may not be trivial and will often require close integration of the knowledge from the development programme for the adult indication. These two items will influence the timing, contents and cost of all subsequent actions to generate evidence on pharmacokinetics, efficacy and safety data. The development of formulations and assessment of corresponding bioavailability and bioequivalence will often rely on data from adult (healthy) subjects. The information required to characterise pharmacokinetic-pharmacodynamic (PKPD) relationships and scale doses across populations will also depend upon the availability of a well-designed clinical plan in adults. Lastly, the use of juvenile toxicology studies must be linked to further understanding of biomarkers, disease and species differences. Inaccurate interpretation of such findings may jeopardise the selection of the appropriate dosing regimen and subsequently lead to failure of the programme.

7 Limitations of Paediatric Legislation

The paediatric legislation alone is unlikely to change the directions of paediatric research, discovery and drug development. As long as pharmaceutical R&D remains dependent upon economical drivers, individual organisations will not be able to make decisions regarding what to develop or not based primarily on value proposition for patients. In fact, those who choose for a different strategy may not survive. Furthermore, the recent approval by the United States of new health care legislation indicates that health care systems are changing even in areas of stronghold of free market. Access to and reimbursement of pharmaceuticals and biologicals are part of a much wider network, and as such cannot be evaluated in isolation. Of particular importance is the impact of ageing in Western countries and the increasing need to address chronic degenerative diseases.

Another shortcoming in the current regulation is the extent to which it is applicable. Whilst gathering of formal evidence for the efficacy and safety is undisputable, the need to consider a paediatric investigational plan for every new formulation, route of administration or dosage form creates a potential for an excessive number of paediatric clinical trials. This is aggravated by the lack of a procedure to objectively evaluate medical need and by the limited experience of the PDCO [Paediatric Committee] members in drug development.

Despite these limitations, the legislation in the United States and European Union has the merit of ensuring that children are considered as an integral part of the R&D process. Such a strict path has never been created for other special patient populations.

8   Future Perspectives in Regulatory Affairs and Public Health Policies

The paediatric legislation in force in both the United States and European Union has and will have long-lasting implications for the development of medicines for children. Paediatric legislation will evolve further and will certainly not cease to exist in either region. They have introduced processes and procedures which will become an integral part of the drug development pursuit. Companies and organisations that dismiss this shift in paradigm will have to face penalties imposed not only by regulatory authorities on the file-ability of a market authorisation application, but also by the resulting change in medical culture and market perception, which will disfavour off-label use of medicines in children. Most importantly, this change may have consequences to the liability of sponsors and paediatricians to legal action.

It is also important to consider that public understanding of drug development is limited at present. Some facts are well known, e.g. increased life expectancy in Western countries and the role modern pharmaceutical treatment plays in this. Other facts remain unclear, particularly in Europe. There remains a quasi-mystical belief in the medical wisdom and in the role of medical training. The appreciation of the value of clinical trials as a key pillar of therapeutics is much less established. This is exacerbated by media speculation and by the belief that children should not be the subject of clinical experimentation. In general terms, this attitude reflects cultural and historical differences between nations. U.S. citizens, on the other hand, have a stronger scepticism towards authority and are more prepared to tread new paths. Irrespective of these differences, the importance of gathering evidence on efficacy and safety based on controlled, randomised clinical trials will become obvious to parents, society and to many other stakeholders.

The debate will go on with defenders and contenders of governmental control and of entrepreneurial freedom. Albeit difficult to predict what will happen in detail, regulatory authorities become active players in drug development. Regulatory authorities have triggered processes and requirements for demonstrating efficacy and safety. Together with all other stakeholders, they share the responsibility for the advancement of health care. Their defensive or conservative role has influenced drug development in different directions. From the availability of anti-retroviral drugs for HIV to the recent approval of HIN51 flu vaccine, regulators have represented the hurdle or the thrust for patient access to innovative therapeutic options.

9   Foreseeable and Unforeseeable Developments

Personalised medicine is still an evolving concept, which demands a very different approach to diagnosis, therapeutics and prognosis of diseases in adults and children. This is taking place in parallel with the evolution of health technology, which has established criteria for ranking effectiveness and consequently for reimbursement policies. Drug discovery, development, approval and labelling will have to account for the requirements this advancement entails. Moreover, the definition of disease, dysfunction and disorder are also changing. New phenotypes are being identified and increasingly more, rare diseases are described, most of which occur in children. As long as health care institutions can afford the cost of innovation in the diagnosis, treatment and prophylaxis of (new) diseases, it can be anticipated that R&D organisations will prioritise investments for the development of therapeutic agents for rare conditions.

In this landscape, it is likely that new specialised niche companies will arise as suppliers of expertise and technology. Development organisations will become distinct from discovery organisations, with the objective of not only launching new products into the market, but also of ensuring clear value proposition and reimbursement of new treatments. Unfortunately, the incentives for innovation also represent a risk to the optimisation of the therapeutic use of existing, off-patent drugs. Despite the possibility of up to 10-year data protection in exchange for paediatric development in the European Union, it is unlikely that new label recommendations, or novel paediatric formulations will rank sufficiently high to ensure reimbursement against other therapeutic options (e.g. generics).

It is not possible to predict with accuracy to what extent the ongoing technology revolution will translate into immediate changes in health care. For the moment, it is clear that society will have to face the consequences of the developments and changes in society and lifestyle over the last 50 years. A further wave of child obesity with all ensuing sequelae, including hypertension, diabetes, dyslipidaemia and other potential health issues will most likely be the focus of attention.

10   Conclusions

Drug development is not a linear process which can be easily directed by guidelines and policies. It involves numerous, complex iterations, many of which do not depend solely on logical, scientific judgement or criteria. It also depends on medical, economical, ethical and political considerations. Given the nature of the latter factors, consensus in health care priorities, medical needs and reimbursement will remain an additional challenge for all stakeholders in R&D. Society, and in particular children and adolescents, will continue to develop and behave differently from today. They will face other lifestyle challenges and will have access to different therapeutic options than today's generation. In any case, the current regulatory framework shows that legislation will continue to determine or at least influence the directions and future of public health care. The right of access to safe and effective medicines is certainly an achievement which cannot be overturned.

References

Cella M, Knibbe C, Danhof M, Della Pasqua O (2010) What is the right dose for children? Br J Clin Pharmacol 70:597–603. doi:10.1111/j.1365-2125.2009.03591.x

DNDi (Drugs for Neglected Diseases Initiative) (2010) http://www.dndi.org. Accessed 14 Oct 2010

European Medicines Agency (2010) http://www.ema.europa.eu. Accessed 14 Oct 2010

FDA (Food and Drug Administration) (2010) http://www.fda.gov. Accessed 14 Oct 2010

FDAAA (FDA Amendment Acts) (2010) http://www.fda.gov/RegulatoryInformation/Legislation/ FederalFoodDrugandCosmeticActFDCAct/SignificantAmendmentstotheFDCAct/ FoodandDrugAdministrationAmendmentsActof2007/default.htm. Accessed 14 Oct 2010

Gates Foundation (2010) http://www.gatesfoundation.org. Accessed 14 Oct 2010

Hilts PJ (2003) Protecting America's health. Alfred A. Knopf, New York

ICH (2010) International Conference on Harmonisation of technical requirements for registration of pharmaceuticals for human use. http://www.ich.org. Accessed 14 Oct 2010

ICH E11 (2010) ICH tripartite guideline: clinical investigation of medicinal products in the pediatric population. http://www.ich.org/LOB/media/MEDIA487.pdf. Accessed 14 Oct 2010

MMV (Medicines for Malaria Venture) (2010) http://www.mmv.org. Accessed 14 Oct 2010

Rose K, van den Anker J (eds) (2010) Guide to paediatric drug development and clinical research. Karger, Basel, Switzerland, http://content.karger.com/ProdukteDB/produkte.asp?Aktion= showproducts&searchWhat=books&ProduktNr=253804. Accessed 14 Oct 2010. ISBN 978-3-8055-9362-5; e-ISBN: 978-3-8055-9363-2

Stoetter H (2007) Paediatric drug development: historical background of regulatory initiatives. In: Rose K, van den Anker JN (eds) Guide to paediatric clinical research. Karger, Basel, pp 25–32

Taussig HB (1962) A study of the German outbreak of phocomelia. JAMA 180(32):1106–1114

Wax P (1995) Elixirs, diluents, and the passage of the 1938 Federal Food, Drug and Cosmetic Act. Ann Intern Med 122:456–461

WHO (2010) http://www.who.int. Accessed 14 Oct 2010

Study Design and Simulation Approach

Stephanie Läer and Bernd Meibohm

Contents

Abstract Modeling and simulation techniques are a mainstay of clinical drug development and are particularly useful to support clinical trials in children. If a pediatrician wants to use these tools most efficiently, a basic understanding of the principles and methods of classical and novel techniques of modeling and simulation is essential. Key elements comprise the definition and description of terms like deterministic simulation, Monte Carlo simulation, classical "top down" or novel

S. Läer (✉)

Department of Clinical Pharmacy and Pharmacotherapy, Heinrich-Heine-University of Düsseldorf, Universitätsstrasse 1, 40225 Düsseldorf, Germany

e-mail: stephanie.laeer@uni-duesseldorf.de

B. Meibohm

College of Pharmacy, University of Tennessee Health Science Center, 874 Union Avenue, Rm. 5p, Memphis, TN 38163, USA

H.W. Seyberth et al. (eds.), *Pediatric Clinical Pharmacology*,   125
Handbook of Experimental Pharmacology 205,
DOI 10.1007/978-3-642-20195-0_6, © Springer-Verlag Berlin Heidelberg 2011

"bottom up" approach, as well as the term "virtual world simulation." The illustrated examples in this chapter from pediatric clinical trials will help to understand and demonstrate these key elements. The importance of the understanding of developmental physiology and pharmacokinetics will become visible when explaining novel "bottom up" approaches like physiologically based pharmacokinetic simulations which also bridge to current research tools from other areas such as systems biology using mathematical models to describe biological systems.

Keywords Modeling • Simulation • Top-down • Bottom-up • Children

Abbreviations

BSA	Body surface area
CO	Cardiac output
CYP	Cytochrome P450
f_u	Unbound fraction of a drug
GFR	Glomerular filtration rate
K_a	Acid constant
K_m	Michaelis–Menten constant
LogP	Parameter describing lipophilicity of a drug
LOQ	Limit of quantification
M&S	Modeling and simulation
MM	Michaelis–Menten
M_{wt}	Molecular weight
PBPK	Physiology-based pharmacokinetics
PD	Pharmacodynamic
PK	Pharmacokinetic
Q_H	Total hepatic blood flow
QT interval	Section of track of the electrocardiogram
QTc interval	Section of track of the electrocardiogram corrected for heart rate
$t_{1/2}$	Terminal half life
UGT	UDP-glucuronyltransferases
USA	United States of America
V_d	Volume of distribution
V_{max}	The maximum initial velocity or rate of a reaction

1 Introduction

Modeling and simulation techniques are a mainstay of clinical drug development for adults and children. European and international guidelines for the development of medicinal products refer to these techniques. Model-based methods are particularly useful to support pediatric drug development because they provide means to leverage knowledge from adult clinical trials enabling efficient data collection by providing dosing schedules, optimizing and/or minimizing the number of plasma samples required for pharmacokinetic and pharmacodynamic investigations and even minimizing the number of infants and children required in clinical trials.

In this chapter, the principles and methods of modeling and simulation approaches using computers and computer software are explained. The illustrated examples from pediatric clinical trials should help to understand and demonstrate the key elements of classical and novel modeling and simulation tools for pediatric drug development. The specific topics will:

- define the terms deterministic simulation and Monte Carlo simulation.
- describe the classical "top down" and the novel "bottom up" approach of modeling and simulation.
- describe virtual world simulation.
- provide a portfolio of examples of simulations to illustrate the benefits and limitations of simulations.

2 Methods

2.1 *Computer-Based Modeling and Simulation*

In the healthcare environment, numerical simulation utilizes mathematical abstractions of processes representative of isolated organs, tissues, whole body organisms, populations of individuals as well as whole societies combined with computing resources to address real-life medical problems.

Modeling and simulation are two techniques that are so closely related to each other that they are usually mentioned in conjunction as a "modeling and simulation" (M&S) approach. Modeling in this context usually comprises the description of the behavior of a system or process by a set of mathematical expressions that is usually a simplification of certain aspects of reality and focuses only on those factors and processes that are believed to be important. Simulation is then the application of this mathematical model usually over time to explore situations that have not been investigated experimentally, thereby extrapolating beyond the currently available experimental data (Laer et al. 2009).

In the context of pharmacotherapy, the M&S approach can be viewed as one of the three pillars of facilitating the solution to pharmacotherapeutic problems, along with theoretical reasoning and hypothesis building as well as clinical experimentation (Fig. 1). The M&S process visualizes and optimizes the clinical experiment and thus helps fastening the process, utilizing resources including research subjects more efficiently, and even reducing the number of experiments needed to be performed. Thus, the M&S approach holds great promise especially in pediatric drug development and applied pharmacotherapy, where the optimal and ethically acceptable use of limited resources with regard to patients, measurements, and

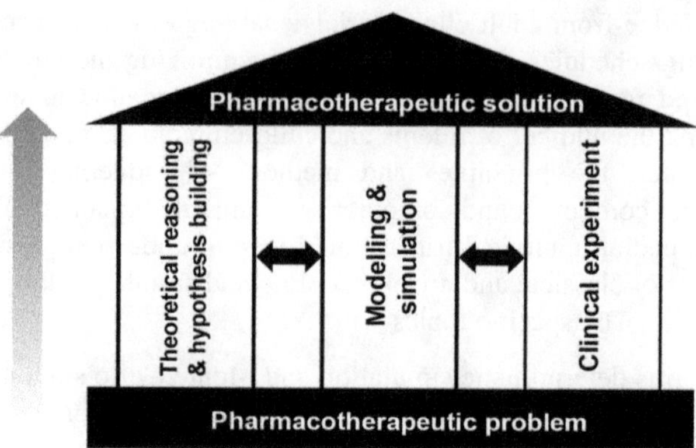

Fig. 1 Modeling and simulation as one of the three pillars of facilitating the solution to pharmacotherapeutic problems, along with theoretical reasoning and hypothesis building and clinical experimentation. The modeling and simulation process visualizes and optimizes the clinical experiment and thus helps fastening the process and even reducing the number of experiments needed to be performed. From Laer et al. (2009)

interventions is even more pressing than in other areas of the healthcare environment.

2.1.1   Deterministic Simulation

Classic approaches in pharmacokinetics and pharmacodynamics usually use deterministic simulations to predict for example time courses of drug concentrations or time courses of drug effect intensities. These deterministic simulations use parameter point estimates for their simulations, which may be considered the "best guesses" for specific parameter values. Thus, one set of parameters for a given model will result in one discrete simulated outcome, for example, a discrete drug concentration vs. time profile in response to a given dose or dosing regimen. The parameters themselves may be dependent on patient specific covariates such as demographic, anthropometric, physiologic or pathophysiologic variables, but each set of parameters will simulate only one specific outcome.

Compartmental pharmacokinetic models applied for individual pediatric patients with discrete data sets, for example, are classic examples of deterministic simulations (Laer et al. 2001). For a given set of parameter point estimates and a specific dose/dosing regimen, they result in one discrete time profile of simulated concentrations. The major advantage of this approach is simplicity and ease of understanding, especially for healthcare professionals not familiar with M&S techniques. A major limitation, however, is the fact that parameter point estimates are given absolute credibility without appreciation of uncertainty related to the estimation process through which they were derived. In addition, only a limited number of patient-specific covariates predictive of drug disposition or response are usually known, and thus patients with even similar known covariates will exhibit a distribution of different parameters, which will subsequently result in variability in drug exposure and/or response. The deterministic modeling approach neglects this uncertainty of the parameter point estimates.

2.1.2 Monte Carlo Simulation

In contrast to deterministic simulations, Monte Carlo simulations are a stochastic simulation technique. Rather than relying on fixed parameter point estimates, Monte Carlo simulations rely upon distributions for each specific parameter that capture the degree of uncertainty in each parameter. Each distribution is defined by a central tendency (e.g., mean or median) and a spread or variability term (e.g., variance or standard deviation). Monte Carlo simulations then use repeated random sampling of parameters from these distributions to simulate the outcome based on the underlying structural model. Thus, Monte Carlo simulations do not result in a discrete outcome, for example, a concentration-time or response-time profile, but in a distribution of outcomes for which again a central tendency (e.g., mean or median) and a distribution (e.g., 90% confidence interval) can be defined (El-Tahtawy et al. 2006). As such, Monte Carlo simulations have the advantage to provide inherently a measure of credibility and likelihood for simulation outcomes that is usually lacking in discrete simulations. A major disadvantage, however, is the increased complexity of the analysis and thus the difficulty in acceptance and understanding of the derived simulations by healthcare professionals not familiar with M&S techniques.

2.2 Models for Simulation

2.2.1 "Top Down" Approach

Modeling approaches in drug development can in general be differentiated into deductive and inductive approaches. Deductive approaches, often also referred to as "top-down" or "analytic" approaches, are based on generalized concepts in medical sciences such as clinical pharmacology. They can be seen as a verification-driven data mining process that allows a modeller to express preconceived facts or theories in model terms, subsequently test their validity within the context of the model system and the available data, and obtain reasons for the validation or invalidation. Thus, the deductive model development process is characterized by a constant rebuilding and refinement of the model given the results of the continuous hypothesis testing. As such, "top-down" modeling is clearly a data-driven process, in which the model is iteratively refined to optimally describe observed data (Laer et al. 2009).

Compartmental pharmacokinetic modeling or the E_{max}-model as a frequently used pharmacodynamic model are clearly empirical models that are derived through the "top down" process and are oftentimes iteratively refined during the model building process through hypothesis testing by evaluation via statistical means whether a modification in the model is actually reflected in an appropriate improved model fit. Albeit largely empirical, "top down" models can still include mechanistic or semi-mechanistic structural model components related to a drug's known pharmacologic mechanism of action and its interplay with physiologic systems.

In pediatric clinical pharmacology, population pharmacokinetic (PK) and population pharmacokinetic/pharmacodynamic (PK/PD) analyses are frequently applied to identify significant determinants of drug disposition and response, and derive and optimize dosing regimens in drug development and applied pharmacotherapy (Bartelink et al. 2006; Meibohm et al. 2005). Population PK/PD analyses are typically performed following a "top down" approach. A population PK/PD model consists of a structural, a stochastic, and a covariate model component. In a first model building step, different structural models, for example. compartmental pharmacokinetic models, are explored in their ability to describe the observed data. Review of goodness-of-fit criteria in visual or numeric form as well as evaluation of statistical summary criteria allows the selection of the most appropriate structural model alternative. In a second step, parameter and error distributions are added in a stochastic model component to differentiate among between-subject variability, between-occasion variability, and unexplained residual variability. In a third step, patient covariates are explored in their ability to predict a fraction of the between-subject variability (Sheiner and Ludden 1992). Thus, the model is sequentially refined using reiterative hypothesis testing, thereby providing a final model that is based on general clinical pharmacology principles and additional details derived from the structure of the available data set.

2.2.2 "Bottom Up" Approach (Physiologically Based Pharmacokinetic Simulation)

In contrast to deductive approaches, inductive modeling approaches, also called "bottom-up" or "synthetic" approaches, synthesize specific available observations, data, and patterns to form broader generalizations and theories. In this modeling approach, individual elements are linked together to form larger subsystems, which then in turn are linked, sometimes in many levels, until a complete top-level model is formed. Physiologically based pharmacokinetic (PBPK) modeling can be seen as an example of inductive modeling. While the "top-down" approach (e.g., via a population pharmacokinetic analysis) aims to partition variation in pharmacokinetics via measured covariates (demographics, biomarker, etc.), the "bottom-up" approach focuses on constructed simulation models consistent with physiologic parameterization of pediatric populations and drug-specific parameters (Khalil and Laer 2011; Willmann et al. 2003).

Concept of Physiologically Based Pharmacokinetic Modeling

The general idea of PBPK modeling is to mathematically describe all physico-chemical and physiological processes that are involved in the determination of substance pharmacokinetics in as much detail as possible. To do this, knowledge in physiology and anatomy will be used to represent the species to be modeled (e.g., human body) or part of it (in case of systems simulation) as a structure composed of physiologically relevant compartments, where each compartment usually represents a single organ or tissue. These compartments will be interconnected, following the anatomical structure of the organism, via the blood circulation loop. Then, mass-balance equations for each compartment describing the fate of the substance within it will be established.

Information for the PBPK model about the different physiological parameters such as organs/tissues/fluids weights and volumes, cardiac output, regional and tissue blood flows, surface area will be obtained from the literature. To make the model complete, the compound-specific parameters are incorporated. These are not static and vary according to the substance under study, most importantly perme-ability and partitioning of the substance between body tissues and the blood/plasma. Tissue/plasma partition coefficients can be obtained either from in vitro experiments, by extrapolating the experimental partition coefficients values from animals to humans, or by calculation/prediction from tissue composition (lipids, proteins, water) and physicochemical properties of the substance in interest. These include molecular weight (M_{wt}), lipophilicity (mostly in term of LogP value), acid dissociation constant (pKa), solubility, blood to plasma concentration ratio and affinity to albumin [in terms of fraction unbound (f_u)].

At the end, the PBPK model employs all these information in order to describe and/or predict the pharmacokinetics of a drug in certain individuals. However, PBPK models can vary in their complexity from simple (basic) to advanced (complex) depending on the model purpose and can range from partial-body models, where only certain systems are included, to whole-body models, where all the important organs and tissues are included. Because some specialized PBPK model software (e.g., PK-Sim®) has additional incorporated modules such as scaling clearance from adults to children and a population pharmacokinetic module, which extend its function and use, these are of importance in the simulation of pharmacokinetics for children. A representative schematic drawing illustrates this concept (Fig. 2 modified from Willmann et al. 2003).

Physiology-Based Pharmacokinetic Modeling in Children

For the integration of physiological data occurring in childhood, age-dependent processes of organs, blood flow, and biochemical processes are incorporated from databases or represented by a variety of regression functions in the PBPK models. These include physiological characteristics of organs, tissues, and blood flows as described by Johnson et al. (2006) (Table 1, Fig. 3 modified from Johnson et al.

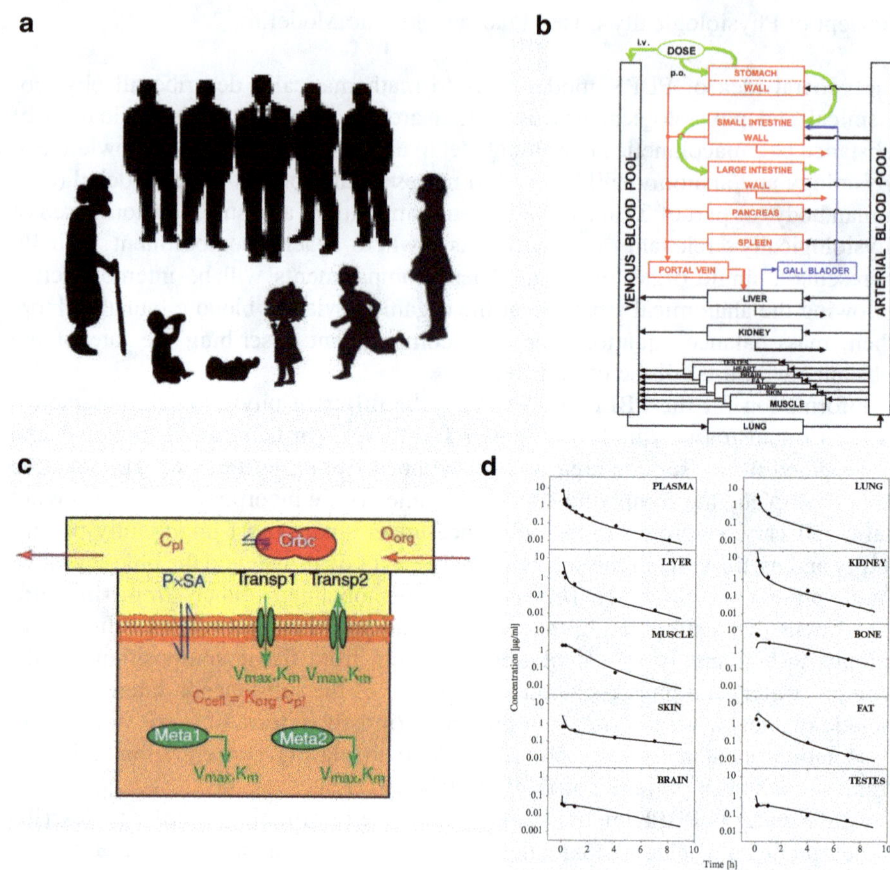

Fig. 2 Illustration of the concept for building a physiologically based pharmacokinetic model modified according to Willmann et al. (2003). (**a**) Organisms, e.g., human beings of different ages or populations are the basis for the model. (**b**) The organism is divided into a number of compartments, each representing a single organ. To describe the distribution of compounds in the body the organs are connected via their arteries and veins to the arterial and venous blood pool. Inter-compartmental mass transport occurs via organ-specific blood flow rates. The organs are mathematically connected. (**c**) Division of each organ into three sub-compartments representing the vascular (with blood cells), interstitial, and cellular space. The interstitial space is assumed to be in direct contact with the plasma. The exchange of substances between the cellular and interstitial compartment can occur by permeation across the membranes via passive diffusion as well as active influx and efflux transport processes by saturable Michaelis–Menten (MM) kinetics (parameters: V_{max}, K_m). Metabolization of substances (Meta1, Meta2) occurs via active enzymes (MM-kinetics). Finally, the model consists of a large number of coupled differential equations. (**d**) Output of the model: Concentration time curves for the substances. Shown are simulated and observed ciprofloxacin concentrations in various organs after intravenously applied ciprofloxacin 5 mg/kg to a rat

Table 1 Body and tissue weights (kg), cardiac output (L/min) as function of age according to Björkman (2004)

Tissue	Neonate	6 months	1 year	2 years	5 years	10 years	15 years	Adult
Body	3.55	8.03	10.2	12.6	19.7	31.4	56.7	73.0
Lung	0.06	0.12	0.16	0.24	0.34	0.43	0.90	1.20
Liver	0.12	0.27	0.36	0.48	0.59	0.87	1.35	1.80
Kidney	0.03	0.05	0.06	0.09	0.11	0.18	0.25	0.31
Gut	0.05	0.09	0.14	0.19	0.34	0.58	0.82	1.02
Muscle	0.80	1.35	1.90	2.83	5.60	11.0	24.0	29.0
Adipose	0.89	2.97	3.64	3.76	5.0	7.50	9.50	14.5
CO	0.58	1.35	1.68	2.06	2.88	3.90	5.77	6.79
Q_H	0.22	0.38	0.45	0.53	0.72	1.04	1.55	1.72

CO cardiac output, Q_H total hepatic blood flow

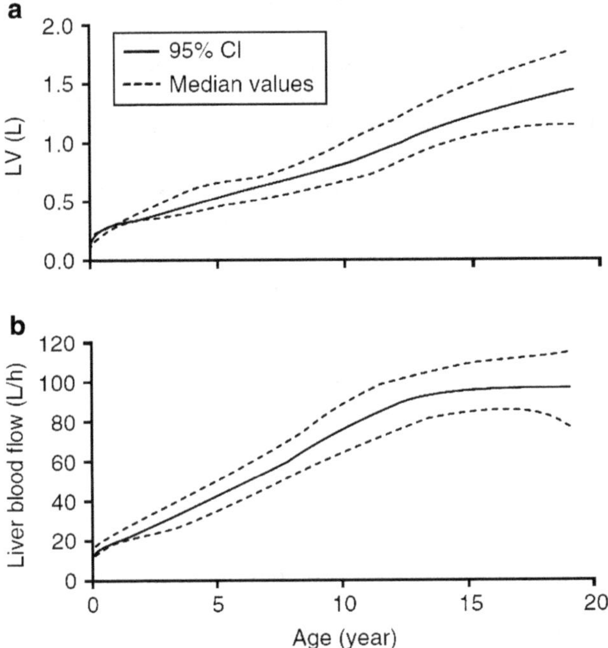

Fig. 3 Changes in liver volume (LV) (**a**) and liver blood flow (**b**) as function of age according to Johnson et al. (2006)

2006), the fraction of vascular and interstitial space, changes in total body water and adipose tissue content, plasma protein concentration especially of albumin and alpha glycoprotein, and renal and hepatic elimination.

There are numerous reports about developmental changes in metabolizing enzymes from birth to adolescence (van der Marel et al. 2003; Bouwmeester et al. 2004; see also Table 2). Nearly each CYP450 isoform shows a different pattern of maturation, and might influence the drug clearance with respect to specific age

Table 2 Enzyme activities (expressed as fraction of adult values) as function of age Edginton et al. (2006)

Enzyme	Neonate	1 month	3 months	6 months	1 years	10 years
Cyp3A4	0.24	0.5	0.7	1.1	1.3	1
Cyp1A2	0.1	0.2	0.25	0.29	0.35	1
Cyp2E1	0.32	0.4	0.46	0.46	1	1
UGT2B7	0.064	0.1	0.3	0.7	1	1

groups. The most abundant hepatic CYP450, the CYPs 3A4 and 3A7, which belong to the subfamily CYP3A, show a different evolution with time: CYP3A7 is the major active isoform in neonates and young infants but there is a progressive shift from CYP3A7 toward CYP3A4 in the first weeks of life. And, although these enzymes share at least 85% sequence identity, they exhibit large differences in substrate specificity and catalytic activities (Hines 2008).

Similar to enzyme systems, the integration of the maturation of renal excretion in a PBPK model is highly relevant because of its impact on the pharmacokinetics of compounds with renal clearance as major elimination pathway (Alcorn and McNamara 2003; Morselli et al. 1980; Yared and Ichikara 1994). Both, glomerular filtration rate and tubular secretion, undergo developmental changes (Arant 1978). Glomerular filtration rate increases rapidly in the first weeks to reach adult values between 2 and 6 months because of an increase in cardiac blood flow, a decrease in arteriolar resistance and an increase in the surface area and the pore size of the glomerular membrane. The tubular secretion increases at a slower rate than the glomerular filtration rate (GFR), particularly because of the delay in the maturation of active transporters, but also due to the smaller size of the tubulus and a smaller mass of functioning tubular cells in children. The maturation of tubular secretion takes about 1 year.

PBPK Modeling Methodologies and Software

Several commercial software tools for the development of physiologically based pharmacokinetic models are available on the market. It is important to distinguish between general mathematical and engineering modeling software packages, and specialized PBPK modeling software packages. General modeling software packages, such as MATLAB®, ModelMaker®, Berkeley Madonna™, and ACSL®, provide a programming language for the model code, routines to solve the differential equations with differential equations integrator and a graphical output of the simulation results. This software offers the greatest flexibility to the PBPK model developer. Easier to use, however, are specialized PBPK modeling software packages. They provide either a click-and-drag assembly of the model structure or have already built one and require less mathematical background and modeling experience. These can either simulate particular PK-relevant processes (e.g., intestinal absorption or metabolic processes) or constitute generic whole body PBPK models. Examples for such software are PK-Sim®, Simcyp®, and

GastroPlus™. Nevertheless, the use of PBPK modeling software relies on expert knowledge in pharmacokinetics, physiological, pathophysiological, and developmental pharmacological processes as well as sufficient experience in the development of pharmacokinetic models using modeling software.

Implementations of PBPK Modeling

Through their enhanced ability to integrate relevant information (physiologically relevant, substance dependent) generated from various sources, PBPK models have gained attention in the fields of pharmacology and drug development and are more and more competitive to empirical pharmacokinetic models. The following list provides some applications of PBPK modeling. Some examples for pediatric applications are given under Section "Examples of 'Bottom Up' Simulations for Deriving Dosing Recommendations".

(a) PBPK modeling can be used to describe and/or predict drug pharmacokinetic profiles through simulation of different dosing regimens, which allows the evaluation and optimization of already established dosing-regimens.
(b) A PBPK model enables the quantification of the exposure in remote and/or inaccessible compartments, such as brain or tumor tissues.
(c) A PBPK model can be used to describe the pharmacokinetics of small-molecule compounds, but also for large proteins and even nano-particles.
(d) PBPK modeling is useful as a learning tool to gain more information about the different processes that are involved in determining drug disposition in tissues as well as the magnitude of the influence of separate parameters on drug pharmacokinetic behavior.
(e) PBPK models are used to describe and/or predict drug pharmacokinetics under different physiological and pharmacological conditions, e.g., in individuals with diseases or altered physiology. The effects of aging, rest, and physical efforts have been explored by PBPK modeling technique.
(f) In case of the pediatric population, PBPK is used to predict drug pharmacokinetics in children (prediction of volume of distribution, clearance values, etc.) and thus may help in the selection of the first dose in different pediatric age groups as illustrated in Fig. 4 with an example for sildenafil (Hsien 2010). This helps to provide information for conducting pediatric clinical trials in optimized form (Fig. 4). PBPK modeling allows the suggestion of a first dose as well as efficient sampling times, giving the opportunity of reducing the number of children required for the clinical study.

Limitations of Physiology-Based Pharmacokinetic Modeling

PBPK modeling requires comprehensive data on the physico-chemical, physiological, and biochemical processes of the organism and the drug. In case of PBPK for

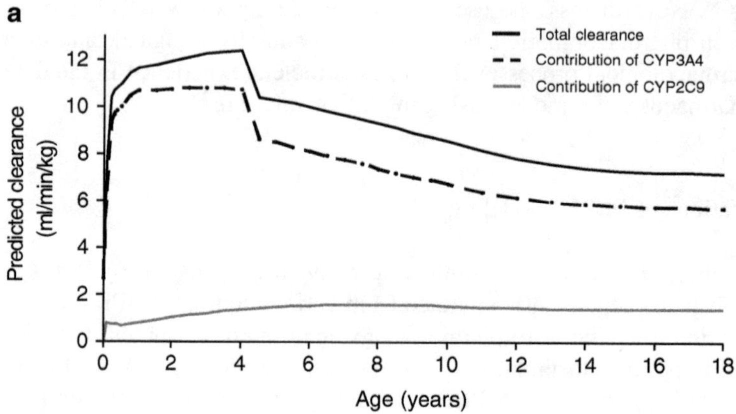

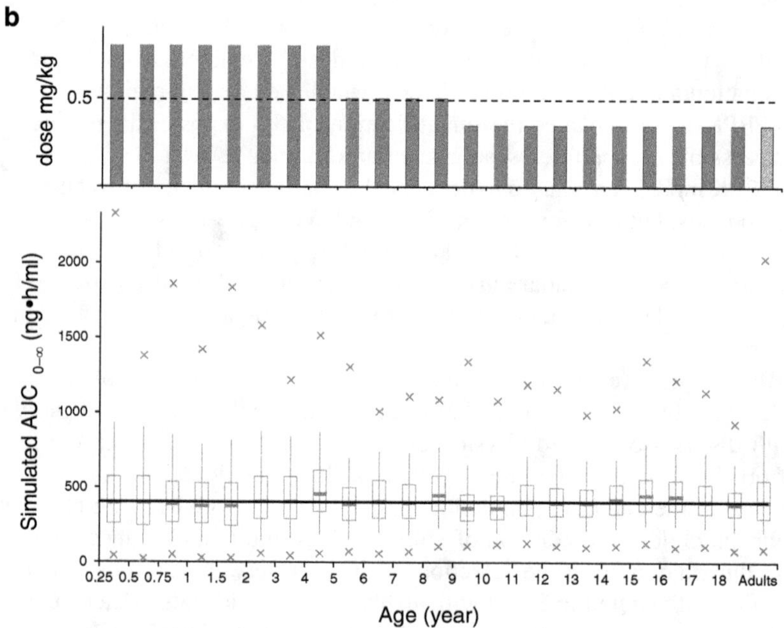

Fig. 4 Simulation results of a PBPK model for sildenafil for children using the PK-Sim®.software module (Hsien 2010). (**a**) Predicted age-dependent sildenafil hepatic clearance across the different pediatric ages based on the clearance scaling module in PK-Sim®. (**b**) Age-related doses for oral sildenafil in children depending on the simulated age-related exposure (not shown) of sildenafil in a virtual pediatric population and the estimated exposure of the estimated doses of sildenafil in children between 3 months and 18 years of age. Potential pediatric doses on the basis of the simulations for sildenafil in order to achieve adult exposure: Infants and younger children from 3 months to 4 years: 0.8 mg/kg, children from 5 to 8 years 0.5 mg/kg and children older than 8 years 0.35 mg/kg similar than in adults. Box plots represent median, 25th and 75th percentiles (*box*), 5th and 95th percentiles (*error bar*) and maximum and minimum values (x) of AUC 0–∞ from 1,000 simulations in each age

children data on the ontogeny of these parameters are not always available and/or they are not available from only one source. This may lead to some confusion and to a problem in establishing a reliable source of accurate and consistent information. In addition, some gaps may be present in fully or accurately describing some physiological process especially in young children, which in turn may lead to an inability of the model to successfully describe the pharmacokinetics of certain drugs in this age group.

2.3 Clinical Trial Simulation

Clinical trial simulation is one of the more complex current applications of M&S techniques and is an example that frequently combines model components derived through inductive as well as deductive analysis approaches (Bonate 2000). Trial simulation uses numerical simulation techniques to assess in silico how a clinical study is likely to perform based on simulation of the behavior of its individual participants and prior knowledge and assumptions for underlying distributions and mechanisms (Girard 2005). As such, trial simulations may include a variety of sub-models. It does not only include a structural dose–exposure–response/toxicity relationship (PK/PD-model) that was derived using the "top-down" or "bottom-up" approach, but also includes model components that capture access to patient populations including patient demographics, study design, enrolment criteria, natural progression of the disease, response to placebo, adherence to the pharmacotherapeutic regimen, and drop-outs from the study. Each of these model components contains one of multiple deterministic as well as stochastic elements. With these model components, clinical trial simulation is able to run many virtual repetitions of a trial. The multiple stochastic elements may affect trial outcome differently in each repetition. With hundreds or thousands of virtual repetitions for the trial execution, clinical trial simulation allows establishing a likelihood profile of trial outcomes that provides the investigator information about the chance of achieving the primary outcome of a study given a specific study design and trial execution environment if only one real-life study is performed. Thus, clinical trial simulation is an excellent tool to optimize study designs, especially in pediatric populations where appropriate study populations are oftentimes scarce and study performance is limited by ethical and logistical constraints. For this reason, the U.S. Food and Drug Administration recommends to perform clinical trial simulation as a routine approach to assess the appropriateness of trial designs in pediatric drug development (Gobburu 2010).

2.4 Virtual World Simulation

An expansion of clinical trial simulations are so-called virtual world simulations. In this approach virtual patients with discrete physiological and pathophysiological characteristics are simulated in a virtual environment, where patient behavior, access to healthcare, healthcare provider interventions, and lifestyle behavior are all integrated. The Archimedes model is a prime example for virtual world simulations (Schlessinger and Eddy 2002). This modeling approach integrates human physiology, diseases, behaviors, interventions, and healthcare systems to predict outcomes including quality of life for the individual patient, whole patient groups with similar characteristics, as well as healthcare resource utilization and healthcare costs. Hundreds of mathematical expressions are the core of the model and represent human physiology and the effects of diseases relevant to the specific condition. Attached to these are additional equations and algorithms that realistically simulate the healthcare system including processes such as tests, treatments, admissions, and physician behaviors. Together with population data, the equations are integrated into a single, large-scale simulation model that accurately represents what happens to real people in real healthcare systems (http://www.archimedes.com). The Archimedes model has been established for several chronic diseases, including diabetes, cardiovascular disease and colon, breast and lung cancer. It is utilized by healthcare providers and insurance organizations such as Kaiser Permanente to assess the cost/benefit ratio of medical interventions. The American Diabetes Association has adopted the Archimedes model as a risk assessment tool for individual patients to assess the impact of lifestyle changes and healthcare interventions (Eddy and Schlessinger 2003). It is freely accessible on the association's website under Diabetes PHD (personal health decisions) at http://www.diabetes.org.

3 Improving Dosing Strategies by Simulations

3.1 Examples of "Top Down" Simulations for Deriving Dosing Recommendations

3.1.1 Dosing Recommendations Based on Pharmacokinetic Simulations

The development of pediatric dosing recommendations based on the simulation of plasma concentration-time profiles makes the assumption that the concentration–effect relationship is independent of age and thus similar between children and adults. In such a situation, dosing regimens that result in similar systemic exposure to the drug should also result in similar efficacy. Antibiotics are a class of therapeutics for which this assumption can often be made, as the concentration–effect relationship is driven by the susceptibility of the pathogen to the antibiotic, especially if the infection is localized in well-perfused tissues and the access of the drug to the pathogen is not limited. In such a situation, variability in drug exposure in the host is a major driving force for differences in efficacy.

Li and co-workers (Li et al. 2010) used this approach to derive dosing recommendations for levofloxacin for the chemotherapy of postexposure inhalational anthrax in children. As efficacy studies with inhalational anthrax are ethically prohibitive, a population pharmacokinetic model for levofloxacin was developed based on an adult data set ($n = 47$) with concentration-time data after a single dose of 500 or 750 mg/kg levofloxacin, given either intravenously or orally, and a pediatric data set with 90 patients (0.5–16 years) receiving different intravenously and oral dose levels. A covariate analysis identified body weight as significant predictor for levofloxacin clearance and volume of distribution. In addition, developmental changes in renal function in children under 2 years of age was a major determinant of clearance as expected from the fact that renal excretion is a major elimination pathway for levofloxacin with 70–80% excreted unchanged in urine.

In subsequent simulation exercises, this population pharmacokinetic model was used to explore different dosing approaches in children that would results into a systemic exposure to levoflocacin similar to the daily dose of 500 mg approved for this indication in adults. This exposure had been shown in animal experiments to prevent the progression of pulmonary anthrax after inhalation exposure. These simulations led to a recommended dose of 8 mg/kg twice a day for children below 50 kg body weight, and 500 mg daily for children with a higher body weight.

3.1.2 Dosing Recommendations Based on PK and PD Simulations

If the pharmacodynamics or concentration–effect relationship for a therapeutic agent is not constant with age, then developmental changes in pharmacokinetics and pharmacodynamics have to be considered simultaneously to develop dosage recommendations for pediatric patients. The development of dosage recommendations for the antiarrhythmic drug sotalol for the treatment of supraventricular tachycardia in children is an example where pharmacodynamic data for safety and efficacy were combined with pharmacokinetic information to derive dosing recommendations (Laer et al. 2005).

Based on pharmacokinetic data for sotalol in 76 pediatric patients between 1 day and 17 years of age, including 12 neonates, 33 infants and toddlers, 26 children, and 5 adolescents, a population pharmacokinetic model was derived that identified weight as significant predictor of clearance and volume, and age as a significant additional predictor for clearance in neonates and infants younger than 1 year of age. The latter was interpreted as the effect of maturation of glomerular filtration and active tubular secretion during the first year of life, since sotalol is exclusively eliminated by renal excretion. In a second step, the age-dependency of cardiac QT-interval prolongation was assessed as safety biomarker. A population PK/PD analysis in a subgroup of 32 pediatric patients revealed an age-dependency of the slope for QT interval prolongation vs. sotalol plasma concentration, suggesting a higher sensitivity toward QTc prolongation in neonates compared to older patient groups. Finally, in a third step, a PD analysis was performed in 15 patients to characterize the relationship between sotalol plasma concentration and conversion into sinus rhythm as efficacy measure. The analysis predicted a 50% probability to convert into sinus rhythm for a sotalol plasma concentration of 0.4 µg/ml, and a more than 95% probability for 1.0 µg/ml, with no indication of an age-dependent difference in antiarrhythmic efficacy.

All three analysis components were subsequently combined to derive dosing recommendations via Monte Carlo simulations for five age groups, neonates, infants under 6 months, infants 6 months to 2 years, children 2–6 years, and children 6–12 years. For start and target dose simulations the treatment goal was defined to achieve a 50% probability (start dose) and more than 95% probability (target dose) to respond to sotalol therapy. An 8-h dosing interval was chosen to ensure a similar

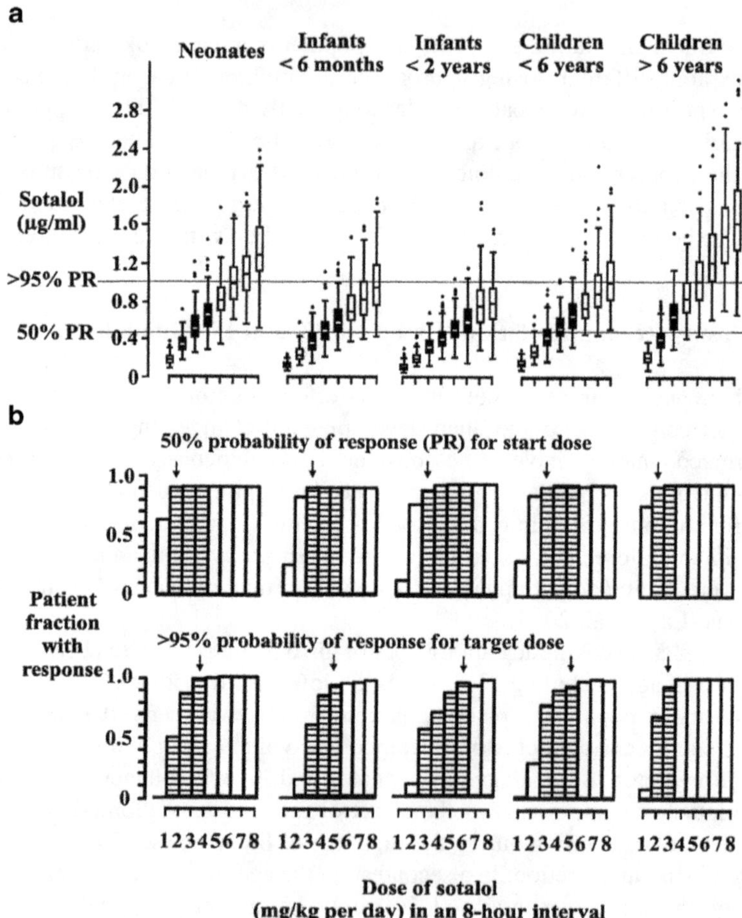

Fig. 5 Simulation results for sotalol dosing recommendation development: (a) Simulated sotalol trough concentrations (125 patients per group and dose level) for pediatric patients with supraventricular tachycardia. *Lines* indicate 50% and more than 95% efficacy. (b) Patient fraction with 50% and more than 95% probability of arrhythmia suppression. *Black box plots* and *hatched bars* indicate recommended dosing range. *Arrows* indicate start and target doses. From Laer et al. (2005)

degree of fluctuation between peak and trough sotalol concentrations in children compared to adults. Dosing recommendations derived from these simulations for different age groups were a starting dose and target dose of 2 and 4 mg/kg/day for neonates, 3 and 6 mg/kg/day for infants and children <6 years, and 2 and 4 mg/kg/day for children >6 years (Fig. 5). Since the higher sensitivity of QT interval prolongation and the higher sotalol exposure in the neonatal age group increase the risk of potential life-threatening rhythm disturbances, however, sotalol should in general not be used in neonates due to these safety concerns (Laer et al. 2005).

3.2 Examples of "Bottom Up" Simulations for Deriving Dosing Recommendations

3.2.1 Physiology-Based Simulations in Individuals with Diseases and/or Altered Physiology

Physiological changes associated with certain pathological conditions such as liver cirrhosis or renal insufficiency affect drug pharmacokinetic behavior. PBPK modeling emerges as an ideal technique to predict drug pharmacokinetics in patients with altered physiology. One successful example is the study published by Edginton and Willmann (2008). The objective of the study was to extend an existing whole-body PBPK model in order to predict drug pharmacokinetics in liver cirrhosis, so that the model was altered to incorporate physiological differences between healthy individuals and patients (e.g., changes in blood flows, reduction in plasma protein synthesis thus an increase in the drug fraction unbound, reduced hepatic function, etc.). In order to do so, the literature was searched for quantitative measures of the physiological changes associated with liver cirrhosis and then these data were incorporated in the modified model. The parameters that were included were the organ blood flows, cardiac index, plasma-binding proteins, hematocrit, functional liver volume, hepatic enzymatic activity, and glomerular filtration rate. Finally, the pharmacokinetic profiles and parameters for four compounds, namely, alfentanil, lidocaine, theophylline, and levetiracetam were predicted and then compared with literature data. The simulation results were found to be adequate when compared with observed data and the model could serve as a building block for creating a generic/global whole-body PBPK model for the progressive disease of liver cirrhosis. Figure 6 illustrates predicted and observed arithmetic mean plasma concentration time curves of alfentanil from patients with liver cirrhosis according to the classification of Child-Pugh compared to healthy controls.

PBPK models were also successfully applied to describe compound pharmacokinetics during pregnancy both in rat and human. Andrew et al. (2008) built a PBPK model for the disposition of midazolam in pregnant women.

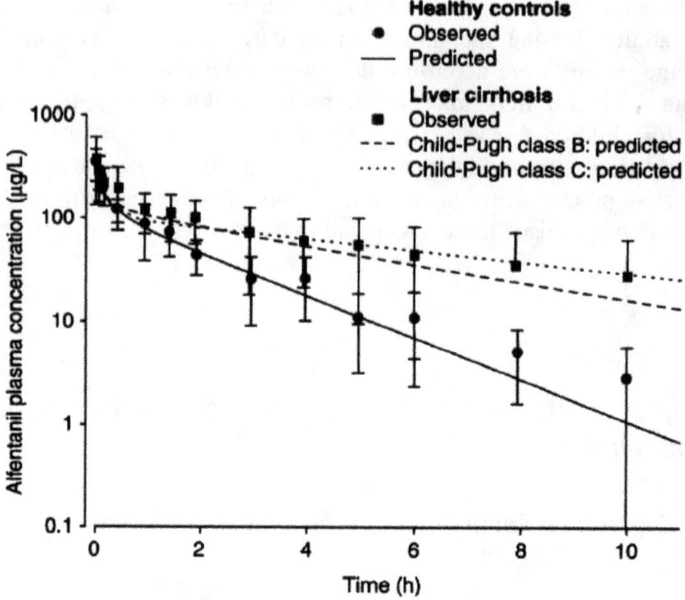

Fig. 6 Predicted and observed arithmetic mean (±SD) plasma concentration time curves of alfentanil in healthy controls and patients with liver cirrhoses according to Edginton and Willmann (2008)

3.2.2 Physiology-Based Pharmacokinetic Simulations for Deriving Dosing Regimens: Prediction of Drug Pharmacokinetics in Different Pediatric Age Groups

Björkman (2004) presented an example for the prediction of drug pharmacokinetics in different pediatric age groups. The aim of the study was to create a general PBPK model for drug disposition in infants and children (neonates, 6 months, 1, 2, 3, 10, and 15 years old) and to evaluate it with two model drugs with different physicochemical and pharmacokinetic characteristics, namely, theophylline and midazolam administered as intravenous application. The model was created using MATLAB software, including about 13 organs/tissues in addition to the arterial and venous blood. Data about the various physiological and drug-dependent parameters for children were incorporated in the model and were obtained either from literature, scaled from rat to human or calculated from adult values using body surface area or an age factor. Age-related changes in clearance pathways were also included and the accuracy and precision of the predictions were assessed via comparison with the corresponding parameter values obtained from the literature. The results of the simulation were considered to be adequate. Figure 7 illustrates the predicted pharmacokinetic parameters for theophylline volume of distribution, clearance, and terminal half life as function of age, together with literature data.

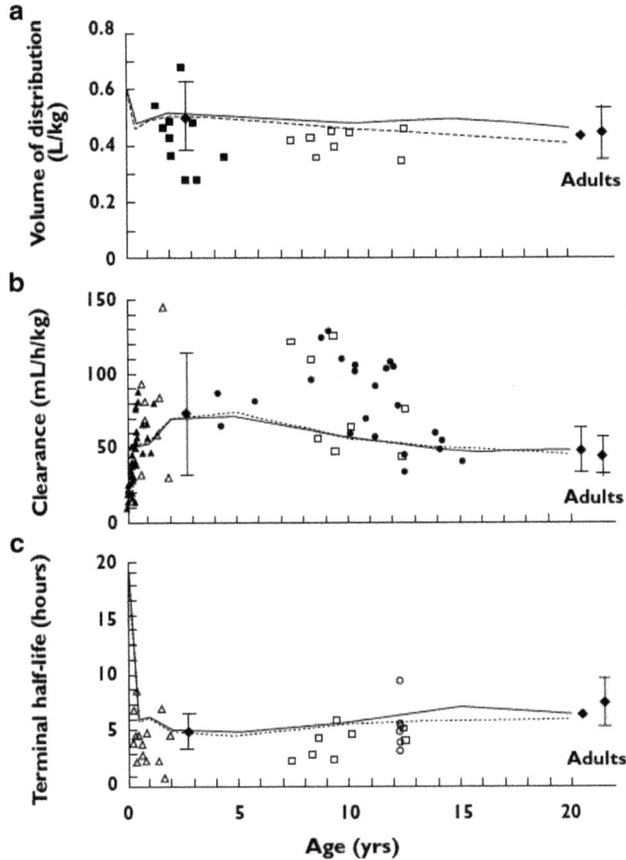

Fig. 7 Predicted pharmacokinetic parameters for volume of distribution, clearance, and terminal half-life of theophylline as function of age, together with literature data according to Björkman (2004)

Another example was presented in Edginton et al. (2006). The goal of this study was to extend an existing adult PBPK model in order to reflect the age-related physiological changes in children from birth to 18 years old. Information about age dependencies of the relevant physiological parameters in children were gathered from the literature and the simulations were carried out using PK-Sim® in conjugation with a previously developed age-specific clearance model. To evaluate the accuracy of plasma profiles prediction in children by the developed pediatric model, a group of five drugs (paracetamol, alfentanil, morphine, theophylline, and levofloxacin) was used. These drugs were selected based on the availability of concentration-time data in the literature for both adults and children. At the beginning, the pharmacokinetic profile of these drugs was simulated in adults and was then compared with observed data for evaluation. When the simulated curves in adults matched the observed data with sufficient accuracy, a predicted pediatric clearance value for each drug was generated using the clearance model mentioned previously and pediatric simulations were done. The simulated plasma concentrations–time curves and pharmacokinetic parameters were then compared with the corresponding observed values and the pediatric simulations were evaluated for appropriateness. The overlap between predicted and observed data was satisfying. As already illustrated in Fig. 4, predicted clearance values can be used to calculate drug exposure and dosing regimens, for example, in specific age groups of children.

4 Improving Clinical Trial Design by Simulations

4.1 Fastening Timelines of Clinical Trials

Unfortunately, many pediatric efficacy trials are still performed with devastating limitations and design flaws, resulting in a high frequency of trial failures. Benjamin and co-workers (2008) analyzed these failures in a recent publication on antihypertensive trials. The authors examined six antihypertensive dose-ranging trials with enalapril, liniopril, losartan, amlodipine, fosinopril, and irbesartan. They could show that trial failures were largely related to poor dose selection, with widely overlapping responses for different dose levels. In contrast, successful studies used wider dose ranges resulting in less overlap in responses. In addition, these studies used diastolic blood pressure rather than systolic blood pressure, which is more reflective of systolic hypertension which is more common in elderly, but not in pediatric populations.

Modeling and simulation approaches, including clinical trial simulation, can contribute to overcome some of these trial limitations by allowing to explore in silico different dose levels, dosing regimens, and efficacy biomarkers if the respective drug- as well as system-specific parameters are available. For antihypertensive drugs, some of these system-specific parameters may be derived from already published trials in this indication and population, for example, the typical variability in systolic and diastolic blood pressure assessment in pediatric populations.

The pharmacometrics team at the US Food and Drug administration recently published a related example where prior knowledge from an investigational antihypertensive drug together with pediatric data from a drug with similar mechanism of action and approved indication in pediatric patients were used to perform clinical trial simulations to explore the optimal choice of dose range, sample size endpoints, and other design elements (Jadhav et al. 2009).

In another example, Mouksassi et al. (2009) applied clinical trial simulation to develop a clinical trial design for a pediatric multiple-dose phase I study to determine the safety, efficacy, and pharmacokinetics of teduglutide, a glucagon-like peptide-2 analogue indicated for the treatment of short-bowel syndrome and Crohn's disease. In this analysis, specific emphasis was put on a realistic simulation of demographic covariates to obtain an accurate assessment of the variability in the expected response. This was accomplished with a generalized additive modeling for location, scale and shape, and qualified with an external age-weight data set. The analysis allowed to optimize the phase I dosing strategy and the likelihood of achieving target exposure and therapeutic effect.

4.2 Optimizing Sample Size and Selection of Pharmacokinetic Sampling Time Points for Pediatric Trials

Willmann (2009) reported an example of using a physiologically based pharmacokinetic model for the determination of optimal sampling times in children. Physiologically based pharmacokinetic simulations show special value when the question arises when to sample plasma in children treated with a drug for the first time. In this situation, the pediatric pharmacokinetic simulations predict the plasma concentration time curve according to the developmental pharmacology of the specific drug. The expected plasma concentration range can be balanced with the limit of quantification (LOQ) of the analytical drug assay. In this way, it might avoid unnecessary sampling at time points where plasma concentrations are out of the assay range. A conceptual example is demonstrated in Fig. 8. If we were willing to conduct a pediatric clinical trial and assuming in which only three blood samples were allowed to be withdrawn from each child, the sampling times were first chosen based on the implied adult concentration-time profile (dark arrows). The three time points were chosen in respect to the limit of quantification of the analytical assay in a way that the first sample was around the peak concentration, and the remaining two in the elimination phase in order to make a conclusion about elimination kinetics. Subsequently, a plasma concentration vs. time profile for a virtual 4-year-old child was simulated with PBPK modeling software PK-SIM®. The simulation showed an accelerated elimination of the same administered weight-normalized dose and thus a different time course of the plasma concentration-time profile. If the same sampling times, determined previously based on adult data, were applied here for this child, the last sample would be below the detection range, i.e., drug concentration could not be quantified, the pharmacokinetic analysis would be impossible, and the child would be exposed to unnecessary strain. However, the simulation allowed to determine optimized sampling times for children of this age group.

5   Conclusion

Modeling and simulation techniques used either as "top down" or "bottom up" approaches are deeply interwoven with pediatric drug development. Within the three pillars mentioned earlier (see Fig. 1), the modeling and simulation pillar is a tool that fastens knowledge gaining and helps to understand the pharmacological properties of the drug in the pediatric population. The idea that modeling and

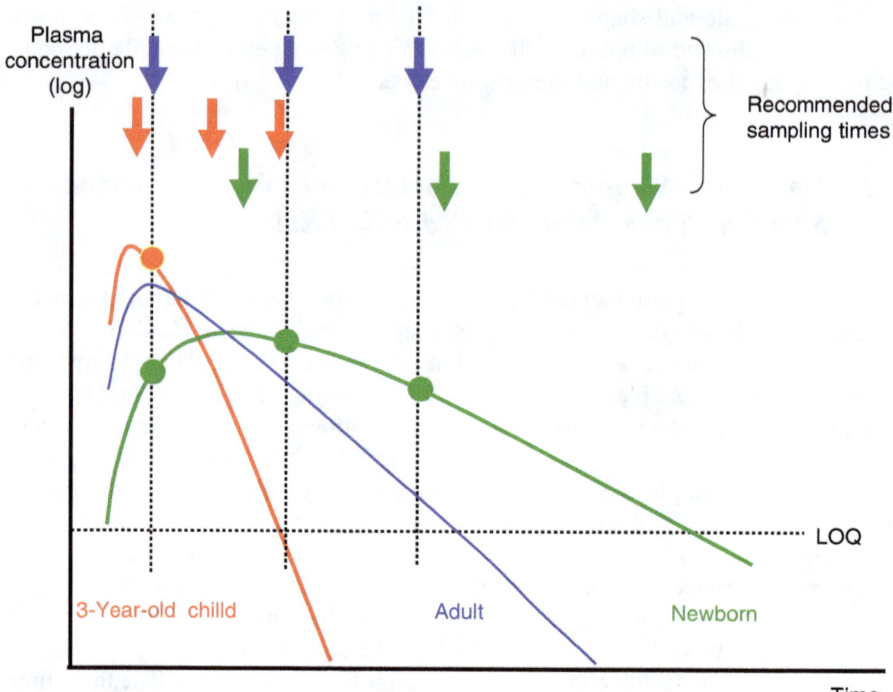

Fig. 8 Schematic drawing of a potential application of physiology-based pharmacokinetic simulations for children of different ages to find optimal blood sampling time points for the pharmacokinetic investigations in a future pediatric trial according to Willmann (2009). *Arrows* indicate optimal sampling time for a 3-year-old child, a newborn, and an adult. *LOQ* Limit of quantification

simulation alone might be sufficient to solve a pharmacotherapeutic problem without relying on the proof of the clinical experiment is highly attractive as it would save substantial costs in the drug development process. Given the complexity, however, of the interaction between human beings and chemical entities, the complete substitution of clinical trials by simulations if there is no severe constraint to perform the clinical trial is not a near future scenario. Nevertheless, it is realistic to assume that simulations can avoid suboptimal trials and can help to reduce the number of pediatric patients to be included if a qualified model is used to simulate a range of different dosing regimens and help to decide which doses are most likely to reach a therapeutic target range.

Unfortunately, up to now software to perform modeling and simulation for the untrained pediatrician is not available. Therefore, the full value of modeling and simulation stick to those who are willing to train themselves. For the future, easier to use software of modeling and simulation for the pediatrician is highly warranted and would be an excellent tool to achieve a deeper and closer involvement of pediatric clinical pharmacology and consequently to better treat the pediatric patient.

Acknowledgement The authors want to thank Feras Khalil from the Department of Clinical Pharmacy and Pharmacotherapy at the Heinrich-Heine University of Düsseldorf for some literature review and comments about the physiologically based pharmacokinetics (see also Khalil and Laer 2011).

References

Alcorn J, McNamara PJ (2003) Pharmacokinetics in the newborn. Adv Drug Deliv Rev 55:667–686

Andrew MA, Hebert MF, Vicini P (2008) Physiologically based pharmacokinetic model of midazolam disposition during pregnancy. Conf Proc IEEE Eng Med Biol Soc 54:54–57

Arant BS Jr (1978) Developmental patterns of renal functional maturation compared in the human neonate. J Pediatr 92:705–712

Bartelink IH, Rademaker CM, Schobben AF et al (2006) Guidelines on paediatric dosing on the basis of developmental physiology and pharmacokinetic considerations. Clin Pharmacokinet 45:1077–1097

Benjamin DK Jr, Smith PB, Jadhav P et al (2008) Pediatric antihypertensive trial failures: analysis of end points and dose range. Hypertension 51:834–840

Björkman S (2004) Prediction of drug disposition in infants and children by means of physiologically based pharmacokinetic (PBPK) modelling: theophylline and midazolam as model drugs. Br J Clin Pharmacol 59:691–704

Bonate PL (2000) Clinical trial simulation in drug development. Pharm Res 17:252–256

Bouwmeester NJ, Anderson BJ, Tibboel D et al (2004) Developmental pharmacokinetics of morphine and its metabolites in neonates, infants and young children. Br J Anaesth 92:208–217

Eddy DM, Schlessinger L (2003) Validation of the Archimedes diabetes model. Diabetes Care 26:3102–3110

Edginton A, Willmann S (2008) Physiology-based simulations of a pathological condition: prediction of pharmacokinetics in patients with liver cirrhosis. Clin Pharmacokinet 47:743–752

Edginton A, Schmitt W, Willmann S (2006) Development and evaluation of a generic physiologically based pharmacokinetic model for children. Clin Pharmacokinet 45:1013–1034

El-Tahtawy A, Kokki H, Reidenberg BE (2006) Population pharmacokinetics of oxycodone in children 6 months to 7 years old. J Clin Pharmacol 46:433–442

Girard P (2005) Clinical trial simulation: a tool for understanding study failures and preventing them. Basic Clin Pharmacol Toxicol 96:228–234

Gobburu JV (2010) How to double success rate of pediatric trials? U.S. Food and Drug Administration, Office of Clinical Pharmacology, Silver Spring, MD, http://www.slideshare.net/JogaGobburu/how-to-double-success-rate-of-pediatric-trials. Accessed 17 Jun 2010

Hines RN (2008) The ontogeny of drug metabolism enzymes and implications for adverse drug events. Pharmacol Ther 118:250–267

Hsien L (2010) Identifying paediatric needs in cardiology and the prediction of sildenafil exposure in children with pulmonary arterial hypertension. PhD thesis at the Faculty of Mathematics and Sciences, University of Düsseldorf, Germany

Jadhav PR, Zhang J, Gobburu JV (2009) Leveraging prior quantitative knowledge in guiding pediatric drug development: a case study. Pharm Stat 8:216–224

Johnson TN, Rostami-Hodjegan A, Tucker GT (2006) Prediction of the clearance of eleven drugs and associated variability in neonates, infants and children. Clin Pharmacokinet 45:931–956

Khalil F, Laer S (2011) Physiologically based pharmacokinetic modeling: Methodology, applications, and limitations with a focus on its role in pediatric drug development. J Biomed Biotechnol. In press

Laer S, Wauer I, Behn F et al (2001) Pharmacokinetics of sotalol in different age groups of children with tachycardia. J Pediatr Pharmacol Ther 6:50–59

Laer S, Elshoff JP, Meibohm B et al (2005) Development of a safe and effective pediatric dosing regimen for sotalol based on population pharmacokinetics and pharmacodynamics in children with supraventricular tachycardia. J Am Coll Cardiol 46:1322–1330

Laer S, Barrett JS, Meibohm B (2009) The in silico child: using simulation to guide pediatric drug development and manage pediatric pharmacotherapy. J Clin Pharmacol 49:889–904

Li F, Nandy P, Chien S et al (2010) Pharmacometrics-based dose selection of levofloxacin as a treatment for postexposure inhalational anthrax in children. Antimicrob Agents Chemother 54:375–379

Meibohm B, Laer S, Panetta JC et al (2005) Population pharmacokinetic studies in pediatrics: issues in design and analysis. AAPS J 7:E475–E487

Morselli PL, Morselli-Franco R, Bossi L (1980) Clinical pharmacokinetics in newborns and infants. Clin Pharmacokinet 5:485–527

Mouksassi MS, Marier JF, Cyran J et al (2009) Clinical trial simulations in pediatric patients using realistic covariates: application to teduglutide, a glucagon-like peptide-2 analog in neonates and infants with short-bowel syndrome. Clin Pharmacol Ther 86:667–671

Schlessinger L, Eddy DM (2002) Archimedes: a new model for simulating health care systems – the mathematical formulation. J Biomed Inform 35:37–50

Sheiner LB, Ludden TM (1992) Population pharmacokinetics/dynamics. Ann Rev Pharmacol Toxicol 32:185–209

van der Marel CD, Anderson BJ, van Lingen RA et al (2003) Paracetamol and metabolite pharmacokinetics in infants. Eur J Clin Pharmacol 59:243–251

Willlmann S (2009) The in silico child. Can computer simulations replace clinical pharmacokinetic studies? Pharm Unserer Zeit 38:62–67

Willmann S, Lippert J, Sevestre M et al (2003) PK-Sim®: a physiologically based pharmacokinetic "whole-body" model. Biosilico 1:121–124

Yared A, Ichikara I (1994) Glomerular circulation and function in paediatric nephrology. Williams and Wilkins, Baltimore

Efficacy Assessment in Paediatric Studies

Siri Wang and Pirjo Laitinen-Parkkonen

Contents

Abstract Even though the regulatory authorities to some extent accept the extrapolation of efficacy data from adults to paediatric patients, it is often the case that differences in the disease process and the developmental stage of the children prevent the extrapolation of efficacy in these populations. Where efficacy studies are needed, the development, validation, and employment of different endpoints for specific age and developmental subgroups become necessary. Children are in continuous development and any measure to assess the efficacy of an intervention should take carefully into account how this development affects the endpoints, including the performance capacity of the child and differences in the condition and symptoms presented. Clinical endpoints that are used in the adult trials to evaluate

S. Wang (✉)
Norwegian Medicines Agency, Tønsberg Hospital Pharmacy, Sven Oftedalsvei 6, N-0950 Oslo, Norway
e-mail: siri.wang@noma.no

P. Laitinen-Parkkonen
Health Care and Social Services, City of Hyvinkää, Suutarinkatu 2 C, 05801 Hyvinkää, Finland
e-mail: pirjo.laitinen-parkkonen@hyvinkaa.fi

H.W. Seyberth et al. (eds.), *Pediatric Clinical Pharmacology*,
Handbook of Experimental Pharmacology 205,
DOI 10.1007/978-3-642-20195-0_7, © Springer-Verlag Berlin Heidelberg 2011

treatment effect may not be suitable in paediatric studies. The development of surrogate endpoints for benefit and risk assessment in children is necessary. Collaboration between the academic researchers, pharmaceutical industry, and regulatory authorities is needed to meet the challenges in proper validation of biomarkers and surrogate endpoints in paediatric trials.

Keywords Efficacy • Assessment • Paediatric studies • Clinical endpoints • Biomarkers • Surrogate endpoints • Validation • Standardisation • Outcome measures

1 Introduction

The regulatory authorities accept to some extent the extrapolation of efficacy data from adult data to paediatric patients in the case the disease process and the expected outcome of the therapy are comparable to that of the adults (ICH E 11 2001). However, it is often the case that differences in the disease process and the developmental stage of the children prevent the extrapolation of efficacy in these populations. Especially, extrapolation of the efficacy data from older children and adults to neonate population is rare. Where efficacy studies are needed, it may be necessary to develop, validate, and employ different endpoints for specific age and developmental subgroups.

The progress in the legislation regarding the development of medicinal products based on adequate and well-controlled studies also in paediatric population in the USA and in EU, such as the Best Pharmaceuticals for Children Act in 2002, Paediatric Research Equity Act in 2003, and Paediatric Regulation in 2006, has encouraged the stakeholders to find alternative ways to measure the magnitude of the treatment response in paediatric population (Regulation EC 2006). Therefore, the interest on assessing development-appropriate endpoints and developing biomarkers and surrogate endpoints suitable to paediatric studies has increased.

2 Setting the Scene for Evaluation of Endpoints

The increasing interest on biomarkers has led the working group of National Institute of Health to provide discussion and definitions for clinical endpoints, biomarkers, and surrogate endpoints.

A clinical endpoint is defined as a variable reflecting how the patient feels, functions, or survives. Biomarkers are defined as biological characteristics that can be objectively measured and evaluated as an indicator of normal biological process, pathogenic process, or pharmacological response to a therapeutic evaluation (Biomarkers Definitions Working Group 2001). Biomarkers can be further classified into Type 0 biomarkers, which are markers of the natural history of a disease that correlates longitudinally with known clinical indices, and Type I biomarkers, which capture the effects of a therapeutic intervention in accordance with its mechanism of action (Puntman 2009). A surrogate endpoint, defined as a biomarker intended to substitute a clinical endpoint, is not directly measuring clinical impact, but is believed to adequately reflect the clinical benefit or harm based on epidemiologic, pathophysiologic, other scientific evidence, or on therapeutic effect (Biomarkers Definitions Working Group 2001).

The most robust way to define the clinical impact of the therapeutic intervention is to use well-defined clinical endpoints in the randomised controlled trials. The clinical endpoints selected for the trial should provide the clinically relevant and scientifically sound evidence to support the primary objectives of the study (FDA 1998). The clinical endpoints can be further categorised into intermediate endpoints, which is not the ultimate outcome, but of clinical benefit such as exercise tolerance, and into ultimate outcome, such as survival or symptomatic response that captures the benefits and risks of an intervention (Lesko and Atkinson 2001).

Clinical endpoints that are conventionally used in the adult trials to evaluate treatment effect may not be suitable in paediatric trials. The experience accumulated from earlier adult studies for a certain indication may not be applicable in the paediatric population (Della Pasqua et al. 2007). Additionally, in a recent systematic review, very few paediatric studies even address the choice of outcomes for clinical research in children (Sinha et al. 2008).

Outcome variables should ideally be measured without bias in a reliable manner using validated instruments with adequate sensitivity to detect real change in patient's health status. The validation process generally assesses this link between changes in the instrument's score and the actual clinical benefit and should be sensitive to treatment effects as well as be clinically relevant (Redmond and Colton 2001). The instrument's validity might be tested through larger clinical trials, or through meta-analysis. For children, the challenge will be the feasibility of large clinical trials and the lack of standardised clinical trial methodology in many paediatric areas, leaving the validation process potentially even more challenging than for adults.

Biomarkers and surrogate endpoints frequently used are physiological and laboratory measurements. The classical examples are the effect of lipid-lowering drugs on LDL-cholesterol levels as surrogate of the cardiovascular health and the effect of antihypertensive drugs on blood pressure as surrogate of the stroke. Biomarkers such as these have traditionally been identified through pathophysiological and epidemiological studies, and some confirmed with clinical trails. Despite the current acceptance of cholesterol lowering as a surrogate endpoint, not all treatment effects can be captured by a single biomarker (Lesko and Atkinson 2001). New developments in molecular science and sophisticated imaging technologies have increasingly facilitated the industrialised process of biomarker discovery, supported by standardised paradigms of biomarker validation (Puntman 2009; Dancey et al. 2010; EMEA 2009a). There is an ongoing discussion between the European regulatory authorities, academia and pharmaceutical industry, on the development and validation of new biomarkers and surrogate endpoints (EMEA 2006a).

The use of surrogate endpoints may facilitate the clinical trials in several ways. For example, a surrogate endpoint may be more sensitive for detection than the "golden standard" endpoint enabling the early intervention. The time required to perform the trial and cost may be reduced (Fleming 2005). A new therapeutical innovation may also be approved earlier by the regulatory authorities due to the reduced duration of the trial (ICH E8 1997; FDA 2003, 2009a; Molenberghs and Orman 2009). These advantages would be welcomed also in the paediatric research. Accelerated approval and conditional approval processes have been implemented by the US and European authorities to provide earlier access to new interventions for diseases with major public health interest when there is an unmet medical need (FDA 2009b; Regulation EC 2004).

In evaluation of biomarkers, the clinical relevance based on mechanistic or biochemical connection in the causal chain leading to the clinical endpoint should be established. Sensitivity and specificity of the treatment effects, defined as the ability to detect the measurement or change, and assay quality and variability for quantitating the biomarker need to be explored. However, it should be noted that the diseases often have multiple causal pathways, and the intervention may lead to intended as well as unintended actions. Additionally, the measurement should be as non-invasive and simple as possible (Lesko and Atkinson 2001). The use of biomarkers as surrogate endpoints further requires the specification of the clinical endpoints that are being substituted, class of therapeutic intervention being applied, and characteristics of the population and disease state in which the substitution is being made (Biomarkers Definitions Working group 2001). The marker must be correlated with the clinical endpoint, but also fully capture the net effect of the intervention on the clinical efficacy endpoint. Validation of surrogate endpoint requires often analysis of many randomised controlled trials to determine the consistency of effects of the intervention across the drug classes and different stages of the disease (Fleming 2005; Lesko and Atkinson 2001). This might be challenging in paediatric population.

The past use of surrogate endpoints in some adult trials has underlined the need for robust evidence on the association of the surrogate endpoint and the effect. The results of the CAST study (Cardiac Arrhythmia Suppression Trial) showed that suppression of ventricular arrhythmias cannot substitute for survival in the evaluation of antiarrhythmic drugs (Echt et al. 1991). The nitric oxide synthase inhibitor, NG-methyl-L-arginine, promoted the resolution of shock, but was associated with increased mortality in adults with septic shock (Bakker et al. 2004; Watson et al. 2004; López et al. 2004). On the other hand, in the trial studying interferon gamma in prevention of infection in chronic granulomatous disease, the surrogate endpoint did not reveal a therapeutic effect, but showed clinical benefit on reduction of serious infections (The ICGDC Study Group 1991). These examples emphasise that a biomarker may reflect only one aspect of the disease process and not the entire complexity of the disease.

The determination of the clinical benefit related to the surrogate endpoint is challenging in the children. The development and validation of biomarkers and surrogate endpoints even in the adult population is still evolving and the reliability of the surrogates in prediction for long-term benefit and risk in children undergoing interventions early in life is not known. However, there is a need to develop sound surrogate endpoints for benefit and risk assessment in paediatric population, which could be collected using as much non-invasive methods as possible.

3 Aspects on Determining Endpoints in Paediatric Clinical Trials

Children are in continuous development and any measure to assess the efficacy of an intervention should take carefully into account how this development affects the endpoints. For example, in patients with chronic diseases, the response to a medicinal product may vary among patients not only because of the duration of the disease and its chronic effects but also because of the developmental stage of the patient. Measurement of subjective symptoms such as pain requires different assessment instruments for patients of different ages, as children may not be able to comply with the endpoints used in adult trials (ICH 2001).

In neonates, either preterm or full term, symptoms, diseases, and management might differ significantly from that seen in older children. Thus, when evaluating medicinal products in neonates, the endpoints should be carefully chosen, linked to the condition and the degree of prematurity. There is a need for establishing appropriate surrogate endpoints in this age group. The known complications and sequelae of prematurity (e.g. intracerebral/intraventricular haemorrhage, necrotising enterocolitis, retinopathy of prematurity, and bronchopulmonary dysplasia) as well as survival should be evaluated at least as secondary endpoints in trials that include the neonatal population (EMEA 2008a).

When patient reporting-based endpoints are used for defining the magnitude of treatment benefits, pre-defined age-appropriate instruments are needed (EMEA 2004; Rothman and Kleinman 2009). The current guidance provided by the FDA on the use of patient reporting-based instruments in children highlights the importance of age-related vocabulary, language comprehension, comprehension of the health concept measured, and duration of recall when developing and using such tools. Instrument development within fairly narrow age groupings is important to account for developmental differences and to determine the lower age limit at which children can understand the questions and provide reliable and valid responses that can be compared across age categories. The proxy-reported outcome measures for this population are not recommended. For patients who cannot respond for themselves (e.g. infants), observer reports that include only those events or behaviours that can be observed are encouraged (FDA 2009c).

This section illustrates some paediatric-specific issues on assessing efficacy in clinical studies. Examples given are not intended to cover all aspects or areas, nor intended as complete scientific or regulatory guidance, but aim to reflect some of the challenges in assessing efficacy in paediatric trials. Many endpoints might be simultaneously influenced by developmental stage, disease variants, and differences in symptoms and performance capacity in the relevant population. The referred paediatric guidelines and addendums provided by the EMA may not necessarily be fully reported.

3.1 Endpoints Affected by Development and Performance Capacity

Treatment of *obesity* could serve as a simple but nevertheless illustrative example on how growth might have a direct effect on the efficacy endpoint. The adult standard goal being weight reduction would not necessarily be as relevant in a paediatric obesity study. Thus, halting abnormal or excess weight gain or decreasing the rate of weight gain could be important goals in a growing child and as well serve as endpoints (EMEA 2008b), whereas they would not be considered appropriate endpoints in adults.

Sometimes the standard methods to measure the degree of symptoms might differ significantly between adults and children, regardless of whether the disease and the symptoms per se might be considered the same as in older subjects. This is particularly relevant when "performance tests" are used as efficacy measures. Measuring *lung function* is one of the obvious endpoints in asthma studies. However, the use of spirometry and other measures recommended for older children and adult such as airway responsiveness and markers of inflammation might be difficult in infants and pre-school children, as it requires complex equipment and/or coordination and cooperation beyond that can be given by children in this age group for appropriate reproducibility and accuracy. The actual lower age group in which adequate tests can be performed is being discussed and might depend significantly on training of the individual child (Crenesse et al. 2001). Spirometry could be considered feasible in children over 3 years, but its usefulness is the lower age group will depend on thorough training. Although so far limited used in clinical trials, either $FEV_{0.5}$ or $FEV_{0.75}$ might be a better measure than FEV_1 (CPMP, 2009; Beydon et al. 2007). Specific airway resistance (sRaw) measured by plethysmography or other validated methods, combined with clinical symptom scores, can be used in children aged 2–6 years (CPMP, 2009). The aspects of appropriate endpoints add to other challenges in many paediatric asthma studies: the difficulties in precisely diagnosing asthma in the youngest cohorts, uncertainties regarding severity classifications, and the practical aspects of age-appropriate formulations and devices. As the need for and possibilities of early and more precise asthma diagnosis and treatment evolve, the search for appropriate endpoints in infants and pre-school children is considered of great importance.

Even more evident is this need for appropriate lung function tests in cystic fibrosis, where diagnosis can easily be done at an early stage and treatment effect could be significant in the first years. Currently, the primary goal of cystic fibrosis therapy is supportive and includes slowing the decline in lung function by clearing airways of mucus and controlling respiratory infections and inflammation to improve or maintain respiratory function. As in asthma, FEV1 is the recommended primary endpoint, but similarly sub-optimal or potentially inappropriate in children beyond 5–6 years. As stated in the recently updated EMA guideline (EMEA 2009b), respiratory function tests in young children can be performed in specialised centres able to promote standardised methods. Tests currently used include plethysmography and RVRTC (compression technique) (Davis et al. 2010; Rosenfeld 2007), but these procedures most often require sedation, partly depending on age group (Davis et al. 2007). Measuring lung clearance index (LCI) by multiple breath washouts might show to be a useful method for appropriate lung function testing in younger children. However, these alternative measures still need to be further validated.

Although paediatric *pulmonary arterial hypertension* (PAH) differs in physiology, progression rate, and treatment response compared to the adult type, the definition of PAH is basically the same (EMA 2010) and the symptoms are similar although with potential different severity (Haworth and Beghetti 2010). However, the traditional endpoint used in adult studies of pulmonary hypertension, the 6-min walking test (6MWT), is of questionable value in younger children (<6 years), obviously inappropriate in the very youngest infants, but considered valid at least in adolescents. In the age group 7–11 years, this test needs further validation (Li et al. 2005). Additionally, its predictive value on the long-term improvement of the disease is not established in the adult population, questioning its usefulness in the paediatric population >6 years (EMEA 2009c).

Time to clinical worsening (TTCW) is probably a more appropriate endpoint to assess disease progression, and is also used in adults. Of note, the definition of the composite endpoint of clinical worsening in children will have to be done carefully. In particular, there is a need for paediatric-specific endpoints that could be used in intervention studies in the early phase of the disease to prevent the fast deterioration seen in many children. TTCW could be such an endpoint (Haworth and Beghetti 2010).

Data on vascular resistance, obtained by invasive haemodynamic measurements or by non-invasive techniques such as echocardiography, could potentially serve as a surrogate endpoint and should be studied as additional endpoint to assess the correlation to final clinical outcome in paediatric studies.

Even more limited data are available regarding relevant endpoints in the field of persistent pulmonary hypertension of the neonate (PPHN), having different aetiology and management and being considered a different clinical entity. At present, several potential endpoints might be useful; however, all-cause mortality and the need for membrane oxygenation (ECMO) are considered the less disputable ones (EMA 2010).

Another example of challenges in assessing efficacy in children is the evaluation of *pain*. According to the International Association of study of pain (IASP), pain includes an unpleasant sensory and emotional experience associated with actual or potential tissue damage, or described in terms of such damage (Merskey and Bogduk 1994). In children, there are differences across the paediatric age span in the causes and the experience of acute pain (Jacobson 2007; Fradet et al. 1990). In chronic and recurrent pain conditions, such as migraine and tension headache, the incidence increases with the onset of puberty (see also section "EndPoints Depending on Different Symptoms in Adult and Pediatric Population"). The incidence and course of neuropathic pain can vary substantially, depending on the contextual factors (Walco et al. 2010). In addition, the spectrum of cognitive, emotional, and physical capabilities, all related to the pain experience, is changing during the childhood (Hain 1997; McGrath et al. 2008).

The pain intensity is the core outcome domain in pain trials. The regulatory guidelines recommend the use of rating scales in the evaluation of time-specific pain intensity difference and pain relief endpoints in trials for nociceptive pain in adult trials whenever it is possible, including responder rates. Other endpoints, such as patient global assessments, functional performance indicators, and validated questionnaire scores should also be considered in accordance with the intended indications and study designs (EMEA 2002). In paediatric acute pain consensus statement, the pain intensity, global judgement of satisfaction with treatment, symptoms, and adverse events, physical recovery, emotional response, and economical factors are proposed as the core outcome domains in children older than 3 years. In chronic and recurrent pain, physical, role, and emotional functioning and sleep are suggested to be added as the core outcome domains, depending on the specific aims of the trial (McGrath et al. 2008).

The main approaches to measure pain in children are the use of self-reports, observational or behavioural, and physiological measures (Walco et al. 2005). Despite the recognition of the multidimensional nature of pain, self-reporting of the pain intensity is commonly used in paediatric clinical pain trials. The developmental factors related to the ability of the child to provide self-assessment are not fully described (Champion et al. 1998; Stinson et al. 2006; Stanford et al. 2006). For the moment, there is no single tool to evaluate the pain intensity with self-reports across the age span and different types of pain. For procedure-related and postoperative pain, the use of Poker Chip Tool (pieces of hurt) has been recommended in children from 3 to 4 years and Visual Analog Scale from 8 years on. The Faces Pain Scale – Revised has been recommended in children from 4 to 12 years old also in disease-related chronic pain. In pre-school-aged children, the inclusion of observational measures as secondary outcome might be needed due to the wide variability in young children's ability to use the self-report tools (Stinson et al. 2006). Further studies on validation of Numerical Rating Scale have suggested its usefulness in self-reporting in children of 8 years and older (von Baeyer et al. 2009)

The observational measures of pain are needed for children who are too young to understand and use a self-report scale or too distressed to use it. In addition, the cognitive and communicative impairment may preclude the use of self-reporting tools. Mechanical ventilation, sedative drugs, restrictive bandages etc. also affect the ability of the child to comply with the self-rating measurements (von Baeyer and Spagrud 2007). From 1 year and above, the FLACC (Face, Legs, Arms, Cry,

Consolability) tool is recommended for procedural and postoperative pains in hospital (Merkel and Voepel-Lewis 1997; Nilsson et al. 2008). In addition, the CHEOPS tool (Children's Hospital of Eastern Ontario Pain Scale) could be used (von Baeyer and Spagrud 2007). The COMFORT scale is recommended for children aged 1 year and above undergoing critical care (van Dijk et al. 2000). Additionally, measures for pain evaluation at home, the Parent's Postoperative Pain Measure, are available.

For the moment, more information on observational tools in chronic pain conditions as well in children with cognitive impairment is warranted.

The validation of other outcome measures proposed for paediatric pain trials is largely missing. Multidimensional assessment tools such as Paediatric Quality of Life (PedsQL) may be used (Varni et al. 1999). Recently, new composite measure of chronic pain, the Bath Adolescent Pain Questionnaire, has been developed, but further studies are needed on the subscales (Eccleston et al. 2005). For emotional responses, tools for assessing the perioperative anxiety as a part of the pain experience have been developed, but further research is needed to establish their use (Bringuier et al. 2009).

In neonates and infants, many behavioural and physiological assessment tools are available, but few are fully validated (Grunau et al. 1998; Debillon et al. 2001; Loizzo 2009). The behaviour of infants having a large number of procedures may become habituated or sensitised depending on the temporal proximity of repeated procedures, motor development, and previous handling. Overlap with manifestations of other states of distress and confounding clinical factors can further reduce the specificity of behavioural and physiological responses (Walker 2008) The widely used premature infant pain profile (PIPP), for example, measures behaviours such as sleep state and change in facial expression to produce a age-weighted composite pain score (Stevens et al. 1996). Such scores have become the major outcome measure despite the fact that they might reflect the activation of subcortical somatic and autonomic motor pathways and may not be reliably linked to central sensory or emotional processing in the brain (Anand et al. 2004). Biomarkers such as non-invasive near-infrared spectroscopy measurements, which are reflecting the functional activation of the cortex, have recently been proposed to be used in evaluation of pain assessment tools with respect to the sensory input and establish whether the resultant PIPP scores reflect cortical pain processing (Slater et al. 2008). The development of new markers is needed, but whether they can be used as endpoints warrants further investigation.

3.2 Endpoints Influenced by Differences in the Condition

As disease course as well as consequences might not necessarily be the same for different paediatric variants of a condition, the aims of the treatment might vary and this could also affect the endpoints. For example, for *incontinence* in children, while the goal for all children would be continence, in neurogenic detrusor overactivity (NDO), as compared to overactive bladder (OAB), reducing renal pressure per se is also a major goal to minimise the risk of renal effects. Thus, urodynamic measures such as cystometric capacity should be assessed in NDO studies but will not be meaningful in OAB studies. Again, the ability of the children to "perform" reflects the appropriate endpoints: while adult incontinence studies would focus on both urgency and incontinence, younger children would have difficulties indicating and expressing bladder sensation differences and only incontinence would be a useful endpoint.

The pathophysiology of *sepsis* is a complex disturbance in the equilibrium between pro-inflammatory response and concomitant anti-inflammatory mechanisms, and the ways to modulate it to improve patient outcomes are not yet fully understood even in adult population. The mortality rates reported in paediatric severe sepsis range from about 4 to 20%, and it is even higher in patients with underlying co-morbidities and organ dysfunction and in children in developing countries, remaining a major health and resource burden (Watson and Carcillo 2005; Inwald et al. 2009; de Oliveira et al. 2008; Odetola et al. 2007). In paediatric patients, the developmental changes in preterm and term neonates, infants, and children and the haemodynamic reserves available complicate the definition of endpoints in the paediatric sepsis trials. Haemodynamic responses of premature neonates with septic shock are least understood (Goldstein et al. 2005; Brierley et al. 2009).

Currently, there is no consensus on basic measures for conducting trials in paediatric severe sepsis and the outcome definitions. For the time being, the main variables defined to direct treatment of paediatric septic shock are the clinical, oxygen utilisation-related, and haemodynamic variables, but there is no agreement on the use of cellular variables (Carcillo et al. 2002; Brierley et al. 2009). Due to the reasonably low mortality rate in paediatric sepsis, the use of mortality endpoints which are widely agreed in the adult population would need a large number of paediatric subjects to demonstrate differences between the treatment modalities (EMEA 2006b; Vincent 2004). Many children have underlying diseases different from adults, and mortality is not reflecting the increasing morbidity after the sepsis event. The use of endpoints such as organ failure-free days, organ failure resolution time, ICU-free days, and progression of the disease has been proposed as primary endpoints. Validated organ failure scores for neonates are lacking for the moment, even though scores for older children have been developed. The external validation of many of the scores is lacking. Health consequences and health-related quality of life should also be considered as endpoints (Goldstein et al. 2005; Buysse et al. 2008; Varni et al. 2001; Curley and Zimmerman 2005).

Assessing degree of disease and treatment effects is particularly challenging in complex diseases such as *JIA* (juvenile idiopathic arthritis). Extrapolation from efficacy results in adult RA is mostly inappropriate since JIA represents a group of different diseases divided into several categories with different prognoses and variable clinical presentation also within the paediatric population (CPMP 2007)

In JIA, both assessment of disease severity and quantification of disease activity over time are important for optimal evaluation of the effectiveness of antirheumatic drugs. A variety of instruments are available for measuring disease activity; however, no single measure would be considered optimal for all patients. Therefore, a core set of parameters has been established by the American College of Rheumatology (ACR) that includes physician scoring, parent assessment, affected joint counts, functional assessment, and laboratory measures, particularly tailored for the paediatric condition (ACR Pedi 30, Pedi 50 and Pedi 70). These tools focus on individual changes in disease activity over time and as such are useful for assessing the effect of an intervention. However, comparison of absolute disease activity between individuals and group comparison is not optimal with this scoring system. Thus, a composite disease activity score for JIA has been developed, called the Juvenile Arthritis Disease Activity Score (JADAS), enabling a single continuous measure of disease activity (Consolaro et al. 2009). The score has been developed and validated by the Paediatric Rheumatology International Trials Organisation (PRINTO) and could be of significant value both in standard clinical care and particularly in clinical trials, potentially minimising inter-centre variations and thereby reducing the sample size required in clinical trials.

The establishment of international networks within the area of paediatric rheumatic diseases has significantly contributed to the standardisation of the evaluation of response to therapy in juvenile idiopathic arthritis (JIA), juvenile systemic lupus erythematosus (JSLE), and juvenile dermatomyositis (Ruperto et al. 2006).

It should be noted that even if a disease differ between adults and children this may not necessarily have impact on the choice of endpoint, as for some conditions the same endpoints might be appropriate, although the disease is not to be considered entirely the same. In these cases, separate studies could be needed or at least provide more meaningful data, since the effect of the intervention could differ for the separate subtypes of the diseases and significantly influence the outcome of the trials.

3.3 Endpoints Depending on Different Symptoms in Adult and Paediatric Population

Sometimes symptoms of a condition might be different in children compared to adults. Thus, these symptoms are relevant as endpoints in adult studies but would not be considered optimal for children, and therefore specific paediatric symptoms will have to be considered as potential endpoints in the paediatric study.

Migraine with or without aura in early childhood is rare, but the prevalence rate is increasing with age up to 5–10%, being even higher and comparable to that of adults in the onset of adolescence (Mortimer et al. 1992; Abu-Afereh and Russel 1994). Due to different disease characteristics in paediatric population, the extrapolation of adult study results in this population is difficult (EMEA 2007b). Additionally, the disease characteristics may change according to the age and maturation stage of the patient (Crawfordt et al. 2009). According to the International

Headache Society (IHS) standards, the definition of the attack differs in pre- and post-pubertal children (IHS 2004).

Several investigators have observed the high and variable placebo response observed in many migraine trials in paediatric population, which makes it difficult to assess efficacy (Winner et al. 2007; Hämäläinen et al. 1997; Ahonen et al. 2004, 2006; Rothner et al. 2006). The reasons for the high placebo response in children are not fully understood. The proposed underlying reasons include differences in presentation of the disease, such as the shorter attacks in children, especially in adolescents, compared to adults, and the different baseline severity of attacks. The trial design-related issues (such as cross-over versus parallel group) and site selection may also affect the placebo response as well as communication and expectancy of the caregivers (Evers et al. 2008; Rothner et al. 2006). Additionally, the sensitivity of the pain rating scales to distinguish the differences in the pain intensity in children should be confirmed (Lewis et al. 2005).

The European regulatory guidelines recommend the percent of patients being pain-free at 2 h after administration of the study agent as primary endpoints in acute paediatric migraine treatment trials similarly as in adults. Recommended secondary endpoints are, for example, the percent of patients pain-free at 2 h after administration of the study product with no use of rescue medication and no relapse within 48 h after administration of the study agent, percentage of subjects with partial relief (including children asleep in 2 h), use of rescue medication, global evaluation by patient and/or parents, and functional disability at 2 h and other time points (e.g. using behavioural scales). In prophylaxis studies, the frequency of the attacks and the speed of effect should be monitored (EMEA 2007b).

It has been suggested to explore other primary endpoints as well, such as the migraine-free primary endpoint (pain-free and symptom-free composite endpoint), 1-h headache response, coupled with the 2-h sustained response and the 24-h sustained headache, and pain-free response to handle the outcome challenge (Lewis et al. 2005; Lewis 2007; Winner et al. 2007). New approaches in the study design are warranted to meet the challenges of efficacy assessment in developmental age migraine.

Studies on antihypertensive treatment with ACE inhibitors and ARBs for *paediatric hypertension* have revealed diverging results. Attempts to analyse the different factors influencing success or failure of these trials have shown that in addition to trial design, dose ranges tested, and dosing accuracy, the choice of primary endpoint might also be relevant (Benjamin et al. 2008). Using change in diastolic blood pressure (DBP) instead of sitting systolic blood pressure (sSBP) as the primary endpoint seemed to give a closer relationship between dosage and blood pressure reduction, probably related to the less variability seen for DBP measures compared to SBP, underlining the potential importance of the inherent characteristics of the endpoint of choice. Another aspect would be that these two endpoints, when used as tools for inclusion, could select different population subsets and thereby affect outcome of the trials. Which endpoint that best correlate to hard cardiac endpoints in children is a vital question. Discussion is ongoing on which endpoint to be considered optimal, also taking into account the different prevalence of the two hypertension subtypes (EMEA 2008c). It is proposed that using mean arterial pressure as a primary endpoint, incorporating both SBP and DBP values, might prove advantageous, and this possibility should be explored in future trials. Perhaps even more beneficial would be the use of ambulatory BP monitoring in paediatric clinical trials for antihypertensive medications (Li et al. 2010).

In acute *heart failure* in adults, dyspnoe is the most commonly reported symptom and useful scores exists for adult studies. However, dyspnoe is not an equally significant symptom in children. In addition, the assessment, including communication, of this symptom might be challenging. In infants, heart failure often presents with breathing trouble, poor feeding, poor growth, excessive sweating, or even low blood pressure. No clinical trials in acute heart failure have evaluated dyspnoe as an endpoint in children. Although scales exist for grading the severity of congestive heart failure in infants (Ross et al. 1992), their usefulness as a single endpoint in clinical trials are limited. Obviously, because death is a relatively rare outcome - in clinical trials – in children with heart failure, alternative endpoints as rate of weight gain, length of hospital stay, and surgical morbidities might be useful (Madriago and Silberbach 2010).

Few studies have yet been performed in children with heart failure and no composite endpoints have been validated for heart failure studies in children. One study, reporting of carvedilol, failed to show efficacy of medical intervention. A composite clinical outcome measure was used as primary endpoint, including death, hospitalisation, need for intravenous medication, worsening of severity and of global assessment score. However, its appropriateness has been debated. The authors conclude that "The inherent heterogeneity of paediatric patients with heart failure and their high rate of spontaneous improvement make the definition of suitable clinical endpoints with a feasible sample size and sufficient statistical power a challenge for future trials in this population" (Shaddy et al. 2007). Plasma brain natriuretic peptide (BNP) levels have been discussed and also used as secondary endpoint in paediatric trials; however, as the BNP levels seem quite low in this population compared to adults, its usefulness might be limited (Shaddy et al. 2007).

As some of these examples show, different disease symptoms would call for specific paediatric endpoints even if the disease is considered the same from a pathophysiological point of view. In some of such cases, however, extrapolation of efficacy from data in adults could be possible, even though the adult endpoints would not have been appropriate if used in a paediatric study.

4 Relationship Between Efficacy Measures and Diagnostic Tools

As briefly mentioned in the examples of lung function tests in asthma, the possibility to make an appropriate diagnosis in children is often hampered by the lack of relevant measures to properly define the condition. Consequently, further research on diagnosis-related pathophysiological measures and severity classification of diseases would also be relevant for further measures of drug efficacy, as the same methods might be valid for both appropriate diagnoses and appropriate endpoints for measuring any effect of intervention.

The development of biomarkers may also facilitate the understanding of disease mechanisms and natural history, expedite the development of new diagnostic tools, and assist the clinical practice (Lesko and Atkinson 2001).

5   Standardisation of Outcome Measures

For many paediatric diseases, performance of meaningful clinical trials is made difficult because of the small number of eligible patients and heterogeneity of the patient group. In these cases, the fact that different trial uses different inclusion criteria and especially a variety of outcome measures makes it hard to optimally assess the effect of interventions. Obviously, the use of wrong or inappropriate endpoint in paediatric studies implies waste of resources and potentially misleading information though the risk of under- or overestimating the effects of an intervention. Also, using non-standardised criteria for either inclusion or assessment of clinical response would make meta-analysis and comparison of different studies difficult.

As previously mentioned, very few paediatric studies address the choice of outcomes for clinical research in children (Sinha et al. 2008). There are initiatives for development and application of agreed standard sets of outcomes, such as OMERACT, IMMPACT, PedIMMPACT, and COMET (Tugwell and Boers 1993; Dworkin et al. 2005; McGrath et al. 2008; University of Liverpool 2010). Such initiatives are of particular relevance in paediatrics where limited numbers of children are included in the trials, the total number of trials is small, and significant effort should be made to avoid unnecessary studies.

6   Conclusions and Future Developments

In this chapter, we have discussed the challenges in assessing efficacy in paediatric trials. In spite of recent developments in legislation and in science, there are still significant unmet medical needs in the paediatric population. This is most prominent in neonates.

Further research on age- and disease-appropriate endpoints for children is necessary. The use of surrogate endpoints is particularly intriguing for paediatric clinical trials, enabling indication of long-term patient outcome by short-term measures of response, and thereby avoiding unnecessary studies. Inevitably, understanding the paediatric variant of a condition and its potential differences compared to adults is crucial in selecting the appropriate surrogate endpoints for paediatric trials. The challenges in proper validation of biomarkers and surrogate endpoints are obvious and significant focus should be put on these aspects to facilitate optimal clinical trials in children. Collaboration and sharing the advances between academia, pharmaceutical industry, and regulatory authorities are of paramount importance.

Disclaimer. The views expressed here are the personal views of the authors and may not be understood or quoted as being made on behalf of the Paediatric Committee or reflecting the position of the Paediatric Committee.

References

Abu-Afereh I, Russel G (1994) Prevalence of headache and migraine in school children. BMJ 309:765–769

Ahonen K, Hämäläinen ML, Rantala H, Hoppu K (2004) Nasal sumatriptan is effective in treatment of migraine attacks in children: a randomized trial. Neurology 62:883–887

Ahonen K, Hämäläinen ML, Eerola M, Hoppu K (2006) A randomized trial of rizatriptan in migraine attacks in children. Neurology 67:1135–1140

Anand KJ, Hall RW, Desai N, Shepard B, Bergqvist LL, Young TE, Boyle EM, Carbajal R, Bhutani VK, Moore MB, Kronsberg SS (2004) NEOPAIN Trial Investigators Group. Effects of morphine analgesia in ventilated preterm neonates: primary outcomes from the NEOPAIN randomised trial. Lancet 363:1673–1682

Bakker J, Grover R, McLuckie A, Holzapfel L, Andersson J, Lodato R, Watson D, Grossman S, Donaldson J, Glaxo Wellcome International Septic Shock Study Group (2004) Administration of the nitric oxide synthase inhibitor NG-methyl L-arginine hydrochloride (546C88) by intravenous infusion for up to 72 hours can promote resolution of shock in patients with severe sepsis: results of a randomized, double-blind, placebo-controlled multicenter study (study no 144-002). Crit Care Med 32:1–12

Benjamin DK Jr, Smith PB, Jadhav P, Gobburu JV, Murphy MD, Hasselblad V, Baker-Smith C, Califf RM, Li JS (2008) Paediatric antihypertensive trial failures: analysis of endpoints and dose range. Hypertension 51:834–840

Best Pharmaceuticals for children Act (2002) Public Law No 107–109

Beydon N, on behalf of the American Thoracic Society/European Respiratory Society Working Group on Infant and Young Children Pulmonary Function Testing et al (2007) An official American Thoracic Society/European Respiratory Society statement: pulmonary function testing in preschool children. Am J Respir Crit Care Med 175:1304–1345

Biomarkers Definitions Working Group (2001) Biomarkers and surrogate endpoints: preferred definitions and conceptual framework. Clin Pharmacol Ther 69:89–95

Brierley J et al (2009) Clinical practice parameters for hemodynamic support of pediatric and neonatal septic shock: 2007 update from the American College of Critical Care Medicine. Crit Care Med 37:666–688

Bringuier S, Dadure C, Raux O, Dubois A, Picot M-C, Capdevila X (2009) The perioperative validity of the visual analog anxiety scale in children: a discriminant and useful instrument in routine clinical practice to optimize postoperative pain management. Anesth Analg 109:737–744

Buysse CM, Raat H, Hazelzet JA, Hop WC, Maliepaard M, Joosten KFM (2008) Surviving meningococcal septic shock: health consequences and quality of life in children and their parents up to 2 years after pediatric intensive care unit discharge. Crit Care Med 36:596–602

Carcillo JA, Fields AI, Task force committee members (2002) Clinical practice parameters for hemodynamic support of paediatric an neonatal patients in septic shock. Crit Care Med 30:1365–1378

Champion GD, Goodenough B, von Baeyer CL, Thomas W (1998) Measurement of pain by self-report. In: Finley GA, McGrath PJ (eds) Measurement of pain in infants and children. IASP, Seattle, WA, pp 123–160

Consolaro A, Ruperto N, Bazso A, Pistorio A, Magni-Manzoni S, Filocamo G, Malattia C, Viola S, Martini A, Ravelli A, for the Pediatric Rheumatology International Trials Organisation (2009) Development and validation of a composite disease activity score for juvenile idiopathic arthritis. Arthritis Rheum 61(5):658–666

CPMP/EWP/4151/00 (2009) Rev. 1. Guideline on the requirements for clinical documentation for Orally Inhaled Products (OIP) including the requirements for demonstration of therapeutic equivalence between two inhaled products for use in the treatment of Asthma and Chronic Obstructive Pulmonary Disease (COPD) in adults and for use in the treatment of Asthma in children and adolescents

CPMP/EWP/422/04 (2007) Guideline on clinical investigation of medicinal products for the treatment of juvenile idiopathic arthritis

Crawfordt MJ, Lehman L, Slater S, Kabbouche MA, LeCates SL, Segers A, Manning P, Powers SW, Hershey AD (2009) Menstrual migraine in adolescents. Headache 49:341–347

Crenesse D, Berlioz M, Bourrier T, Albertini M (2001) Spirometry in children aged 3 to 5 years: reliability of forced expiratory maneuvers. Pediatr Pulmonol 32:56–61

Curley MA, Zimmerman JL (2005) Alternative outcome measures for pediatric clinical sepsis trials. Pediatr Crit Care Med 6(Suppl):S150–S156

Dancey JE, Dobbin KK, Groshen S, Milburn Jessup J, Hruszkewycz AH, Koehler M, Parchment R, Ratain MJ, Shankar LK, Stadler WM, True LD, Gravell A, Grever MR, On behalf of the Biomarkers Task Force of the NCI Investigational Drug Steering Committee (2010) Guidelines for the development and incorporation of biomarker studies in early clinical trials of novel agents. Clin Cancer Res 16:1745–1755

Davis SD, Brody AS, Emond MJ, Brumback LC, Rosenfeld M (2007) Endpoints for clinical trials in young children with cystic fibrosis. Proc Am Thorac Soc 4:418–430

Davis SD, Rosenfeld M, Kerby GS, Brumback L, Kloster MH, Acton JD, Colin AA, Conrad CK, Hart MA, Hiatt PW, Mogayzel PJ, Johnson RC, Wilcox SL, Castile RG (2010) Multicenter evaluation of infant lung function tests as cystic fibrosis clinical trial endpoints. Am J Respir Crit Care Med 182(11):1387–1397

de Oliveira CF, de Oliveira DSF, Gottschald AFC, Moura JDG, Costa GA, Ventura AC, Fernandes JC, Vaz FAC, Carcillo JA, Rivers EP, Troster EJ (2008) ACCM/PALS haemodynamic support guidelines for paediatric septic shock: an outcomes comparison with and without monitoring central venous oxygen saturation. Intensive Care Med 34:1065–1075

Debillon T, Zupan V, Ravault N, Magny J-F, Dehan M (2001) Development and initial validation of the EDIN scale, a new tool for assessing prolonged pain in preterm infants. Arch Dis Child Fetal Neonatal Ed 85:F36–F41

Della Pasqua O, Zimmerhackl L-B, Rose K (2007) Study protocol design for paediatric patients of different ages. In: Rose K, van den Acker JN (eds) Guide to paediatric clinical research. Basel, Karger, pp 87–107

Dworkin RH, Turk DC, Farrar JT, Haythornthwaite JA, Jensen MP, Katz NP, Kerns RD, Stucki G, Allen RR, Bellamy N, Carr DB, Chandler J, Cowan P, Dionne R, Galer BS, Hertz S, Jadad AR, Kramer LD, Manning DC, Martin S, McGormick GC, Mc Dermott MP, McGrath P, Quessy S, Rappaport BA, Robbins W, Robinson JP, Rothman M, Royal MA, Simon L, Stauffer JW, Stein W, Tollet J, Wernicke J, Witter J (2005) Core outcome measures for chronic pain trials: IMMPACT recommendations. Pain 113:9–19

Eccleston C, Jordan A, McCracken LM, Sleed M, Connell H, Clinch J (2005) The Bath Adolescent Pain Questionnaire (BAPQ): development and preliminary psychometric evaluation of an instrument to assess the impact of chronic pain on adolescents. Pain 118:263–270

Echt BS, Liebson PR, Mitchell LB (1991) Mortality and morbidity in patients receiving ecainide, flecainide or placebo. The cardiac arrhythmia suppression trial. N Engl J Med 324:781–788

EMA/CHMP/EWP/213972/2010 (2010) Paediatric addendum to CHMP guideline on the clinical investigations of medicinal products for the treatment of pulmonary arterial hypertension

EMEA/522496/2006 (2006a) Report on the EMEA/CHMP biomarkers workshop

EMEA/536810/08 (2008a) Guideline on the Investigation of medicinal products in the term and preterm neonate

EMEA/CHMP/EWP/139391/2004 (2004) Reflection paper on the regulatory guidance for the use of health-related quality of life (HRQL) measures in the evaluation of medicinal products

EMEA/CHMP/EWP/4713/03 (2006b) Guideline on clinical investigation of medicinal products for the treatment of sepsis

EMEA/CHMP/EWP/517497/2007 (2008b) Guideline on clinical evaluation of medicinal products used in weight control (cpmp/ewp/281/96 rev. 1) Addendum on weight control in children

EMEA/CHMP/EWP/545456/2008 (2008c) Concept paper on the need for the development of a paediatric addendum to the note for guidance on the clinical investigation on medicinal products in the treatment of hypertension

EMEA/CHMP/EWP/644261/2008 (2009c) Concept paper on the need for the development of a paediatric addendum to the CHMP guideline on the clinical investigations of medicinal products for the treatment of pulmonary arterial hypertension

EMEA/CHMP/EWP/9147/2008 (2009b) Guideline on the clinical development of medicinal products for the treatment of cystic fibrosis

EMEA/CHMP/ICH/380636/2009 (2009a) Note for guidance on genomic biomarkers related to drug response: context, structure and format of qualification submissions

EMEA/CPMP/EWP/612/00 (2002) Note for guidance on clinical investigation of medicinal products for treatment of nociceptive pain

EMEA/CPMP/EWP/788/01 (2007) Rev. 1. Guideline on clinical investigation of medicinal products for the treatment of migraine

Evers S, Marziniak M, Frese A, Gralow I (2008) Placebo efficacy in childhood and adolescence migraine: an analysis of double-blind and placebo-controlled studies. Cephalgia 29:436–444

Fleming TR, DeMets DL (1996) Surrogate endpoints in clinical trials: are we being misled? Ann Intern Med 125:605–613

Food and Drug Administration (1998) US Departmentof Health and Human Services. Guidance for industry; E9 statistical principles for clinical trials. Office of Training and Communications, Rockville, MD

Food and Drug Administration (2003) Code of Federal Regulations 601.40

Food and Drug Administration (2009a) Code of Federal Regulations 21 314.50

Food and Drug Administration (2009b) Accelerated approval of new drugs for serious or life-threatening illnesses. Code of Federal Regulations, Title 21, Volume 5, revised

Food and Drug Administration (2009c) Guidance for industry. Patient-reported outcome measures: use in medicinal product development to support labeling claims

Fradet C, McGarth PJ, Kay J, Adams S (1990) A prospective survey of reactions to blood test by children and adolescents. Pain 40:53–60

Goldstein B, Giror B, Randolph A, and the Members of the International Consensus Conference of Pediatric Sepsis (2005) International pediatric sepsis consensus conference: Definitions for sepsis and organ dysfunction in pediatrics. Pediatr Crit Care Med 6:2–8

Grunau RE, Oberlander T, Holsti L, Whitfield MF (1998) Bedside application of the Neonatal Facial Coding System in pain assessment of premature neonates. Pain 76:277–286

Hain RGW (1997) Pain scales in children: review. Palliat Med 11:341–350

Hämäläinen ML, Hoppu K, Santavuori P (1997) Sumatriptan for migraine attacks in children: a randomized placebo-controlled study. Do children with migraine respond to oral sumatriptan differently from adults? Neurology 48:1100–1103

Haworth SG, Beghetti M (2010) Assessment of endpoints in the pediatric population: congenital heart disease and idiopathic pulmonary arterial hypertension. Curr Opin Pulm Med 16(Suppl 1): S35–S41

International Conference for Harmonisation (1997) General considerations for Clinical Trials E 8

International Conference for Harmonisation (2001) Clinical investigation of medicinal products in the paediatric population E 11. CPMP/ICH/2711/99

International Headache Society Headache Classification Subcommittee (2004) International classification of headache disorders, 2nd edition. Cephalgia 24(Suppl 1):9–160

Inwald DP, Tasker RC, Peters MJ, on behalf of the Paediatric Intensive Care Society Study Group (PIGS-SG) (2009) Emergency management of children with severe sepsis in the United Kingdom: the results of the Paediatric Intensive Care Society sepsis audit. Arch Dis Child 94:348–353

Jacobson S (2007) Common medical pains. Paediatr Child Health 12:105–109

Lesko JJ, Atkinson AJ Jr (2001) Use of biomarkers and surrogate endpoints in drug development and regulatory decision making: criteria, validation, strategies. Annu Rev Pharmacol Toxicol 41:347–366

Lewis DW, Winner P, Wasiewski W (2005) The placebo responder rate in children and adolescents. Headache 45:232–239

Lewis DW, Paul Winner P, Hershey AD, Warren W, Wasiewski WW, on behalf of the Adolescent Migraine Steering Committee (2007) Efficacy of zolmitriptan nasal spray in adolescent migraine. Pediatrics 120:390–396

Li AM et al (2005) The six-minute walk test in healthy children: reliability and validity. Eur Respir J 25:1057–1060

Li JS, Benjamin DK Jr, Severin T, Portman RJ (2010) Paediatric anti-hypertensive clinical trials and various factors influencing trial success or failure. In: Rose K, van den Anker JN (eds) Guide to paediatric drug development and clinical research. Karger, Basel, pp 196–205

Loizzo A, Stefano Loizzo S, Capasso A (2009) Neurobiology of pain in children: an overview. Open Biochem J 3:18–25

López A, Lorente JA, Steingrub J, Bakker J, McLuckie A, Willatts S, Brockway M, Anzueto A, Holzapfel L, Breen D, Silverman MS, Takala J, Donaldson J, Arneson C, Grove G, Grossman S, Grover R (2004) Multiple-center, randomized, placebo-controlled, double-blind study of the nitric oxide synthase inhibitor 546C88: effect on survival in patients with septic shock. Crit Care Med 32:21–30

Madriago E, Silberbach M (2010) Heart failure in infants and children. Pediatr Rev 31(1):4–11

McGrath PJ, Walco GA, Turk DC, Dworkin RH, Brown MT, Davidson K, Eccleston C, Finley GA, Goldschneider K, Haverkos L, Hertz SH, Ljungman G, Palermo T, Rappaport BA, Rhodes T, Schechter N, Scott J, Sethna N, Svensson OK, Stinson J, von Bayer CL, Walker L, Weisman S, White RE, Zajick A, Zeltzer L (2008) Core outcome domains and measures for pediatric acute and chronic/recurrent pain clinical trials: PedIMMPACT recommendations. J Pain 9:771–783

Merkel SI, Voepel-Lewis T (1997) The FLACC: a behavioural scale for scoring postoperative pain in young children. Pediatr Nurs 23:293–297

Merskey H, Bogduk N (eds) (1994). Part III: pain terms, a current list with definitions and notes on usage. In: Classification of chronic pain, 2nd edn. IASP Task Force on Taxonomy. IASP Press, Seattle WA, pp 209–214

Molenberghs G, Orman C (2009) Surrogate endpoints: application in pediatric clinical trials. In: Mulberg A, Silber S, vand der Acker JN (eds) Pediatric drug development, concepts and applications. Wiley-Blackwell, Hoboken, NJ, pp 501–511

Mortimer MJ, Kay J, Jaron A (1992) Childhood migraine in general practice: clinical features and characteristics. Cephalgia 12:238–253

Nilsson S, Finnström B, Kosinky E (2008) The FLACC behavioural scale for procedural pain assessment in children aged 5–16 years. Pediatr Anesth 18:767–774

Odetola FO, Gebremariam A, Freed GL (2007) Patient and hospital correlates of clinical outcomes and resource utilization in severe pediatric sepsis. Pediatrics 119:487–494

Paediatric Research Equity Act (2003) Public Law No 108–155

Puntman VO (2009) How-to guide on biomarkers: biomarker definitons, validation and applications with examples from cardiovascular disease. Postgrad Med J 85:538–545

Redmond C, Colton T (eds) (2001) Biostatistics in clinical trials, Wiley reference series in biostatistics., p 322, Outcome measure

Regulation (EC) (2006) No 1901/2006 On medicinal products for paediatric use

Regulation (EC) No 726/2004 (2004) On conditional approval of medicinal products

Rosenfeld M (2007) An overview of endpoints for cystic fibrosis clinical trials: one size does not fit all. Proc Am Thorac Soc 4:299–301

Ross RD, Bollinger RO, Pinsky WW (1992) Grading the severity of congestive heart failure in infants. Pediatr Cardiol 13(2):72–75

Rothman M, Kleinman L (2009) Patient-reported outcomes in paediatric drug development. In: Mulberg A, Silber S, der Acker JN (eds) Pediatric drug development, concepts and applications. Wiley-Blackwell, Hoboken, NJ, pp 513–524

Rothner AD, Wasiewski W, Winner P, Lewis D, Stankowski J (2006) Zolmitriptan oral tablet in migraine treatment: high placebo responses in adolescents. Headache 46:101–109

Ruperto N, for the Pediatric Rheumatology International trials Organisation (PRINTO) and the Pediatric Rheumatology Collaborative Study Group (PRCGS) et al (2006) The pediatric rheumatology international trials organization/American college of rheumatology provisional criteria for the evaluation of response to therapy in juvenile systemic lupus erythematosus: prospective validation of the definition of improvement. Arthritis Rheum (Arthritis Care Res) 55(3):355–363

Shaddy RE, for the Pediatric Carvedilol Study Group et al (2007) Carvedilol for children and adolescents with heart failure. JAMA 298(10):1171–1179

Sinha I, Jones L, Smyth RL, Williamson PR (2008) A systematic review of studies that aim to determine which outcomes to measure in clinical trials in children. PLoS Med 5:e96

Slater R, Cantarella A, Franck L, Meek J, Fitzgerald M (2008) How well do clinical pain assessment tools reflect pain in infants? PLoS Med 6:e129

Stanford EA, Chambers CT, Graig KD (2006) The role of developmental factors in predicting young children's use of self-report scale for pain. Pain 120:16–23

Stevens B, Johnston C, Petryshen P, Taddio A (1996) Premature infant pain profile: development and initial validation. Clin J Pain 12:13–22

Stinson JN, Kabanagh T, Yamada J, Gill N, Stevens B (2006) Systematic review of the psychometric properties, interpretability and feasibility of self-report pain intensity measures for use in clinical trials in children and adolescents. Pain 125:143–157

The International Chronic Granulomatous Disease Cooperative Study Group (1991) A controlled trial of interferon gamma to prevent infection in chronic granulomatous disease. N Engl J Med 324:509–516

Tugwell P, Boers M (1993) OMERACT conference on outcome measures in RA clinical trials: introduction. J Rheumatol 20:528–530

University of Liverpool (2010) Core Outcome Measures in Effectiveness Trials (COMET). http://www.liv.ac.uk/nwhtmr/comet/comet.htm

van Dijk M, de Boer JB, Koot HM, Tibboel D, Passchier J, Duivenvoorden HJ (2000) The reliability and validity of the COMFORT scale as a postoperative pain instrument in 0 to 3 year-old infants. Pain 84:367–377

Varni JW, Seid M, Rode CA (1999) The PEdsQL: measurement model for the Pediatric Quality of Life Inventory. Med Care 37:126–139

Varni JW, Seid M, Kurtin PS (2001) PedQL 4.0: reliability and validity of the Pediatric Quality of life Inventory version 4.0 generic core scales in healthy and patient populations. Med Care 39:800–812

Vincent JL (2004) Endpoints in sepsis trials. More than just 28 day mortality? Crit Care Med 32 (Suppl):S209–S213

von Baeyer CL, Spagrud LJ (2007) Systematic review of observational (behavioral) measures of pain for children and adolescents aged 3 to 18 years. Pain 127:140–150

von Baeyer CL, Spagrud LJ, McCormick JC, Choo E, Neville K, Connelly MA (2009) Three new datasets supporting the use of the Numerical Rating Scale (NRS-11) for children's self-reports on pain intensity. Pain 143:223–227

Walco GA, Conte PM, Labay LE, Engel R, Zeltzer LK (2005) Procedural distress in children with cancer: self-report, behavioral observations, and physiological parameters. Clin J Pain 21:484–490

Walco G, Dworkin RH, Krane EJ, LeBel AA, Treede R-D (2010) Neuropathic pain in children: special considerations. Mayo Clin Proc 85(Suppl):S33–S41

Walker SM (2008) Pain in children: recent advances and ongoing challenges. Br J Anaesth 101:101–110

Watson RS, Carcillo JA (2005) Scope and epidemiology in pediatric sepsis. Pediatr Crit Care Med 6(Suppl):S3–S5

Watson D, Grover R, Anzueto A, Lorente J, Smithies M, Bellomo R, Guntupalli K, Grossman S, Donaldson J, Glaxo Wellcome International Septic Shock Study Group (2004) Cardiovascular effects of the nitric oxide synthase inhibitor NG-methyl L-arginine hydrochloride (546C88) in patients with septic schock: results of a randomized, double-blind, placebo-controlled multicenter study (study no 144–002). Crit Care Med 32:13–20

Winner P, Linder SL, Lipton RB, Almas M, Parsons B, Pitman V (2007) Eletriptan for acute treatment of migraine in adolescents: results of a double-blind placebo-controlled trial. Headache 47:511–518

Safety Assessment in Pediatric Studies

Gideon Koren, Abdelbasset Elzagallaai, and Fatma Etwel

Contents

Abstract It typically takes many years before an association of a drug with a rare, serious adverse reaction is established. As related to pediatric drug use, evidence is even more erratic, as most drugs are used off labels. To enhance child safety, there is an urgent need to develop robust and rapid methods to identify such associations in as timely a manner as possible. In this chapter, several novel methods, both clinically based pharmacoepidemiological approaches and laboratory-based methods, are described.

Keywords Adverse drug reactions • Children • Neonates • Side effects

G. Koren (✉)
The Motherisk Program, Division of Clinical Pharmacology and Toxicology, Hospital for Sick Children, University Avenue 555, Toronto M5G 1X8, ON, Canada
e-mail: gidiup_2000@yahoo.com

A. Elzagallaai • F. Etwel
Division of Clinical Pharmacology and Toxicology, Hospital for Sick Children, University Avenue 555, Toronto M5G 1X8, ON, Canada

H.W. Seyberth et al. (eds.), *Pediatric Clinical Pharmacology*,
Handbook of Experimental Pharmacology 205,
DOI 10.1007/978-3-642-20195-0_8, © Springer-Verlag Berlin Heidelberg 2011

1 Introduction

Each year prescription drugs cause fatal adverse drug reactions (ADR) to 100,000 individuals in the USA, making prescription drugs between the fourth and sixth leading cause of death, after heart disease, cancer, stroke, pulmonary disease, and accidents (Lazarou et al. 1998).

Before a pharmaceutical product is marketed, the manufacturer must prove that it is both effective and safe by performing extensive studies in animals and in human clinical trials. However, premarketing studies cannot guarantee product safety as they are limited by the small numbers of patients (between 1,000 and 3,000 subjects). Importantly, serious ADRs (e.g., agranulocytosis) occur at a rate of between 1:1,000 and 1:10,000 patients. Additionally, clinical trials typically exclude vulnerable populations such as pregnant women, children, elderly people, those with complicated diseases, or those taking other medications. Hence, uncommon adverse effects, delayed effects, or consequences of long-term drug administration often are not observed before the drug has been marketed (Stricker and Psaty 2004). While the more common type A ADRs (reactions that are an augmentation of the normal pharmacological actions of the drug) may already have been identified by the time of licensing (Pirmohamed et al. 1998), type B ADRs (idiosyncratic or bizarre reactions that cannot be predicted from the known pharmacology of the drug) will only be detected after licensing through postmarketing surveillance (Meyboom et al. 1997).

Postmarketing studies are based on collecting spontaneous case reports of ADRs. There are two systems where clinical observers can use to address their voluntary reporting of ADRs. The first is the published medical literature, which is a highly efficient warning system for new adverse reactions, and often recognizes rare events and people at high risk (Begaud et al. 1994). The second consists of national and international adverse drug reaction monitoring centers, such as the Food and Drug Administration (FDA). In the USA, the FDA started a voluntary reporting system in the late 1960s, receiving reports from health care providers, consumers, and pharmaceutical companies. Unlike health care providers and consumers, the manufacturers have a regulated duty to report to the FDA on any ADR. The system had been criticized in the 1970s for its delay in sending reports of the newly identified ADRs to the Physicians Desk Reference (Zielinskin 2005). The FDA system is probably overwhelmed by ADR reports from all interested parties, as the experts at the Agency have insufficient time to analyze all incoming reports in depth. Moreover, the FDA does not have the regulated authority to mandate drug manufacturers to conduct directed postmarketing surveillance studies (Millichap 1976), which could help in detecting uncommon serious ADRs.

2 Pharmacoepidemiological Approaches

Over the last few years, we have developed a novel detection method to allow regulatory agencies and manufacturers to create a rapid signal for an association between the drug and the corresponding ADRs, in the postmarketing period. This method can allow early identification of rise in the incidence rate of severe organ failure associated with the medication. This method can help to protecting the public from unexpected harmful effects of new drugs. Herein, we will use the pemoline-associated acute liver failure (ALF) as a model for the development of this novel system.

3 Pemoline-Index Case

Pemoline (phenylisohydantoin, Cylert™) is a mild central nervous system stimulant that has been approved in 1975 for children with attention-deficit hyperactivity disorder (ADHD) (Stevenson and Wolraich 1989; Berkovitch et al. 1995). In 1995, we reported the case of a 14-year-old boy diagnosed with ADHD (Berkovitch et al. 1995) who had been previously healthy and had received concomitant pemoline, 37.5 mg a day, for 16 months and methylphenidate, 20 mg a day for 2 months, to control his symptoms. He was hospitalized due to jaundice, which progressed into ALF. A liver biopsy was suggestive of drug toxicity. He underwent liver transplant which failed and the child died. All known causes of liver failure were ruled out including infection, metabolic disease, tumor, or chemicals. We found two previous published fatal cases due to ALF associated with pemoline both from the USA. At that time, the USA, FDA, and the manufacturer were not aware of additional cases. We estimated that a child receiving pemoline has a relative risk of development of liver failure of 45.3 (95% confidence interval, 4.1–510) and urged others to report on similar cases. This highly significant association ($p < 0.001$) suggested causation. After this report, other investigators around the world reported more cases of liver failure associated with pemoline. A black box warning was added to the labeling in the USA in December 1996, and a "Dear Doctor" letter was mailed out by the manufacturer to all US physicians to use the drug as a last resort, but physicians continued to use pemoline as a first-line therapy. In September 1999, Health Canada withdrew pemoline from the Canadian market (more cases of pemoline liver toxicity were reported, and pressure on the FDA increased to ban the drug). In May, 2005, the manufacturer chose to stop sales and marketing of Cylert™ in the US Cylert™ would remain available through pharmacies and wholesalers until supplies are exhausted; no additional product would be available. In November 2005, pemoline was finally removed from the US market.

From these events, it is evident that there was a 25-year delay in identifying pemoline-associated ALF, leading to a delay in withdrawing the drug from the market and putting children at risk for fatal drug-related injury.

We hypothesized that using available data one could predict pemoline-associated ALF several years after its marketing, without the protracted delay of 25 years.

The study was a postmarketing surveillance of pemoline hepatotoxicity based on cases reported to either the FDA and/or in the medical literature. The population for the study consisted of children in the USA and Canada. For each calendar year after 1975 when pemoline was approved to be marketed as a treatment for ADHD, the number of children who were on pemoline was estimated as was the number of reported cases of ALF associated with pemoline.

After obtaining the yearly number of children on pemoline and the yearly number of children who developed ALF while on pemoline, a comparison was made between these data and the background incidence rate of idiopathic ALF in children in the general population. This comparison was made year by year to define the earliest year when the rate of serious ALF due to pemoline was significantly higher than predicted in the general population.

Data were synthesized from systematic review of the published literature. Only studies calculating the rate of ALF in children and their etiologies, including idiopathic liver failure, were included.

Information regarding the number of children on pemoline in Canada per year was obtained from IMS (International Medical Statistics, Montreal Quebec). The IMS is a holder of statistical medical information that can be accessed by researchers, academics, and government. For US data, we gathered the information by synthesizing available published data, by systematic review of Medline EMBASE and Scopus, and by obtaining all articles that reported on the number of children prescribed pemoline.

The annual number of children on pemoline in the USA and Canada who developed ALF was obtained from the FDA under the Freedom of Information Act. All pemoline cases reported to the FDA between 1975 and 1999 were analyzed. The criteria for selection of liver injury cases were age between 0 and 18 years, any report of irreversible damage to the liver, and children who received the dose schedule recommended for its primary indication. We excluded cases reporting increased liver enzyme levels that returned to normal once pemoline was discontinued. Some of these cases have also been published in the literature and articles were obtained. We used the same criteria for selection of the literature cases as was used in the FDA cases. All the published cases were subjected to causality assessment using the Naranjo ADR probability Scale (Naranjo et al. 1981). The Naranjo ADR probability scale is a tool widely used to determine the likelihood that an ADR is caused by the implicated medication. Ten questions are answered and assigned a weighted score of +2 to −2. Where there were insufficient data available, the particular question receives a score of 0. Based on the Naranjo criteria 15, each case is scored between ($<$1 and $>$9) and assigned a likelihood of causing an ADR from doubtful, possible, probable, to highly probable.

Based on a recent large comprehensive study of fulminant hepatic failure, approximately 230 children are estimated to be afflicted each year in the USA (Liu et al. 2001). The number of children who lived in the USA has been estimated at 73,043,506 (Children Defense fund), and hence the overall rate of ALF in children is estimated at 1:300,000.

Based on all available studies, 16% of the cases of ALF were due to unknown reasons (idiopathic). Hence, we estimated that the rate of idiopathic liver failure in North American children is 1:2,000,000.

We identified all papers that surveyed the prevalence of medication use to treat children with ADHD in the USA and they were used to calculate the yearly number of American school children on ADHD medication from 1975 through 1993. For any missing year for which no publication was available, we calculated the mean value from the closest years before and after. The percentage of children receiving treatment with stimulant medication for ADHD ranged between 2.1 and 6%. The percentage of reported pemoline use among ADHD children was 1% in 1975 and increased gradually to 6% in 1987. Between 1987 and 1993, there was no data available on the percentage of pemoline use among ADHD children, so we assumed that the percentage was not changed since 1987. The overall number of school children in the USA was obtained from international statistics. Based on the above number, we estimated the number of children taking pemoline in the USA.

We estimated that a total of 45,404 Canadian children years were treated with pemoline from 1978 to 2004. In Canada, the marketing of pemoline started only in the 1980s. The Canadian Drug Identification Codes are drug product database books published annually. The first time pemoline was included in these databases was in 1981 (the first time pemoline was included in the Compendium of Pharmaceuticals and Specialties was in 1986) (Canadian Pharmaceutical Association and Canadian Pharmacists Association 1986).

3.1 Pediatric ALF Cases Receiving Pemoline and Reported to the FDA

Thirty cases of children who were on pemoline therapy and who developed irreversible ALF were reported to the FDA. The first case was in 1977.

3.2 Calculating Relative Risk of Pemoline Associated with ALF

Using the FDA reports, each year after introducing pemoline the relative risk of children on pemoline developing ALF was high, ranging between 9.12 and 24.08. The highest RR was detected in 1978. All these RR were statistically significant (Etwel et al. 2008).

Using pemoline as a model, we were able to show that employing existing data at the time one could estimate the incidence rate of serious ADRs early in the marketing cycle.

Hence, as early as 1978, a significant signal existed indicating that pemoline is associated with ALF, 16 years before the first published suggestion by Berkovitch and colleagues (1995), 22 years before removal of the medication from the Canadian market, and 28 years before removal from US market. While we present analysis related to ALF, similar population-based statistics are available for all other adverse events, from agranulocytosis to pulmonary fibrosis. This method should enable researchers, clinicians, drug companies, and regulators to identify uncommon adverse drug reactions, associated with new medications, earlier in the course of marketing and thus quantify serious ADRs and identify patient populations at special risk.

4 Laboratory-Based Methods of Predicting Serious Adverse Reactions in Children

The concept of developing laboratory tests that can predict rare, but potentially fatal, adverse drug reactions is ideally exemplified in the case of the anticonvulsant hypersensitivity syndrome (AHS).

We will review critically the usefulness of available in vitro tests in the diagnosis of AHS.

Anticonvulsant hypersensitivity syndrome (AHS), also known as drug hypersensitivity syndrome or drug rash with eosinophilia and systemic symptoms (DRESS), is a type B ("bizarre") adverse drug reaction (ADR) that develops in susceptible patients following exposure to certain drugs, including aromatic anticonvulsants (Shear and Spielberg 1988; Zaccara et al. 2007) Although lacking a defined clinical picture, AHS is typically associated with the development of skin rash, fever, and internal organ dysfunction that may include blood dyscrasias, hepatitis, nephritis, myocarditis, thyroiditis, and interstitial pneumonitis and encephalitis (Peyriere et al. 2006). The pathophysiological mechanisms underlying AHS are not well understood; however, it is believed to be immune mediated in general and involve generation of electrophilic reactive metabolites that react covalently with macromolecules to form immunogenic adducts able to activate the immune system (Shapiro and Shear 1996; Spielberg et al. 1981a, b). The accurate incidence of AHS is unknown due to underreporting, but it has been estimated to range from 1 in 1,000 to 1 in 10,000 in patients newly exposed to aromatic anticonvulsants (Tennis and Stern 1997). While the disorder is rare, it is potentially fatal and represents a clinical dilemma to treating doctors. Diagnosis of AHS is challenging, as a reliable and safe diagnostic test is not available to confirm causality or identify the culprit drug. A number of in vivo and in vitro tests have been devised and used to aid the diagnosis of AHS. These include skin tests (patch test, prick test, and intradermal test), the lymphocyte transformation test (LTT), and the lymphocyte toxicity assay (LTA) (Pourpak et al. 2008).

In vitro diagnostic tests have the advantage over in vivo tests (patch test and rechallenge) of bearing no potential harm to patients. A number of in vitro diagnostic tests have been used to aid the diagnosis of delayed-type drug hypersensitivity reactions (Naranjo et al. 1992; Beeler and Pichler 2007; Lan et al. 2006); however, their true value is yet to be defined. Among these tests are those that utilize peripheral blood mononuclear cells (PBMCs) as target cells, including the LTT and the LTA. Unfortunately, these techniques require expensive equipment and sophisticated laboratories as well as specialized experience with biochemical and molecular methods, so only a few centers are sufficiently equipped to perform them. Hence, these methods, although successfully employed as research tools, have not been successfully translated into diagnostic tests (Wu et al. 2006; Beeler et al. 2006).

Leukocytes are present in peripheral blood at densities of 5–7 × 10^3 cells/mm^3; 20–50% of these cells are lymphocytes, whereas 2–10% are monocytes. Lymphocytes are favored as a model for investigation of immune-mediated diseases because of their unique characteristics, which include that (1) they are easily obtained at adequate density; (2) they play a key role in the immune system by orchestrating different elements of the immune response and thus represent the state of the immune system in the specific patient; (3) they are metabolically active and express most of the enzymes required for drug detoxication; and (4) individual genetically based defects in the expression or activity of these detoxication enzymes are phenotypically expressed in lymphocytes.

4.1   The Lymphocyte Transformation Test

The in vitro lymphocyte transformation phenomenon was first described during the late 1950s. In short, human peripheral blood leukocytes (PBLs) differentiate in short-term primary cultures, forming plasts. This effect was later attributed to the presence of a constituent [phytohemagglutinin (PHA)] of a plant extract from red kidney beans (*Phaseolus vulgaris*) that is used to isolate blood peripheral leukocytes (Rigas and Osgood 1955). PHA causes erythrocytes to aggregate and sediment, allowing leukocytes to separate from whole blood preparations. In a later report, Nowell (1960) demonstrated that PHA also initiates mitotic activity (transformation) in cultured human leukocytes. To show that lymphocyte behavior in vitro has an immunological basis, Pearmain et al. (1963) exposed PBLs isolated from both tuberculin-sensitive and tuberculin-nonsensitive patients to tuberculin in vitro. Only PBLs from tuberculin-sensitive patients showed mitotic activity, whereas cells from patients not previously exposed to the antigen showed no mitosis.

One of the first reports of using the LTT for diagnosis of drug allergy was by Holland and Mauer (1964) who evaluated the effect of phenytoin on cultured lymphocytes isolated from patients sensitive to the drug and nonsensitive (control) subjects. In these experiments, PHA used as a positive control showed nonspecific stimulation of all cells sampled, whereas phenytoin stimulated only the cells from phenytoin-sensitive patients. When tested with peripheral lymphocytes isolated from a sulfadiazine-sensitive patient and incubated with the culprit drug in vitro, this effect was found to be concentration-dependent.

The procedure includes incubation of PBMCs isolated from drug-hypersensitive patients with the incriminated agent at nontoxic concentrations and observation of any increase in the rate of cell proliferation measured by [^{3}H]thymidine incorporation. The increase in cell proliferation is expressed as a ratio between proliferation of cells incubated with and without the drug (vehicle alone; control). This ratio is defined as the stimulation index (SI) and it is calculated as follows (1):

$$SI = \frac{[^3H]\ \text{thymidine uptake in the presence ofthedrug}}{[^3H]\ \text{thymidine uptake in the absense of the drug}} \qquad (1)$$

where [^{3}H]thymidine uptake is expressed in counts per minute.

Cell cultures from drug-exposed and unexposed nonsensitive individuals are also used to confirm the specificity of a potential drug effect. The final result of the test depends on several factors such as the value of background cell proliferation and the type of the drug; however, an SI of >3 is always considered indicative of a positive reaction. Other end points for measurement of T-cell activation, such as elevation of released cytokines (using an enzyme-linked immunosorbent assay [ELISA]), have been proposed and could be a more sensitive method for detection of T-cell activation than measurement of the rate of cell proliferation.

The LTT has been used by some investigators for diagnosis of potential drug allergy cases for more than 20 years. However, its value in diagnosis and prediction of AHS remains controversial.

4.2 The Lymphocyte Toxicity Assay

Introduced by Spielberg and colleagues (1980), the LTA is an in vitro test that utilizes isolated PBMCs to investigate the mechanistic pathogenesis of idiosyn-cratic drug reactions. The test is based on the hypothesis that drug hypersensitivity develops as a result of imbalance between generation of toxic reactive metabolites (metabolic activation or toxication) and detoxication capacity that leads to accu-mulation of toxic metabolites (the "reactive metabolite" hypothesis). In this test, lymphocytes are used not as immunogenic cells but rather as easy-to-obtain surro-gate target cells. The procedure of the test entails incubation of PBMCs isolated from the patient with the culprit drug in the presence of Phenobarbital-induced mouse, rat, or rabbit liver microsomal $19{,}000 \times g$ supernatant fraction (S9), as a source of cytochrome P450 (CYP) mono-oxygenase activity.

CYP activity in the rodent (or sometimes human) liver preparation is hypothesized to oxidize drug to its active (cytotoxic) metabolite(s). Lymphocytes contain enzymes that are required for drug detoxication, including epoxide hydrolases and glutathione S-transferases, and any genetic defect in the function of these enzymes is phenotypically expressed in these cells. The percentage of cell death is then determined using different methods for assessing cell death [e.g., trypan blue exclusion or with a tetrazolium dye; for example, by the MTT (3-(4,5-dimethylthiazol-2-yl)-2,5-diphenyltetrazolium bromide) method]. Cell death is assumed to reflect the vulnerability of the cells to the toxic effects of the drug, which is hypothesized to indicate the susceptibility of the patient to develop hypersensitivity reactions to the parent drug and its reactive metabolite(s), presum-ably via differences in detoxication capacity and immune processing.

Aromatic anticonvulsants are excellent examples of metabolically activated cytotoxicants, metabolized primarily by hepatic CYP isozymes into reactive electrophilic arene oxide metabolites (Begaud et al. 1994). These unstable and highly reactive intermediate metabolites are readily detoxified by epoxide hydrolase and/or glutathione *S*-transferase enzymes, usually to non-electrophilic products (dihydrodiols and *S*-glutathione conjugates, respectively).

Although the same cell model (isolated PBMCs) is used in both types of assay, LTT and LTA are completely different approaches to the diagnosis of AHS. Whereas the former detects the in vivo immunological generation of drug-specific T lymphocytes used as a sign of hypersensitivity, the latter detects genetic defects that lead to accumulation of toxic metabolites, which are assumed to be a major factor in the etiology of drug hypersensitivity in addition to possible differences in cell death. Because the two tests use the same cell model and have similar nomenclature, it is not uncommon for individuals to confuse the LTT for the LTA or vice versa, or to use different nomenclature to describe these tests.

Retrieved publications were manually reviewed and the following selection criteria were applied: (1) original article written in English; (2) study performed in human subjects; (3) LTA or LTT used to diagnose AHS due to one or more aromatic anticonvulsant drug(s); and (4) sufficient technical data for scientific evaluation.

Thirty-one articles from PubMed, 22 articles from MED-LINE, and 28 from EMBASE were found that met our selection criteria. The search results from the three databases were then combined and duplicates were removed. The final number of included articles from the three databases was 48. Thirty-six articles used the LTT and 12 used the LTA for the diagnosis of AHS (Figure 4). Although single case reports were included in the review, none of these reports were used to calculate any of the tests' epidemiological characteristics.

In the systematic review we have conducted recently its use was almost always confined to experienced technicians in well-equipped research centers, primarily for the purpose of investigating the mechanism of T-cell-mediated reactions rather than diagnosis of drug allergy (Elzagallaai et al. 2009). In addition, because of its low laboratory-to-laboratory reproducibility and difficulty in evaluating results, this test cannot be described as user friendly and requires a great deal of experience for interpretation of results. For this reason, the test has not been translated into widespread clinical use. In fact, only a few research groups worldwide use this technique routinely.

In an attempt to determine the sensitivity and specificity of the LTT in the diagnosis of allergy to different drugs, the files of 923 patients with possible hypersensitivity reactions to drugs were studied. These patients were classified based on their medical history, follow-up, and provocation tests into four groups where drug allergies were "definite," "probable," "less probably," or "negative." One hundred cases were considered to have a very high probability of drug allergy, of which 78 had a positive LTT. Only three of these 100 cases were attributed to anticonvulsants (2 to carbamazepine and 1 to phenytoin). The two carbamazepine cases exhibited positive LTTs, whereas for the phenytoin case, the LTT was negative. Although the chemistry of the drug in question appears to play a major role in determining the usefulness of the LTT, the overall specificity and sensitivity of this test in this study were found to be in the range of 85 and 76%, respectively. It is not known whether or not these numbers can be applied to anticonvulsant drugs. However, because many different factors are involved in determining the final result of the LTT as discussed below, one cannot generalize these figures to include all types of drugs taken under various conditions.

Numerous factors have been found to affect the predictive value of the LTT in the diagnosis of drug hypersensitivity reactions. These factors include the timing of the test in relation to the beginning of the reaction, the type of clinical manifestations cause by the drug, the nature of the suspected drug, and the test procedure itself.

4.3 The LTA in the Diagnosis of AHS

The use of the LTA in diagnosing AHS dates back to the early 1980s. However, the lack of large-scale application is quite obvious. Shear and Spielberg (1988) studied 53 patients with a medical history suggesting AHS due to phenytoin, carbamazepine, or phenobarbital, as well as 49 unexposed healthy controls and 10 phenytoin-exposed healthy controls. Symptoms include fever, skin rash (varying in severity from generalized exanthema to TEN), eosinophilia, atypical lymphocytosis, and internal organ involvement (liver, kidney, thyroid, or lung). The performance of the LTA as a diagnostic test in this cohort of patients was excellent, with only two false positives and one false negative result in patients with hypersensitivity reactions to phenobarbital.

AHS is a rare but potentially lethal disorder. One of the most challenging aspects of this disease is the difficulty of establishing a solid diagnosis in a timely manner. Lack of a diagnosis or misdiagnosis may result in increased morbidity, increased mortality, and extended hospitalization. Between 10 and 27% of patients with epilepsy discontinue their first antiepileptic drug because of the development of adverse reactions (Kwan and Brodie 2001). Aromatic anticonvulsant drugs such as phenytoin, carbamazepine, phenobarbital, and lamotrigine are linked to a relatively high risk of development of hypersensitivity reactions. Carbamazepine was found to be the most common cause of severe forms of AHS (i.e., SJS and TEN).

The diagnosis of AHS entails two main processes: first, establishing the diagnosis of the hypersensitivity reaction, usually from a series of clinically similar differential diagnoses; and second, identifying the culprit drug, potentially among a number of other concomitantly prescribed, innocent drugs. Numerous diagnostic tests are available and have been attempted for the diagnosis of drug hypersensitivity reactions; however, their epidemiological qualities are dependent on the type of reaction (immediate vs. delayed reactions) and type of drug, and choosing the best test for a specific drug or drug class can be challenging.

The sensitivity and specificity of the LTT in the diagnosis of drug allergy have been estimated to range from 56 to 78% and from 85 to 93%, respectively, although these estimates are generally based on cases of allergy to β-lactam antibacterials and cannot be extended to other types of drugs. In the diagnosis of AHS due to aromatic anticonvulsants, the LTT has frequently shown a sensitivity between 71 and 100%, but this also ranges as low as 19–40%.

Combined use of pharmacoepidemiological approaches and biological markers is needed to improve the ability to predict adverse drug reactions in children and prevent severe morbidity and mortality.

References

Beeler A, Pichler WJ (2007) *In vitro* tests of T-cell-mediated drug hypersensitivity. In: Pichler WJ (ed) Drug hypersensitivity. Karger, Basel, pp 380–390

Beeler A, Engler O, Gerber BO et al (2006) Long-lasting reactivity and high frequency of drug-specific T cells after severe systemic drug hypersensitivity reactions. J Allergy Clin Immunol 117:455–462

Begaud B, Moride Y, Tubert-Bitter P, Chaslerie A, Haramburu F (1994) False-positives in spontaneous reporting: should we worry about them? Br J Clin Pharmacol 38:401–404

Berkovitch M, Pope E, Phillips J, Koren G (1995) Pemoline-associated fulminant liver failure: testing the evidence for causation. Clin Pharmacol Ther 57:696–698

Canada (1981) Drugs Directorate. Canadian Drug Identification Code

Canadian Pharmaceutical Association and Canadian Pharmacists Association (1986) Compendium of pharmaceuticals and specialties. Canadian Pharmaceutical Association, Toronto

Elzagallaai AA, Knowles SR, Rieder MJ, Bend JR, Shear NH, Koren G (2009) *In vitro* testing for the diagnosis of anticonvulsant hypersensitivity syndrome. Mol Diagn Ther 13:313–330

Etwel FA, Rieder MJ, Bend JR, Koren G (2008) A surveillance method for the early identification of idiosyncratic adverse drug reactions. Drug Saf 31:169–180

Holland P, Mauer AM (1964) Drug-induced *in-vitro* stimulation of peripheral lymphocytes. Lancet 1:1368–1369

Kwan P, Brodie MJ (2001) Effectiveness of first antiepileptic drug. Epilepsia 42:1255–1260

Lan CC, Wu CS, Tsai PC et al (2006) Diagnostic role of soluble fas ligand and secretion by peripheral blood mononuclear cells from patients with previous drug-induced blistering disease: a pilot study. Acta Derm Venereol 86:215–218

Lazarou J, Pomeranz BH, Corey PN (1998) Incidence of adverse drug reactions in hospitalized patients: a meta-analysis of prospective studies. J Am Med Assoc 279:1200–1205

Liu E, Dobyns E, Narkewicz M (2001) Acute hepatic failure in children: a seven year experience at a children's hospital. Hepatology 34:197A

Meyboom RH, Egberts AC, Edwards IR, Hekster YA, de Koning FH, Gribnau FW (1997) Principles of signal detection in pharmacovigilance. Drug Saf Int J Med Toxicol Drug Exp 16:355–365

Millichap JG (1976) The hyperactive child. Practitioner 217:61–65

Naranjo CA, Busto U, Sellers EM (1981) A method for estimating the probability of adverse drug reactions. Clin Pharmacol Ther 30:239–245

Naranjo CA, Sher NH, Lanctot KL (1992) Advances in the diagnosis of adverse drug reactions. J Clin Pharmacol 32:897–904

Nowell PC (1960) Phytohemagglutinin: an initiator of mitosis in cultures of normal human leukocytes. Cancer Res 20:4

Pearmain G, Lycette RR, Fitzgerald PH (1963) Tuberculin-induced mitosis in peripheral blood leucocytes. Lancet 1:637–638

Peyriere H, Dereure O, Breton H et al (2006) Variability in the clinical pattern of cutaneous side-effects of drugs with systemic symptoms: does a DRESS syndrome really exist? Br J Dermatol 155:422–433

Pirmohamed M, Breckenridge AM, Kitteringham NR, Park BK (1998) Fortnightly review: adverse drug reactions. Br Med J 316:1295–1298

Pourpak Z, Fazlollahi MR, Fattahi F (2008) Understanding adverse drug reactions and drug allergies: principles, diagnosis and treatment aspects. Recent Pat Inflamm Allergy Drug Discov 2:24–46

Rigas DA, Osgood EE (1955) Purification and properties of the phytohemagglutinin of *Phaseolus vulgaris*. J Biol Chem 212:607–615

Shapiro LE, Shear NH (1996) Mechanisms of drug reactions: the metabolic track. Semin Cutan Med Surg 15:217–227

Shear NH, Spielberg SP (1988) Anticonvulsants hypersensitivity syndrome: in vitro assessment of risk. J Clin Invest 82:1826–1832

Spielberg SP (1980) Acetaminophen toxicity in human lymphocytes *in vitro*. J Pharmacol Exp Ther 213:395–398

Spielberg SP, Gordon GB, Blake DA et al (1981a) Anticonvulsant toxicity in vitro: possible role of arene oxides. J Pharmacol Exp Ther 217:386–389

Spielberg SP, Gordon GB, Blake DA et al (1981b) Predisposition to phenytoin hepatotoxicity assessed in vitro. N Engl J Med 305:722–727

Stevenson RD, Wolraich ML (1989) Stimulant medication therapy in the treatment of children with attention deficit hyperactivity disorder. Pediatr Clin North Am 36:1183–1197

Stricker BC, Psaty BM (2004) Detection, verification, and quantification of adverse drug reactions. Br Med J 329:44–47

Tennis P, Stern RS (1997) Risk of serious cutaneous disorders after initiation of use of phenytoin, carbamazepine, or sodium valproate: a record linkage study. Neurology 49:542–546

Wu Y, Sanderson JP, Farrell J et al (2006) Activation of T cells by carbamazepine and carbamazepine metabolites. J Allergy Clin Immunol 118:233–241

Zaccara G, Franciotta D, Perucca E (2007) Idiosyncratic adverse reactions to antiepileptic drugs. Epilepsia 48:1223–1244

Zielinskin SL (2005) FDA attempting to overcome major roadblocks in monitoring drug safety. J Natl Cancer Inst 97:872–873

Small Sample Approach, and Statistical and Epidemiological Aspects

Martin Offringa and Hanneke van der Lee

Contents

Abstract In this chapter, the design of pharmacokinetic studies and phase III trials in children is discussed. Classical approaches and relatively novel approaches, which may be more useful in the context of drug research in children, are discussed. The burden of repeated blood sampling in pediatric pharmacokinetic studies may be overcome by the population pharmacokinetics approach using nonlinear mixed effect modeling as the statistical solution to sparse data. Indications and contraindications for phase III trials are discussed: only when there is true "equipoise" in the medical scientific community, it is ethical to conduct a randomized clinical trial. The many reasons why a pediatric trial may fail are illustrated with examples. Inadequate sample sizes lead to inconclusive results. Twelve classical strategies to minimize sample sizes are discussed followed by an introduction to group

M. Offringa (✉) • H. van der Lee
Department of Paediatric Clinical Epidemiology, Emma Children's Hospital, Academic Medical Centre, University of Amsterdam, Meibergdreef 9, 1105 AZ Amsterdam, The Netherlands
e-mail: m.offringa@amc.uva.nl

H.W. Seyberth et al. (eds.), *Pediatric Clinical Pharmacology*,
Handbook of Experimental Pharmacology 205,
DOI 10.1007/978-3-642-20195-0_9, © Springer-Verlag Berlin Heidelberg 2011

sequential design, boundaries design, and adaptive design. The evidence that these designs reduce sample sized between 35 and 70% is reviewed. The advantages and disadvantages of the different approaches are highlighted to give the reader a broad idea of the design types that can be considered. Finally, working with DMCs during the conduct of trials is introduced. The evidence regarding DMC activities, interim analysis results, and early termination of pediatric trials is presented. So far reporting is incomplete and heterogeneous, and users of trial reports may be misled by the results. A proposal for a checklist for the reporting of DMC issues, interim analyses, and early stopping is presented.

Keywords Pharmacokinetics • Sample size • Power • Phase III trial • Pediatrics • Child • Data Monitoring Committees • Interim analysis • Sequential design • Triangular test

1 Part 1: Design of Pharmacokinetic Studies

1.1 Pharmacokinetics Trials, the Classical Approach

The goal of pharmacokinetic (PK) studies is to obtain generalizable information about Absorption, Distribution, Metabolism, and Excretion (ADME) to make rational dosing and administration decisions. For many drugs, PK information is available from adults, but the question is whether this information can be extrapolated to children. For many drugs, we know that this is not the case. Children differ from adults with regard to the ADME characteristics in various ways, and, moreover, within the wide age range from premature to adolescent there is no linear development. Thus, PK studies need to be performed in various age groups. The choice of these groups and the priority between age categories depend on clinical, pathophysiological, and pharmacological considerations.

The classical approach of a PK study is a dose-escalation study. Participants are randomized to receive either a prespecified dose or placebo; blood is drawn after, e.g., 0.5, 1, 2, 4, 6, 8, 12, 16, and 24 h. Several dosages are specified in advance and investigated simultaneously or sequentially. When dosages are investigated sequentially, an interim analysis is performed after each dose has been tested in a prespecified number of individuals. If there are no reasons to stop the study (either because there is no relevant difference with the former dose or because of safety), the next higher dose is investigated in the next group of participants. As an example, the results are shown of a PK study of lisdexamfetamine dimesylate in children with attention-deficit/hyperactivity disorder (ADHD) aged 6–12 (Boellner et al. 2010) (Table 1).

The number of participants in a classical PK study is usually based on earlier information about the variability of results. Typically between 10 and 20 participants are included for each dosage to be studied.

Table 1 PK study of lisdexamfetamine dimesylate in children with attention-deficit/hyperactivity disorder (reprinted with permission from Boellner et al. 2010)

	LDX dose (mg)		
Pharmacokinetic parameter	30 ($n = 16^{\mathrm{a}}$)	50 ($n = 17$)	70 ($n = 17$)
C_{max}, ng/mL Mean (SD)[*], %CV	53.2 (9.62), 18.1	93.3 (18.2), 19.5	134 (26.1), 19.4
T_{max}, h Mean (SD), %CV	3.41 (1.09), 31.9	3.58 (1.18), 33.0	3.46 (1.34), 38.6
$t_{1/2}$, h Mean (SD), %CV	8.90 (1.33), 15.0	8.61 (1.04), 12.1	8.64 (1.32), 15.3
$AUC_{0-\infty}$, ng/mL/h Mean (SD)[*], %CV	844.6 (116.7), 13.8	1,510.0 (241.6), 16.0	2,157.0 (383.3), 17.8
AUC_{0-t}, ng/mL/h Mean (SD)[*], %CV	745.3 (129.3), 17.4	1,448.0 (246.7), 17.0	2,088.0 (394.0), 18.9

[a]Pharmacokinetic data were unavailable in one patient at the 30-mg dose; this patient was excluded from the analysis
[*]$P < 0.001$ (ANOVA)

In a sequential dose-escalation study, sometimes dose finding is approached by "continual reassessment" methods, in which the next dosage is defined based on the results of the earlier steps. According to the Efficacy Working Party of the European Medicines Agency (EMA) Committee for Medicinal Products for Human Use (CHMP): "The properties of such methods far outstrip those of conventional 'up and down' dose finding designs. They tend to find the optimum (however defined) dose quicker, they treat more patients at the optimum dose, and they estimate the optimum dose more accurately" (CHMP 2006b).

1.2 Population Pharmacokinetics

In pediatric PK studies, the burden of repeated blood sampling is a problem. In the ADHD example, blood samples were taken from an indwelling catheter to minimize pain from multiple hand vein sticks. In younger children, blood sampling may be an even greater challenge. In neonates or premature infants, not only the number of samples, but also the amount of blood that can be withdrawn for each measurement has to be minimized, thus making great demands on the analysis techniques to measure drug levels.

In a population PK study, each individual contributes to the dataset with a small number of (typically 2) samples. By using nonlinear mixed effect modeling, e.g., with the NONMEM program, PK parameters are estimated taking into account the variability within and between individuals (De Cock et al. 2010).

Validation is necessary, first in existing datasets, or in a part of the original dataset in which the PK model was built, and subsequently in prospective studies. Proper validation is reported to have been performed only in a minority of PK studies (De Cock et al. 2010).

For prospective studies, several software packages can help define the optimal number of participants and sampling frame, e.g., WINPOPT and PopED. It should be acknowledged that many factors have to be taken into account (Ogungbenro and Aarons 2008).

2 Part 2: Phase III Clinical Trials: Classic and Novel Designs

2.1 When Is a Phase III Clinical Trial Necessary?

In the Christmas issue of the British Medical Journal of 2003, a paper was published entitled "Parachute use to prevent death and major trauma related to gravitational challenge: systematic review of randomised controlled trials" (Smith and Pell 2003). It is not surprising that the literature search preformed to detect any such RCTs yielded no results. When the natural course of a disease is known, and case reports show clearly and unambiguously that a particular intervention changes the natural course in the preferred direction, it would be unethical to include patients in a randomized clinical trial (Glasziou et al. 2007; Peto and Baigent 1998). Examples of this principle are PGE_1 infusion for ductus patency in newborns with obstructive right heart malformation and indomethacin treatment of newborns with life-threatening polyuric salt-losing tubulopathies (SLTs). The therapeutic advantage of these treatments is beyond any doubt. Only when there is true "equipoise" in the medical scientific community, it is ethical to conduct an RCT (Edwards et al. 1998). In the development of new drugs, RCTs usually cannot be avoided. However, it is not always necessary or ethical to perform these trials in children (Sammons 2011).

2.2 Classical Sample Size Calculations

Imagine a pediatrician who wants to investigate whether a new drug leads to more improvement in a specified outcome than the old drug. How many patients does he or she need to include in the study? The consulted statistician will explain that the required sample size is defined by the power of the study, the significance level, whether a one- or two-sided test is required, the variance of the outcome in the study population, and the expected or clinically relevant difference in the outcome between the two intervention groups to be detected.

2.2.1 Sample Size Calculation and Power

Sample size calculations are necessary to minimize the risk of false-negative results. Although often neglected, there is also a risk of a false-positive result in hypothesis testing. When the threshold α for the level of statistical significance is set at 0.05, this means that we accept a false-positive rate of 5%.

The null hypothesis H_0 to be tested states that there is no difference in outcome between the groups and the alternative hypothesis states that there is a difference. In case of a two-sided test, which is usually applied, the difference can either mean superiority or inferiority of the experimental intervention compared to the control intervention.

A one-sided test is applied if inferiority of the experimental intervention is considered very improbable (Knottnerus and Bouter 2001). The result of a one-sided test can either be non-inferiority, i.e., not worse, possibly better than the control intervention, or superiority, i.e., definitely better than the control intervention. When a one-sided test is applied, the null hypothesis states that the effect of the experimental intervention is either worse, in case of a non-inferiority trial, or worse than or equal to the control intervention, in case of a superiority trial. If the data that are obtained in the study are very unlikely under the null hypothesis, so unlikely that the probability to obtain these or more extreme data is smaller than α, we reject the null hypothesis. This leaves a probability of α for a false-positive result or type I error.

If the alternative hypothesis is true, there is a risk, called β, of obtaining data that are not unlikely under the null hypothesis, which leads to a false-negative result or type II error. Usually, the risk of a type II error (false-negative result) is considered to be less undesirable than a type I error. Therefore, β is usually set at 10 or 20%. The power of a study is the probability of rejecting the null hypothesis if the alternative hypothesis is true, i.e., $1 - \beta$. As an example, the general formula for a continuous outcome measure to calculate the required sample size for a T-test is as follows:

$$N = (Z_{\alpha/2} + Z_{(1-\beta)})^2 \times \frac{\sigma^2}{(\mu_1 - \mu_2)^2} \tag{1}$$

$$\sigma^2 = \sigma_1^2 + \sigma_2^2 - 2r\sigma_1\sigma_2 \tag{2}$$

In which N is the number of subjects per group, $Z_{\alpha/2}$ is the value of the standard Normal distribution corresponding with the chosen value of α (two-sided), $Z_{(1-\beta)}$ is its equivalent for the chosen value of β, σ^2 is the variance of the outcome variable in

Table 2 Theoretical probabilities of correct and false conclusions of hypothesis testing

Investigator's conclusion	(Unknown) reality	
	H_0 true	H_0 not true
H_0 not rejected	$1 - \alpha$	β type II error
H_0 rejected	α type I error level of significance	$1 - \beta$ power

H_0 = Null hypothesis

the study population, which is the sum of the variances in the two groups minus two times the product of the standard deviations in the two groups multiplied by the correlation between the observations ($r = 0$: unpaired t-test, $r > 0$ paired t-test), and μ_1 and μ_2 are the estimated means of the outcome variable in the two groups to be compared.

From this formula, it becomes clear that the required sample size increases if we choose a smaller risk of type I (α) or type II errors (β), if the variability σ^2 is larger, or if the difference that we want to be able to detect ($\mu_1 - \mu_2$) is smaller.

These days regulatory authorities and many journal editors request that the results of a study are expressed as point estimates and 95% Confidence Intervals (CIs). The advantage of this presentation, estimation instead of hypothesis testing, is that the size of the effect can be appreciated as well as its statistical significance. Thus, a small effect with a narrow CI may be statistically significant, i.e., the neutral value lies outside the CI, but because of its small size the effect may be considered to be clinically irrelevant, whereas a large effect that is not statistically significant – i.e., $p > 0.05$; neutral value inside CI – may be considered to be important for clinical practice. However, if the CI is wide, more information is needed to get a precise estimate. It is quite possible that the effect found in one small study turns out to be negligible when the study is replicated in a larger sample.

2.2.2 Practical and Ethical Issues

When designing a clinical trial, the probability of finding an effect if there is one in reality, i.e., a true-positive result, should be maximized, irrespective of whether the result will be expressed as estimation or as a hypothesis test. As we have seen, this can be achieved by maximizing the number of subjects included in the study. However, there are practical and ethical restraints to the inclusion of large numbers of subjects, especially in the pediatric population. Usually, the number of children eligible for the study is limited because many conditions are uncommon.

Furthermore, the financial and time resources are always limited. Apart from that, clinicians have an ethical obligation to give the best treatment to their patients. As long as there is equipoise, i.e., the medical scientific community is uncertain which treatment is best, it is justified to include patients in a clinical trial. However, suppose there were no practical limitations to including patients in a trial, and a researcher would continue including patients, at a certain moment the results could be expressed in a very narrow CI. At what moment would equipoise be abandoned? That would be the moment to stop including patients in the trial and to start treating consecutive patients with the optimal intervention mode. Therefore, for each trial it has to be stated in advance when to stop including patients. Usually, this is done by calculating the number of patients needed to get 80 or 90% certainty that if there is an effect of a predefined size, it will be found statistically significant at $\alpha = 0.05$. However, this calculation often leads to required sample sizes that are very hard, or impossible to attain.

2.3 Inadequate Sample Size

Inadequate sample sizes lead to inconclusive results. As an example, from December 1997 to March 2001 data were collected for a multicenter randomized placebo-controlled trial in the Netherlands to evaluate the efficacy of intravenous dexamethasone in young patients mechanically ventilated for respiratory syncytial virus lower respiratory tract infection (van Woensel et al. 2003). Randomization was stratified by center. The number of patients to be included was calculated based on the notion that a between-group reduction in duration of mechanical ventilation of 1.5 days was clinically relevant.

The authors reported a mean difference between the placebo group and the dexamethasone group of 1.6 days; 95% CI $= -0.8$ to $+3.8$ days. Thus, the point estimate showed a clinically relevant difference, but the 95% CI was not narrow enough to reach statistical significance. This 95% CI indicates that dexamethasone may reduce the duration of mechanical ventilation with almost 4 days or it may extend its duration with almost 1 day. It means that, although the difference is not statistically significant, the possibility of a clinically relevant beneficial effect of dexamethasone has not been excluded.

This result could be described as "no evidence of effect" (Tarnow-Mordi and Healy 1999). Clinicians need to make decisions about the administration of treatments, in this case dexamethasone. Inconclusive evidence is better than no evidence at all, but not really helpful in clinical decision-making.

What was the reason that no definitive, statistically significant result was found in this trial? As it turned out, the sample size estimation was based on too optimistic assumptions for the variability of the outcome measure; a flaw that is often encountered (van der Lee et al. 2009; Vickers 2003).

2.4 Classical Strategies to Minimize Sample Sizes

The problem of limited availability of subjects to be included in a trial has led to different strategies used by researchers to improve power. As was stated in the EMA guideline on clinical trials in small populations (CHMP 2006a), "No methods exist that are relevant to small studies that are not also applicable to large studies. However, it may be that in conditions with small and very small populations, less conventional and/or less commonly seen methodological approaches may be acceptable if they help to improve the interpretability of the study results."

We describe 12 possible approaches, i.e., (1) use of one-sided instead of two-sided hypothesis testing, (2) inflation of the minimal clinically relevant difference, (3) composite or (4) surrogate outcomes, (5) improved reproducibility of outcome measurements, (6) repeated measurements, (7) the crossover design, (8) matching or stratification, (9) analysis of covariance instead of simple comparison of outcomes in two groups, (10) response-adaptive design, (11) conducting an underpowered trial for a later meta-analysis, and (12) the prospective meta-analysis approach. Table 3 gives an overview of these approaches, their drawbacks, and their applicability in pediatric drug development trials.

Ad (1) One-sided instead of two-sided testing has been suggested for ethical and efficiency reasons when inferiority of the experimental intervention is considered very improbable (Knottnerus and Bouter 2001). However, other authors are convinced that each randomized trial should also be able to detect harm in terms of a worse outcome due to the experimental intervention (Moye and Tita 2002). Usually, one-sided testing is limited to the non-inferiority design.

Ad (2) The assumptions to be made in advance in the design phase of the study are often arbitrary. Sometimes negotiations take place between the researcher and the statistician. "If we want to detect a 10% difference, we need 132 patients but if we expect the difference to be 15%, we need 52 patients." Since there are no criteria to be used in defining the minimal clinically relevant difference, this is often used as a "closing entry." The number of patients that can be recruited is usually the limiting factor, α and β are more or less predetermined, and the variance in the study population cannot be altered. This leaves the minimal clinically relevant difference as the only input in the power formula that can be adjusted. This procedure has been referred to as a "sample size samba" (Schulz and Grimes 2005).

Ad (3) In the field of AIDS research, the "simple" outcome mortality became less frequent due to advances in treatment. The use of mortality as an outcome variable would have led to an increase in the required sample size. Therefore, composite outcomes were formulated, consisting of a number of possible adverse events, e.g., first symptoms of disease progression expressed as neurological symptoms or growth retardation (McKinney et al. 1998).

Ad (4) Another way of increasing power is to use surrogate outcomes, which allow a smaller size of the study population, for instance, glomerular filtration rate instead of patient or graft survival in renal transplant trials (Filler et al. 2003). An important prerequisite for a surrogate outcome is that its predictive validity or association with the "true clinical outcome" should be established (CHMP 2006a).

Ad (5) If the outcome measure is a continuous variable, it may be possible to improve its reproducibility and in this way reduce the Standard Deviation. Improving the reproducibility typically starts with a clinimetric study, sometimes called a Generalizability study, in which the influence of several possible sources of variability, called "facets," is quantified. Subsequently, approaches are proposed and investigated to improve the reproducibility of the measurement. Depending on the type of measurement, these approaches may consist of better standardization of the measurement process or of the use of a mean value of repeated measurements instead of one single measurement value. The effect of such a mean value,

Table 3 Classical approaches to minimize sample size

Principle	Application (related to approach # in text)	Drawbacks	Recommendation for pediatric drug trials
Enhancing statistical power			
Significance level ↑		Increased risk of type I error	
	One-sided instead of two-sided test (1)	Less convincing, no conclusion about possible harm	+/−
Minimal clinically important difference ↑	"Sample size samba" (2)	Risk of missing a truly relevant effect	−
Variance ↓		In most instances, this cannot be influenced	
	Composite outcomes (3)	Conclusion may be based on less relevant components of the composite outcome	+
	Surrogate outcomes (4)	Validity issue: association with truly relevant outcomes is often insufficient or unknown	+/−
	Improve reproducibility (5)	Practical and logistical constraints	+
	Repeated measurements (6)	Practical, logistical, financial, and ethical constraints	+
	Crossover design (7)	Only possible in chronic conditions for treatments with no carry-over effect; very seldom in children	−
	Restriction, matching, andstratification (8)	Selection of study participants jeopardizes recruitment; limitation of external validity	+/−
	Analysis of covariance (9)	Only applicable when outcome is continuous and can be assessed before randomization and after the intervention	+
Minimizing sample size while preserving power			
	Response-adaptive design (10)	Cumbersome; only for short term outcomes; modest effects on sample size	+/−
Beyond single trials			
	Meta-analysis of several small trials (11)	Often heterogeneity between trials, e.g., variability in inclusion criteria, dosages, comparisons, and outcome measures	−[a]
	Prospective meta-analysis (12)	Organizational challenge; discouraged by publication policies	++

[a]Retrospective meta-analysis is considered very relevant for clinical guideline development, but not for drug development

and the optimal number of repeated measurements, can be investigated in a so-called Decision study, which consists of simulations based on the information from the G-study (Streiner and Norman 2008).

Ad (6) The use of repeated measurements to increase statistical power often has important practical limitations. Nevertheless, in some cases it may be possible to use repeated outcome measures. The number of subjects required is then obtained by multiplying formula (1) with $\{1 + (T - 1)r\}/T$, in which T is the number of measurements and r is the correlation between subsequent measurements in the same subject. For instance, if the number of subjects needed is 60, this can be reduced to 40 by using three measurements instead of one, assuming the correlation between measurements to be 0.5 (Twisk 2003).

Ad (7) In a crossover design, the sample size is reduced because all subjects serve as their own controls and the reduction in sample size is linearly related to the observed correlation (r) between the measurements under the two treatments (see equation 2) (von Goedecke et al. 2005). The correlation between the measurements is usually estimated to be 0.5 in a crossover trial. Thus, a parallel trial, for which 502 children would be required ($\alpha = 0.05$, $\beta = 0.20$, effect size is 0.25), could be replaced by a crossover trial including 126 children. The most important requirement for a crossover design is that there is no carry-over effect, i.e., that the treatment given in the first phase has no influence at all during the second phase of the study (Woods et al. 1989). This requirement is often not convincingly met. Especially in pediatric research this is hard to prove, when the outcome may be influenced by developmental factors. A particular type of crossover design is the N-of-1 trial series, in which several – usually more than 2 – treatment periods of the drugs under investigation are randomized in individual patients. The advantage of this type of trial is that each participant will finally find out which drug is best for him or her. Disadvantages are, apart from the requirements that need to be met for all crossover trials, the limited external validity or generalizability to other patients.

Ad (8) Restriction by using severe inclusion criteria leads to less variability between trial subjects, but limits the external validity of a trial and may hamper recruitment, which is often a limiting factor in the execution of a pediatric trial. Restriction, matching, or stratification makes the analysis more efficient. However, the influence of the matching factors cannot be investigated anymore.

Ad (9) Analysis of covariance including the baseline score as a determinant in the analysis adds information to the analysis and improves the statistical power, as was shown by Vickers and Altman. This approach is comparable to the repeated measurements approach (Vickers and Altman 2001).

Ad (10) Response-adaptive design is a way of treatment allocation aimed at maximizing the power and minimizing the number of patients allocated to the "inferior" treatment while preserving randomization. One of the requirements for this type of design is that outcomes should become available early in the trial. The effect on total sample size is modest (Rosenberger and Huc 2004).

Ad (11) Some scientists state that conducting an underpowered trial is unethical (Freiman et al. 1978). However, given the small numbers of specific diagnoses seen in most pediatric clinics, the only way to obtain a sufficient sample size is by conducting a (international) multicenter study, which is hampered by practical and logistic problems. Therefore, it may be more realistic to perform a small, underpowered trial, the results of which are presented in such a way that they can be incorporated in a meta-analysis (Sackett and Cook 1993).

Ad (12) A recent development is a prospective meta-analysis using individual patient data. This is a type of design which combines some aspects of a multicenter study with a meta-analytic approach (Simes 1995).

2.5 Group Sequential Design, Boundaries Design, and Adaptive Design

The principles of randomized clinical trials were originally derived from agricultural research, in which the statistical methods of analysis of variance and regression analysis were developed (Whitehead 1997). An essential difference between agricultural and clinical trials is the time period during which data are gathered. In an agricultural field trial, all crops are harvested simultaneously at the end of the growth season, whereas in clinical trials it usually takes weeks or months, sometimes even years before all subjects are included, and consequently the gathering of the outcome data is extended over a similarly long time period. Thus, it is possible that before the end of the inclusion phase of a clinical trial enough information has already been assembled, though usually not analyzed, to decide which intervention is superior.

Because subjects will be included and randomized until the sample size that was determined in advance has been reached, this may lead to inefficiency, that is, inappropriate inclusion of subjects, unnecessarily prolonging the trial duration, and, more importantly, to allocation of trial subjects to the "inferior" intervention at a time when the evidence of its inferiority might be available. Some authors have referred to such practices as substandard or unethical (van der Lee et al. 2010; Whitehead 1997). Sequential designs were developed to overcome these problems.

Various sequential procedures exist, and they can be (roughly) divided into two types, namely those derived from the repeated significance test approach, also called group sequential designs, and those derived from the boundaries approach. Because there is no uniform terminology, we make a distinction between "design" and "analysis" (Sebille and Bellissant 2003). Thus, within the boundaries design a distinction can be made between "continuous sequential analysis" and "group sequential analysis." Recently, a modification of the group sequential design has been proposed, called the adaptive design. We will discuss the group sequential design, the boundaries design, and adaptive design in more detail below.

2.5.1 Group Sequential Design, Repeated Significance Testing

In this approach, a series of conventional statistical analyses, so-called interim analyses, are carried out at various predetermined time points on the accumulating data. The basis for this methodology was laid by Armitage in the 1970s (Armitage 1958, 1975). To ensure an overall type I error probability (α), the significant thresholds at the various time points are adjusted to allow for the repetition (α^*). Various methods for α-adjustment have been proposed, either with the same α^* for all analyses, Pocock's method (Pocock 1977), which is seldom used, or with different α^* at each analysis, for example, O'Brien and Fleming (1979), and Haybittle and Peto (Haybittle 1971). As an example, when two analyses are planned, i.e., one interim and one final analysis, the method of O'Brien and Fleming prescribes α^* of 0.0054 and 0.0492 for the interim and the final analysis, respectively. In the same situation, α^* would be 0.0100 and 0.0500 for the interim and the final analysis, respectively, for the Haybittle–Peto method. In contrast to the earlier methods of Pocock, O'Brien and Fleming, and Haybittle–Peto, the so-called α-spending function developed by Lan and De Mets (Lan and DeMets 1983) that characterizes the rate at which the α is spent and thus determines the α^* at each interim analysis only depends on the number of past and current interim analyses and not on the number of future interim analyses. This approach enhances the flexibility of the design, because the number of (interim) analyses does not have to be predetermined. Further modifications included the possibility of stopping early when there is no relevant difference between the intervention groups (stopping for futility) (Emerson and Fleming 1989; Pampallona and Tsiatis 1994).

An example of a useful interim analysis, when the original effect size estimation appeared too conservative in retrospect, is a randomized clinical trial to investigate the difference in incidence of injection pain during intravenous induction of anesthesia in children between a new formulation (Etomidate–[R]Lipuro) and the existing standard of propofol with added lidocaine (Nyman et al. 2006). The required sample size, calculated based on an expected proportion of 25% in the propofol–lidocaine group and 5% in the Etomidate–[R]Lipuro group, α of 0.05, and power of 90%, was reported to be 110. On request of the Ethics Committee, an interim analysis was planned after the inclusion of 80 patients, with a nominal value $\alpha^* = 0.02$. The rationale for the interim analysis was to prevent unnecessary injection pain in children if there was a difference in pain incidence between the two groups. The underlying considerations for the timing and α^* of the interim analysis were not reported. The study was ended when this interim analysis showed a significantly lower incidence of injection pain in the Etomidate–[R]Lipuro group (5%; 95% CI = 0.61–16.9%) than in the propofol–lidocaine group (47.5%; 95% CI = 31.5–63.9%) ($P = 0.0007$) (Nyman et al. 2006).

2.5.2 Boundaries Design

This approach relies on a graphical rule, where a V statistic, representing the amount of information gathered in the course of a trial, is plotted on the X-axis, and a Z statistic, representing the effect size, is plotted on the Y-axis. Prior to the start of the experiment, the boundaries are calculated based on the alternative hypothesis and the desired levels of the type I and II errors (α and β, respectively). Examples of boundaries are shown in Fig. 1.

Tests of this type are descendants of the sequential probability ratio test (SPRT) of Wald (Wald 1947; Whitehead 1997). Initially, these methods could only be used to compare a single proportion or mean to a hypothetical value, or for the comparison of two proportions (paired observations). These restrictions hampered a successful application of these types of tests. After modifications by Whitehead (Whitehead and Jones 1979; Whitehead and Stratton 1983), comparison of two independent groups with respect to continuous, binomial (e.g., alive/dead), or censored outcomes (survival data) was possible, thus increasing the applicability of the methods. In an SPRT, the boundaries are parallel (Fig. 1a), giving an infinite "continuation region." Therefore, it is theoretically possible that a trial requires an almost infinite value of V (and thus n), which renders this test impracticable for clinical trials.

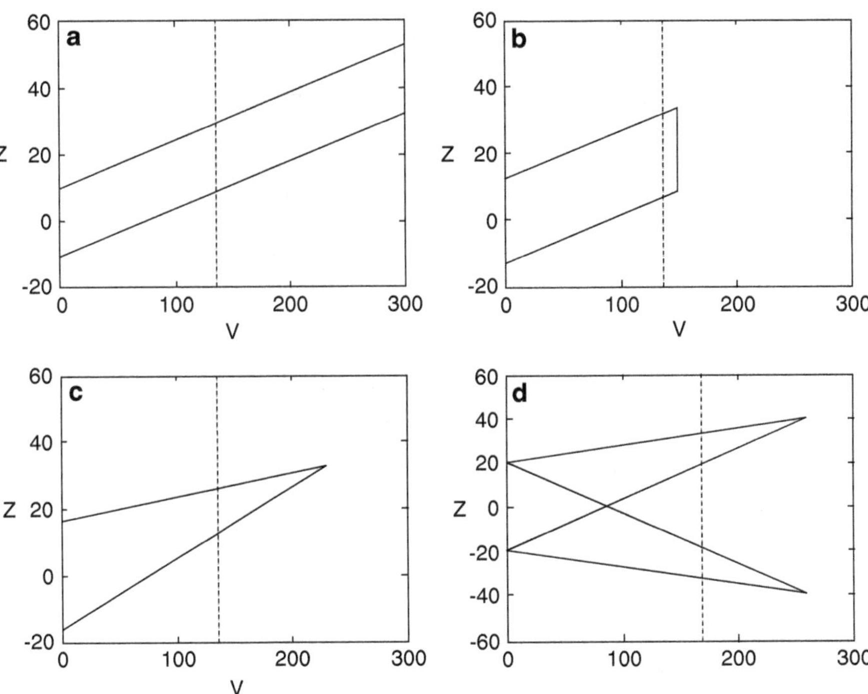

Fig. 1 Boundaries design in four hypothetical cases – see text for details (reprinted with permission from van der Lee et al. 2008)

At each analysis, which can be done after each patient (continuous sequential analysis) or after a fixed or variable number of patients (group sequential analysis), the two statistics Z and V are calculated based on the data accumulated thus far, and plotted, creating a so-called sample path. This is illustrated in Fig. 2.

Inclusion and randomization of subjects are continued as long as the sample path remains between the boundaries (continuation region). A conclusion is reached when a boundary is crossed. In case of a one-sided test, that is, investigating only whether the experimental treatment leads to a better outcome than the control treatment, a single pair of boundaries is plotted (Fig. 1a–c). Crossing of the upper boundary leads to rejection of the null hypothesis; crossing of the lower boundary leads to non-rejection of the null hypothesis.

Two pairs of boundaries are plotted symmetrically around the horizontal axis in case of a two-sided test, in which both possibilities of better and worse outcomes of the experimental compared to the control treatment are investigated (Fig. 1d). Crossing of the upper or lower boundary leads to the conclusion that the experimental treatment is superior or inferior, respectively; crossing of the boundaries between both pairs of boundaries leads to non-rejection of the null hypothesis.

Alternatives that are useful in clinical trials are the truncated SPRT (Fig. 1b) and the triangular test (TT) (Fig. 1c) (Anderson 1960; Whitehead 1997). In the truncated SPRT, a maximum value (L) of V is determined after which the trial stops, irrespective of the result. This truncation point L is chosen more or less arbitrarily, but it has to be beyond the amount of information V_{FIXED} required for the equivalent fixed sample design to correct for multiple hypothesis testing. The space between the parallel boundaries is influenced by the choice of L. In other words, the choice of L has consequences for the sample size. For a given α, β, and effect size, the boundaries are closer to each other with increasing L. In case of the TT (Fig. 1c, d), the boundaries are convergent, resulting in a finite "continuation region." Therefore, the optimal properties of the SPRT and TT differ: the average sample size reduction is larger with the SPRT when the actual effect size is (much) larger than expected and smaller when the actual effect size is smaller than expected (Fig. 1a vs. c) (Sebille and Bellissant 2000). When the actual and expected effect sizes are similar, the expected sample size reductions are about equal. Obviously, it is impossible to predict whether the actual effect size will be smaller or larger than the expected effect size. In practice, in most trials, the actual effect size turns out to be smaller than expected. In those cases, the TT is more efficient (Sebille and Bellissant 2000). In contrast to the classical fixed sample size design, the eventual amount of information, that is, number of patients, needed to complete a trial is unknown at the start of a sequential trial. The choice of design usually depends on the statistician's expertise and the availability of the software.

Although correction for multiple testing results in a larger maximal possible sample size (the amount of information which is represented by the apex of the triangle in Fig. 1c, d), the average sample size needed to complete a trial using a sequential method in simulations was always smaller than that of the corresponding fixed design, irrespective of the effect size or power (Sebille and Bellissant 2000). The 90th percentiles of the sample size distributions of the sequential designs were in the same order of magnitude as the corresponding fixed designs, when the actual effect was close to the expected effect, but larger when the actual effect was smaller than expected, especially for the SPRT. In principle, Z and V can be calculated after each individual patient, but generally Z and V are calculated after the data of a number of patients have become available, that is, group sequential analysis.

Given the possibility that intermediate points, if plotted, could have lain outside the triangular region during long gaps between inspections, and thus opportunities for stopping might have been missed, an adjustment of the stopping boundaries is made, resulting in a so-called Christmas tree shape (Fig. 2). After a boundary has been crossed, an adjusted point estimate and CI of the effect can be calculated with the computer program PEST or EaSt (2004; Cytel Software Corporation 1992). Due to the sequential nature of the analysis, the CIs are wider than those obtained with conventional fixed sample size methods of analysis.

In summary, the advantage of a sequential design is that the inclusion and randomization can be stopped when enough information is available to draw a definite conclusion, of either futility or efficacy, based on statistical significance. For a sequential trial to be feasible, the time from randomization to outcome should be limited relative to the recruitment rate. On average, the number of subjects needed is smaller than in a classical fixed sample size design. However, in a particular trial it may be larger than that. Drawbacks are that the eventual sample size is not exactly known at the start, which hampers logistic and financial planning, and that the 95% Confidence Intervals around the point estimate of the effect size are somewhat wider than when there is only one analysis at the end of the trial.

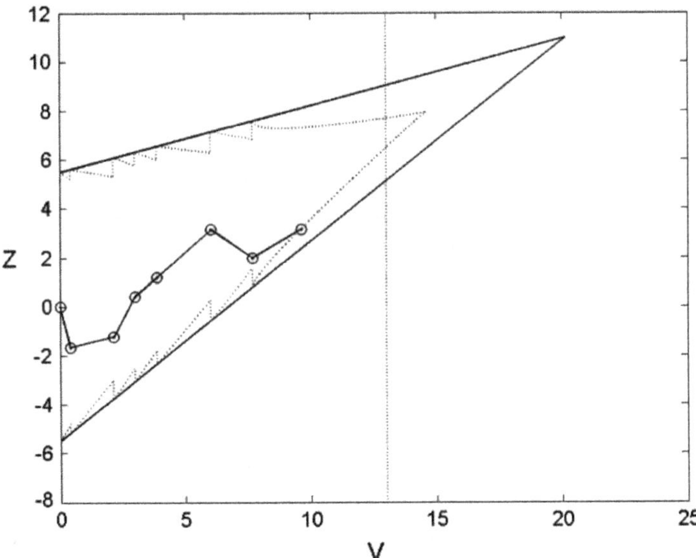

Fig. 2 One-sided superiority triangular test and sample path of a trial (reprinted with permission from van der Lee et al. 2008)

Table 4 Relative benefits and drawbacks of fixed sample size and triangular test

	Fixed sample size	Triangular test
Risk of biased end result	Small if conducted according to well-known standards; if no interim analyses have been planned, analysis can be done by investigators after all trial data have been assembled	Data analysis should be independent from trial performance and masked; important that confidentiality of results is ensured until the end of the trial
Feasibility in a multicenter trial	Logistics are known in advance; planning for a specific number of trial patients; outcome information may be assembled per center and sent to coordinating center later	Number of patients to be included unknown at study onset; planning may be hampered by uncertainties; block-randomization necessary to avoid discrepancies in numbers per arm; outcome information has to be sent to coordinating center immediately when it occurs or is measured
Familiarity, acceptance by funders, editors, peers, and readers	Very well known, generally accepted as the most valid design to answer questions of effects of interventions	Less familiar design; despite unjust suspicion for increased risk of type I errors, final analysis is valid, maintaining type I error and power

In Table 4, the relative benefits and drawbacks of the fixed sample size and triangular test are presented (van der Lee et al. 2009).

Bellissant et al. described a TT to assess the efficacy of metoclopramide on gastroesophageal reflux in infants (Bellissant et al. 1997). The trial was designed to detect a mean benefit on a continuous outcome scale of 0.5 with an expected standard deviation of 0.5 with 95% power and a one-sided α of 0.05. In a fixed design, 23 patients per treatment arm would have to be included. The authors anticipated that recruitment would be difficult and wanted to stop the study as soon as sufficient information was collected and decided, therefore, to use the TT. After 3 years and 9 months and inclusion of 39 children, the trial ended in futility, because the lower boundary was crossed (Fig. 2). The observed benefit of metoclopramide over placebo was approximately 0.2 instead of 0.5.

2.5.3 Adaptive or Flexible Design

Adaptive designs share a number of features with sequential designs, in which the null hypothesis is tested at a sequence of interim analyses (Wassmer 2000). However, in contrast, the design of an adaptive trial can be changed based on full knowledge gained from the interim analyses. When modifications are made, a new phase of trial starts, and data accumulated in (an) earlier phase(s) are no longer combined with data from the new phase. All phases are analyzed separately, and the P-values of the different phases are then combined using a predefined rule.

Examples of combination rules are the product criterion of Fisher (Bauer and Kohne 1994) and the inverse normal method by Lehmacher (Lehmacher and Wassmer 1999). The emphasis in these designs is more on flexibility of the design than on minimization of the average sample size.

Different adaptations are possible including reassessment of sample size (see critical reflection by Jennison and Turnbull 2003), selection of treatments (e.g., Hommel 2001; Kelly et al. 2005), adaptation of end points (e.g., Bauer and Kieser 1999; Kieser et al. 1999), or inserting or deleting interim analyses. See for a more extensive description of this design the tutorial by Bretz et al. (2009). However, many features, for example, definition of stopping rules (van Houwelingen 1999) or interpretation of the results when primary end points have been changed, for instance, are still subject for debate (CHMP 2006b).

The term "adaptive design" is a comprehensive term comprising many possible design adaptations (CHMP 2006b). It should not be confused with the more specific term "response-adaptive design," discussed in section "Inadequate Sample Size", where the allocation ratio can be adapted based on preliminary results from the trial (Coad and Ivanova 2005). To our knowledge, no pediatric trials with an adaptive design have been published so far. Because it maximizes the efficiency of data gathering from individual patients, this approach deserves more attention (Hirtz et al. 2006).

2.5.4 Implications of Sequential and Adaptive Designs

In a systematic review of pediatric trials using a sequential design 24 sequential trials, published between 1963 and 2005, were found (van der Lee et al. 2010). In nine studies, the information about the assumptions was sufficient to calculate a fixed sample size.

The median reduction in included sample size in these trials compared with the fixed sample size calculation was 52 subjects (range: -22 to 229), a reduction of 35% (range: -42 to 90%) of the fixed sample size. The median sample size reduction when considering the number of subjects included in the analysis until crossing of the boundaries was 77% (range: 15–90%). In this review, the number of trials stopped early for benefit (4) equaled the number of trials stopping early because there was enough information not to reject the null hypothesis. In another recent systematic review, the practice of stopping early for benefit was found to lead to inflated effect sizes (Bassler et al. 2010). However, this review did not include information on trials which were stopped early for futility.

Table 5 Proposed minimal set of parameters to be reported about DMC activities, interim analysis and early stopping[a, b]

Data Monitoring Committees and interim analysis[b]

Terminology

Use of the standard nomenclature "Data Monitoring Committee"

Composition of the DMC

Members' name, affiliation, and training

Independence status from research team and sponsor

Tasks of the DMC

Whether the DMC reviewed and accepted the protocol before the start of the trial

Main roles (e.g., monitoring of safety and/or efficacy), and explicit definition of which outcomes were analyzed[c]

Any additional roles (e.g., monitoring recruitment and quality assurance)

To which outcome(s) was the DMC blinded or unblinded

Interim analysis and statistical monitoring methods

Whether the protocol included a predefined statistical monitoring plan

Number of planned interim analyses

Timing of planned interim analyses and parameter defining timing (i.e., participants or person-time recruitment, number of end points, and ad hoc time interval)

Type of analysis planned (i.e., efficacy, harm, futility, and/or sample size adjustment), specific statistical methods used (with references and uniform terminology), description of boundaries (i.e., their symmetry, p-value/confidence interval, and adjustment, if applicable), and outcome (s) to which they were applied (i.e., primary/secondary, any subgroup analysis)

Any formal predefined stopping rules, to which outcome(s) did they apply, and whether they included statistical boundaries and/or other considerations

Whether the statistical monitoring plan was completed as planned; if not, which changes were performed, and their rationale

Adjustment for multiple analysis in final results (i.e., reported p-values and/or confidence intervals)

Recommendations to the sponsor/steering committee

DMC recommendation regarding continuation or termination of the trial (with or without adjustments in protocol)

Rationale (i.e., statistical boundaries and/or other considerations)

Whether the sponsor followed the DMC's recommendations

Early terminated trials

Motive(s) for termination (e.g., efficacy, harm, futility, and recruitment)

All previously stated items, particularly rationale for early termination (including predefined statistical monitoring plan, type of analysis, predefined stopping rules, and DMC recommendation), and adjustment for multiple analysis and early termination in final results

Timing of early termination, i.e., which of the interim analyses led to trial termination, and on which parameter the timing of this interim analysis was based (e.g., number of participants enrolled and predefined number of end points)

Planned and final sample size

Total number of events after which the trial was terminated, including definition of these events

Discussion of implications of early termination (i.e., concerning type I ands II errors)

Report early termination in the abstract of the paper

---

[a]These recommendations are for main reports; further details could be available using other modes of publication (e.g., online appendices, trial design/protocol papers, and web-based repositories), to which the report should refer to; planned items of this minimal set of parameters should be included in prospective trial registries

[b]Based on the book by Ellenberg et al. and the report of the DAMOCLES group (Ellenberg et al. 2002; Grant et al. 2005)

[c]Particularly regarding safety – whether it included adverse events and/or main efficacy outcomes

3 Part 3: Conduct of Trials and Working with DMCs

In a systematic review of 648 pediatric trials published in eight high impact journals, Fernandes et al. concluded that the reporting of DMC activities, interim analysis results, and early termination of pediatric trials is incomplete and heterogeneous (Fernandes et al. 2009). Most of the included trials were, however, designed and conducted before the DAMOCLES standards for DMC use were published in 2005 (Grant et al. 2005). Fernandes et al. proposed a checklist for the reporting of DMC issues, interim analyses, and early stopping, which is shown in Table 5.

4 Conclusion

The goal of trialists in pediatric drug development is to design and conduct trials that are valid, efficient, and safe. Various techniques are available to enhance the efficiency of trials, without compromising their validity and safety. Few of these techniques have been used on a large scale in pediatric drug development. We suggest that experience and knowledge are shared on (internet) forums, such as StaR Child Health (http://www.starchildhealth.org), to improve the standards of pediatric trials and make sure that all children participating in drug trials benefit from these standards (Klassen et al. 2009).

References

(2004) PEST 4.4 operating manual. The University of Reading, Reading

Anderson TW (1960) A modification of the sequential probability ratio test to reduce the sample size. Ann Math Stat 31:165–197

Armitage P (1958) Sequential methods in clinical trials. Am J Public Health 48:1395–1402

Armitage P (1975) Sequential medical trials. Blackwell, Oxford

Bassler D, Briel M, Montori VM, Lane M, Glasziou P, Zhou Q, Heels-Ansdell D, Walter SD, Guyatt GH, Flynn DN, Elamin MB, Murad MH, Abu Elnour NO, Lampropulos JF, Sood A, Mullan RJ, Erwin PJ, Bankhead CR, Perera R, Ruiz CC, You JJ, Mulla SM, Kaur J, Nerenberg KA, Schunemann H, Cook DJ, Lutz K, Ribic CM, Vale N, Malaga G, Akl EA, Ferreira-Gonzalez I, Alonso-Coello P, Urrutia G, Kunz R, Bucher HC, Nordmann AJ, Raatz H, da Silva SA, Tuche F, Strahm B, Djulbegovic B, Adhikari NK, Mills EJ, Gwadry-Sridhar F, Kirpalani H, Soares HP, Karanicolas PJ, Burns KE, Vandvik PO, Coto-Yglesias F, Chrispim PP, Ramsay T (2010) Stopping randomized trials early for benefit and estimation of treatment effects: systematic review and meta-regression analysis. JAMA 303:1180–1187

Bauer P, Kieser M (1999) Combining different phases in the development of medical treatments within a single trial. Stat Med 18:1833–1848

Bauer P, Kohne K (1994) Evaluation of experiments with adaptive interim analyses. Biometrics 50:1029–1041

Bellissant E, Duhamel JF, Guillot M, Pariente-Khayat A, Olive G, Pons G (1997) The triangular test to assess the efficacy of metoclopramide in gastroesophageal reflux. Clin Pharmacol Ther 61:377–384

Boellner SW, Stark JG, Krishnan S, Zhang Y (2010) Pharmacokinetics of lisdexamfetamine dimesylate and its active metabolite, d-amphetamine, with increasing oral doses of lisdexamfetamine dimesylate in children with attention-deficit/hyperactivity disorder: a single-dose, randomized, open-label, crossover study. Clin Ther 32:252–264

Bretz F, Koenig F, Brannath W, Glimm E, Posch M (2009) Adaptive designs for confirmatory clinical trials. Stat Med 28:1181–1217

CHMP (2006a) Guideline on clinical trials in small populations. EMA, London

CHMP (2006b) Reflection paper on methodological issues in confirmatory clinical trials with flexible design and analysis plan. EMA, London

Coad DS, Ivanova A (2005) The use of the triangular test with response-adaptive treatment allocation. Stat Med 24:1483–1493

Cytel Software Corporation (1992) EaSt: a software package for the design and interim monitoring of group sequential clinical trials. Cytel Software Corporation, Cambridge, MA

De Cock RF, Piana C, Krekels EH, Danhof M, Allegaert K, Knibbe CA (2011) The role of population PK-PD modelling in paediatric clinical research. Eur J Clin Pharmacol. 67 Suppl 1:5–16

Edwards SJ, Lilford RJ, Braunholtz DA, Jackson JC, Hewison J, Thornton J (1998) Ethical issues in the design and conduct of randomised controlled trials. Health Technol Assess 2:1–132

Ellenberg SS, Fleming TR, DeMets DL (2002) Data Monitoring Committees in Clinical Trials. Chichester, John Wiley Sons, Ltd

Emerson SS, Fleming TR (1989) Symmetric group sequential test designs. Biometrics 45: 905–923

Fernandes RM, van der Lee JH, Offringa M (2009) A systematic review of the reporting of Data Monitoring Committees' roles, interim analysis and early termination in pediatric clinical trials. BMC Pediatr 9:77

Filler G, Browne R, Seikaly MG (2003) Glomerular filtration rate as a putative 'surrogate endpoint' for renal transplant clinical trials in children. Pediatr Transplant 7:18–24

Freiman JA, Chalmers TC, Smith H Jr, Kuebler RR (1978) The importance of beta, the type II error and sample size in the design and interpretation of the randomized control trial. Survey of 71 "negative" trials. N Engl J Med 299:690–694

Glasziou P, Chalmers I, Rawlins M, McCulloch P (2007) When are randomised trials unnecessary? Picking signal from noise. BMJ 334:349–351

Grant AM, Altman DG, Babiker AB, Campbell MK, Clemens FJ, Darbyshire JH, Elbourne DR, McLeer SK, Parmar MK, Pocock SJ, Spiegelhalter DJ, Sydes MR, Walker AE, Wallace SA (2005) Issues in data monitoring and interim analysis of trials. Health Technol Assess 9:1–238

Haybittle JL (1971) Repeated assessment of results in clinical trials of cancer treatment. Br J Radiol 44:793–797

Hirtz DG, Gilbert PR, Terrill CM, Buckman SY (2006) Clinical trials in children – how are they implemented? Pediatr Neurol 34:436–438

Hommel G (2001) Adaptive modifications of hypotheses after an interim analysis. Biometrical J 43:581–589

Jennison C, Turnbull BW (2003) Mid-course sample size modification in clinical trials based on the observed treatment effect. Stat Med 22:971–993

Kelly PJ, Stallard N, Todd S (2005) An adaptive group sequential design for phase II/III clinical trials that select a single treatment from several. J Biopharm Stat 15:641–658

Kieser M, Bauer P, Lehmacher W (1999) Inference on multiple endpoints in clinical trials with adaptive interim analyses. Biometrical J 41:261–277

Klassen TP, Hartling L, Hamm M, van der Lee JH, Ursum J, Offringa M (2009) StaR Child Health: an initiative for RCTs in children. Lancet 374:1310–1312

Knottnerus JA, Bouter LM (2001) The ethics of sample size: two-sided testing and one-sided thinking. J Clin Epidemiol 54:109–110

Lan KKG, DeMets DL (1983) Discrete sequential boundaries for clinical trials. Biometrika 70:659–663

Lehmacher W, Wassmer G (1999) Adaptive sample size calculations in group sequential trials. Biometrics 55:1286–1290

McKinney RE Jr, Johnson GM, Stanley K, Yong FH, Keller A, O'Donnell KJ, Brouwers P, Mitchell WG, Yogev R, Wara DW, Wiznia A, Mofenson L, McNamara J, Spector SA (1998) A randomized study of combined zidovudine-lamivudine versus didanosine monotherapy in children with symptomatic therapy-naive HIV-1 infection. The Pediatric AIDS Clinical Trials Group Protocol 300 Study Team. J Pediatr 133:500–508

Moye LA, Tita AT (2002) Hypothesis testing complexity in the name of ethics: response to commentary. J Clin Epidemiol 55:209–211

Nyman Y, Von HK, Palm C, Eksborg S, Lonnqvist PA (2006) Etomidate-Lipuro is associated with considerably less injection pain in children compared with propofol with added lidocaine. Br J Anaesth 97:536–539

O'Brien PC, Fleming TR (1979) A multiple testing procedure for clinical trials. Biometrics 35:549–556

Ogungbenro K, Aarons L (2008) How many subjects are necessary for population pharmacokinetic experiments? Confidence interval approach. Eur J Clin Pharmacol 64:705–713

Pampallona S, Tsiatis AA (1994) Group sequential designs for one-sided and two-sided hypothesis testing with provision for early stopping in favor of the null hypothesis. J Stat Plan Infer 42:19–35

Peto R, Baigent C (1998) Trials: the next 50 years. Large scale randomised evidence of moderate benefits. BMJ 317:1170–1171

Pocock SJ (1977) Group sequential methods in the design and analysis of clinical trials. Biometrika 64:191–199

Rosenberger WF, Huc F (2004) Maximizing power and minimizing treatment failures in clinical trials. Clin Trials 1:141–147

Sackett DL, Cook DJ (1993) Can we learn anything from small trials? Ann NY Acad Sci 703:25–31

Sammons HM (2011) Avoiding clinical trials in children. Arch Dis Child 96:291–292

Schulz KF, Grimes DA (2005) Sample size calculations in randomised trials: mandatory and mystical. Lancet 365:1348–1353

Sebille V, Bellissant E (2000) Comparison of four sequential methods allowing for early stopping of comparative clinical trials. Clin Sci (Lond) 98:569–578

Sebille V, Bellissant E (2003) Sequential methods and group sequential designs for comparative clinical trials. Fundam Clin Pharmacol 17:505–516

Simes RJ (1995) Prospective meta-analysis of cholesterol-lowering studies: the Prospective Pravastatin Pooling (PPP) Project and the Cholesterol Treatment Trialists (CTT) Collaboration. Am J Cardiol 76:122C–126C

Smith GC, Pell JP (2003) Parachute use to prevent death and major trauma related to gravitational challenge: systematic review of randomised controlled trials. BMJ 327:1459–1461

Streiner DL, Norman GR (2008) Health Measurement Scales: a practical guide to their development and use. Oxford University Press, Oxford

Tarnow-Mordi WO, Healy MJ (1999) Distinguishing between "no evidence of effect" and "evidence of no effect" in randomised controlled trials and other comparisons. Arch Dis Child 80:210–211

Twisk JWR (2003) Applied longitudinal data analysis for epidemiology; a practical guide. Cambridge University Press, Cambridge van der Lee JH, Wesseling J, Tanck MW, Offringa M (2008) Efficient ways exist to obtain the optimal sample size in clinical trials in rare diseases. J Clin Epidemiol 61:324–330

van der Lee JH, Tanck MW, Wesseling J, Offringa M (2009) Pitfalls in the design and analysis of paediatric clinical trials: a case of a 'failed' multi-centre study, and potential solutions. Acta Paediatr 98:385–391

van der Lee JH, Wesseling J, Tanck MW, Offringa M (2010) Sequential design with boundaries approach in pediatric intervention research reduces sample size. J Clin Epidemiol 63:19–27

van Houwelingen HC (1999) On "Bayesian monitoring...". J Clin Epidemiol 52:713–714

van Woensel JB, van Aalderen WM, de Weerd W, Jansen NJ, van Gestel JP, Markhorst DG, van Vught AJ, Bos AP, Kimpen JL (2003) Dexamethasone for treatment of patients mechanically ventilated for lower respiratory tract infection caused by respiratory syncytial virus. Thorax 58:383–387

Vickers AJ (2003) Underpowering in randomized trials reporting a sample size calculation. J Clin Epidemiol 56:717–720

Vickers AJ, Altman DG (2001) Statistics notes: analysing controlled trials with baseline and follow up measurements. BMJ 323:1123–1124

von Goedecke A, Brimacombe J, Hormann C, Jeske HC, Kleinsasser A, Keller C (2005) Pressure support ventilation versus continuous positive airway pressure ventilation with the ProSeal laryngeal mask airway: a randomized crossover study of anesthetized pediatric patients. Anesth Analg 100:357–360

Wald A (1947) Sequential analysis. Wiley, New York

Wassmer G (2000) Basic concepts of group sequential and adaptive group sequential test procedures. Stat Pap 41:253–279

Whitehead J (1997) The design and analysis of sequential clinical trials. Wiley, Chichester

Whitehead J, Jones DR (1979) The analysis of sequential clinical trials. Biometrika 66: 443–452

Whitehead J, Stratton I (1983) Group sequential clincial trials with triangular continuation regions. Biometrics 39:227–236

Woods JR, Williams JG, Tavel M (1989) The two-period crossover design in medical research. Ann Intern Med 110:560–566

Sample Collection, Biobanking, and Analysis

Maurice J. Ahsman, Dick Tibboel, Ron A.A. Mathot, and Saskia N. de Wildt

Contents

Abstract Pediatric pharmacokinetic studies require sampling of biofluids from neonates and children. Limitations on sampling frequency and sample volume complicate the design of these studies. In addition, strict guidelines, designed to guarantee patient safety, are in place. This chapter describes the practical implications of sample collection and their storage, with special focus on the selection of the appropriate type

M.J. Ahsman • R.A.A. Mathot
Department of Clinical Pharmacy, Erasmus MC, Rotterdam, The Netherlands

D. Tibboel • S.N. de Wildt (✉)
Intensive Care and Department of Pediatric Surgery, Erasmus MC Sophia Children's Hospital,
Dr. Molewaterplein 60, 3015 GJ Rotterdam, The Netherlands
e-mail: s.dewildt@erasmusmc.nl

H.W. Seyberth et al. (eds.), *Pediatric Clinical Pharmacology*,
Handbook of Experimental Pharmacology 205,
DOI 10.1007/978-3-642-20195-0_10, © Springer-Verlag Berlin Heidelberg 2011

of biofluid and withdrawal technique. In addition, we describe appropriate measures for storage of these specimens, for example, in the context of biobanking, and the requirements on drug assay methods that they pose.

Pharmacokinetic studies in children are possible, but they require careful selection of an appropriate sampling method, specimen volume, and assay method. The checklist provided could help prospective researchers with the design of an appropriate study protocol and infrastructure.

Keywords Pediatric • Biobank • Sampling • Blood • Meconium • Saliva • Drug assay

1 Introduction

The ICH guidelines on pediatric drug studies (Anonymous 2000, 2001a) emphasize patient safety, which has consequences for the volume of, and methods for, sampling of biofluids. This has consequences for pharmacokinetic studies in children by imposing challenges upon sample collection and drug analysis. The main questions are as follows:

- Which biological specimen can be used and how can this specimen be collected in the intended study population?
- What are the maximum allowed sample volumes per occasion and per study period?
- By what methods can we store samples and acquire reliable drug concentrations?

In this chapter, we discuss these questions and aim to provide practical solutions and examples to help those planning pharmacokinetic studies in children. The details of designing population PK studies are outside the scope of this chapter and are discussed elsewhere.

2 Sample Types and Collection Techniques

2.1 Blood

Extensive blood sampling for traditional pharmacokinetic analysis is usually not possible in this population for ethical and practical reasons. No official guidelines exist on the maximum amount of blood that can be sampled in pediatric studies. However, several guidelines accept a maximum of 3–5% of the total blood volume per 4 weeks (Anonymous 2004, 2008). In case of simultaneous trials, the recommendation of 3–5% remains the maximum. In addition, repeated blood sampling in children by repeated punctures can be considered nonethical due to associated pain, anxiety, and distress. Safety can be improved by reducing the burden associated with invasive blood sampling and by using methods aimed to reduce the blood volume needed for drug analysis. In children, blood for pharmacokinetic analysis is preferably sampled from indwelling central venous or arterial catheters, already in place for clinical care. Sampling from these catheters is easy, causes only minimal or no discomfort, and allows for sufficient sample volume collections. Risks associated with the use of these catheters are bloodstream-related infections and unintended blood loss. If these catheters are not already in place for clinical purposes, placement of these catheters solely for research purposes is usually not considered acceptable by research ethics committees and/or patients and their family. Alternatively, blood can be sampled from peripherally inserted catheters. Insertion of these catheters solely for research purposes is sometimes acceptable, more specifically in the context of therapeutic drug trials. The main limitation, especially in neonates, is that blood draws are difficult if not impossible from small bore catheters as used in this population. To overcome this problem, blood can be taken from heel prick or venepuncture, the latter being much less painful, preferably when done together with regular blood work. When combining research blood sampling with regular blood work, the burden for the child may be considered acceptable both by children and their parents as well as by research ethics committees. Disadvantages of heel prick samples are the limitation in the volume, timing of blood samples, and painfulness. In general, blood volumes sampled per heel prick are limited to 0.5–0.6 ml, including blood collected for regular clinical blood work. Hence, blood volumes needed for pharmacokinetic analysis should preferably not exceed 0.2–0.3 ml per sample. In addition, timing of sampling is restricted if it needs to coincide with clinical blood sampling. Consequently, extensive and timed sampling for a full pharmacokinetic washout curve is not possible using this method.

A more detailed and practical guide for different blood sampling methods in children and neonates has been published by the UK Medicine for Children Research Network (Hawcutt et al. 2008).

2.2 Urine

For renally cleared drugs, urine sampling may provide an alternative to blood for the estimation of pharmacokinetics. Also, urinary excretion of the drug and its metabolites may provide valuable insight into developmental changes in drug metabolism and excretion (Streetman et al. 2001; Allegaert et al. 2006; Tucker et al. 1998). From a pharmacokinetic standpoint, the preferred method to collect urine is by urinary catheter or by direct collection in older children. Using a catheter facilitates complete urine collection over predefined time periods. A major limitation of the use of urinary catheters in children is the burden and risks associated with insertion of the catheter, such as pain, infection, urethral restriction (mainly in boys), and displacement. Hence, in general, if a catheter is not already in place for clinical purposes, most research ethics boards will not approve its use for research purposes only in children. Adhesive collection bags are also frequently used to collect urine, especially in infants and neonates (Allegaert et al. 2006). In these younger infants, the repeated use of adhesive urinary bags may result in skin abrasion. Skin abrasion is not only painful and causes discomfort; it may also increase the risk of invasive infections in a vulnerable population. The "gauze/cotton ball method" can be used alternatively. A small gauze with cling film (the latter facing the diaper material to prevent urine absorption in the diaper) is put in the diaper and urine is collected by expressing the urine from the gauze (Fell et al. 1997). In a similar fashion, nonabsorbent diapers can be used (Burke 1995). An important limitation of both the bag and gauze/diaper collection methods is that complete urine collection is most often not possible. Urine may leak along the bag into the diaper and not all urine can be expressed from the gauze/diaper. This limitation can be overcome by weighing the diapers to estimate total urine volume and to multiply volume with urine drug concentrations to be able to estimate total urinary drug and/or metabolite excretion.

2.3   Saliva

Saliva can be used as a noninvasive alternative to blood for a significant number of drugs, e.g., caffeine, anti-HIV drugs, anticonvulsants, digoxine, and codeine (Drummer 2006). Saliva can also be used for DNA sampling. First, saliva can be collected by simply asking children to spit in a cup. For DNA sampling, specific cups are available containing anti-DNAse solutions. Understandably, this method is only feasible in older children (>8 years of age) who are capable to understand and follow simple instructions.

Younger children can chew on a gauze, cotton "salivette," or a cotton-cellulose eyespear, from which saliva can be extracted. Citric acid containing products may stimulate saliva production and enhance collection. Several commercially available methods for saliva collection are available (Drummer 2006). In preterm infants, commercially available products, such as salivettes, are difficult to use. First, the cotton swab provided is relatively large to be inserted in the mouth. Also, the saliva volume needed to extract enough saliva from the cotton is considerably higher than can be sampled from preterms. Before deciding to use one of these methods, it is important to validate the intended method by studying the correlation between blood concentrations and saliva concentrations. Saliva drug concentrations may vary according to method used, with or without citric acid (de Wildt et al. 2001; Strazdins et al. 2005).

2.4   Breath Samples

Breath tests using stable or radioactive isotopes are used in the context of drug metabolism studies (Paine et al. 2002; de Wildt et al. 2007). Breath sampling of exhaled labeled CO_2 is easiest when children can follow instructions to breathe in a balloon, from which breath samples can be taken. In younger or critically ill children, this approach is obviously not feasible. The original collection method of respiratory CO_2 used in children, including neonates, occurs via trapping of CO_2 in sodium hydroxide. This method involves a tight-fitting face mask and passing of the expired air through a condenser containing sodium hydroxide (Pons et al. 1988). This is impractical and difficult in neonates. Alternatively, a direct nasopharyngeal sampling technique can be used (van der Schoor et al. 2004). This technique allows for direct sampling from the nasopharynx using a gastric tube attached to a syringe or direct attachment of a syringe to a side-port of the endotracheal tube. During observed expiration, the researcher collects air by pulling the syringe. The collected air is then transferred to a vacuum tube for laboratory analysis.

2.5 Meconium

By accumulating from the 12th gestational week until birth, meconium acts as a reservoir for exogenous compounds, such as drugs and metabolites. Drugs are incorporated into meconium through swallowing drug-contaminated amniotic fluid or via biliary excretion. Meconium analysis is thought to detect maternal drug use during the second and third trimesters. Meconium passage occurs in the first 1–3 days after birth, but may be prolonged in preterm infants. Collection of meconium from diapers is easy, by scraping meconium from the diaper. 0.5–1 g of meconium is usually enough for toxicological, quantitative analysis. Contamination of meconium with urine may occur, which obscures the results. After collection, meconium can be stored at low temperatures ($-20°C$). Storage at room temperature may reduce the concentrations of drug by degradation. Due to its complex composition, consisting of epithelial cells, swallowed amniotic fluid, bile salts, lipids, other endogenous compounds, and xenobiotics until birth, extraction of drugs is difficult (Gray et al. 2009).

2.6 Hair

Drugs can be incorporated in hair through blood supply of the hair, by external exposure (through, e.g., smoke) or through secretion from sweat and sebum adjacent to the hair follicle.

Hair samples are mainly used for toxicological screening in prenatal alcohol and drug exposure.

These samples are best collected from the back of the head. The proximal zone (i.e., the zone which is closer to the root) should be clearly indicated if segmental analysis is to be performed. The sample can then be stored and transported light and moisture protected at room temperature. Since hair grows about 1 cm per month, segmental analysis can be done to estimate the time window of drug exposure (Gallardo and Queiroz 2008).

3 Leftover Material and Biobanking

In addition to freshly collected blood samples in the context of a single pharmacokinetic study, the use of leftover or previously stored blood samples should be considered.

This may significantly reduce the burden to the individual child participating in a trial.

For example, leftover material from regular patient blood work could be used for pharmacokinetic analysis of drugs that the patient is taking therapeutically. As the sample volume available will likely be small, very sensitive analytical techniques, to be described below, are required. This approach has several advantages. First, the pharmacokinetic results will reflect the real-life clinical situation, as the drug is studied in the population that actually needs the drug for treatment. Second, the need for additional blood sampling is limited or nonexistent, which can significantly reduce the burden to individual patients. This may even result in a higher informed consent rate from the child and/or his parents to participate in the study.

Secondly, blood could be sampled routinely for biobanking purposes from all consenting children/parents on a specific ward or with a predefined disease for later studies, provided blood sample volumes are within acceptable limits. In this context, biobanking is defined as collection of biological material and the associated data and information stored in an organized system, for a population or a large subset of a population.

This approach is taken in large-scale pharmacogenetic studies in the adult population. Anonymous linking of clinical data may provide researchers with ample opportunity to study multiple research questions. Ethics committees and subjects will generally be amenable to long-term sample storage for future research, provided that there are sufficient assurances that stringent processes and standards for patient privacy/confidentiality are in place.

When previously collected samples are necessary to perform a new study, it may still be possible to obtain consent from the original participants. However, the consent procedure may vary depending on the source of original data and the intended purpose; see Helgesson et al. (2007) and Hoeyer et al. (2005) for a discussion on the ethical aspects of using these data. Some have advocated the renewal of consent once former study participants reach adulthood, particularly because the sharing of genetic and phenotypic data could have consequences that were unforeseen at the time of parental consent decades earlier (Farin et al. 1999). Although not related to biological fluids, the use of *digital* leftover material, i.e., the combination of existing pharmacokinetic datasets from medical literature, may significantly reduce the need for prospective pharmacokinetic trials. This could, for instance, be used to study the effect of age and other covariates in the pediatric population (Ince et al. 2009; de Wildt and Knibbe 2009).

4 Storage and Shipping

According to the Good Clinical Laboratory Practice (GCLP) guidelines issued by the World Health Organization (Anonymous 2009), samples should be kept "in such a way as to ensure the integrity and accessibility to the material retained." GCP guidelines state that national legislation determines the minimum period during which data records and material should be stored. The samples should be stored to allow (re-) examination, but only for as long as the quality permits evaluation, i.e., for as long as analyte levels can be reliably requantified without excessive degradation. This requires simulation of average and worst-case conditions in sampling, storage, and shipping to see the effects on sample integrity. The consequences of different storage and handling protocols for the analytical results of each type of sample is too big a topic to be discussed in this brief overview; the reader is referred to the excellent review by Mehta regarding preanalytical considerations in drug assays (Mehta 1989).

A major issue in GCP is the protection of subject confidentiality, which should be maintained not only in reports of final results but also in the preceding steps, i.e., during storage, shipping, and drug assay. This requires storage in coded vials, with access to the original subject data restricted to specific individuals (usually the researchers directly involved in sampling, storage, and data extraction). To maintain sample integrity, appropriate measures should be taken to guarantee the right temperature, protection from light, etc., throughout the preassay period. These measures might, for instance, include the use of refrigerators or freezers with continuous temperature registration and should include standard operating procedures (SOP) describing responsibilities of the individuals involved in sampling and shipping.

For more information on the GCLP guidelines, the reader is referred to Ezzelle et al. (2008) and Anonymous (2009). Practical examples of necessary measures can be found in Peakman and Elliott (2008), Elliott and Peakman (2008), Mehta (1989), and Vaught (2006).

5 Drug Assays

Quantification of analytes in pediatric studies is complicated by the limited availability (both in numbers and volume) of biological specimens. The analytical methods should therefore be sensitive enough to quantify compounds in complex mixtures (such as blood, plasma, or cerebrospinal fluid) in sample volumes of 10 to maximum 100 µL. Ideally, these so-called microassays can be used to quantify different analytes of interest in the same sample, e.g., drugs and their metabolites or combinations of coadministered drugs.

5.1 Assay Methods

The required sensitivity can be reached using mass spectrometric techniques such as liquid (LC-MS) or gas (GC-MS) chromatography–mass spectrometry. These techniques rely on chromatographic separation of analytes from each other and from matrix components, followed by ionization and counting of analytes of a selected molecular mass. Compounds of similar mass can be distinguished via mass filters that allow a single analyte to be selected in the presence of other drugs, metabolites, or endogenous compounds. To enhance selectivity even further, the selected compounds can be subsequently fragmented by collision with an inert gas. This leads to molecular fragments that are highly specific for the original drug or metabolite. After selection of one of these fragments via another mass filter, the compound of interest can be quantified. This is called tandem mass spectrometry or MS/MS (Fig. 1). The mass spectrometric techniques carry a distinct advantage over other sensitive assays such as enzyme-linked assay, fluorometric assay, and radioassay. Whereas the latter often suffer from cross-reactivity between structurally related compounds such as drugs and their metabolites or endogenous substrates (Tribut et al. 2005; Moyer et al. 1986; de Paula et al. 1998; Premaud et al. 2006; Tate and Ward 2004), the mass spectrometric methods allow

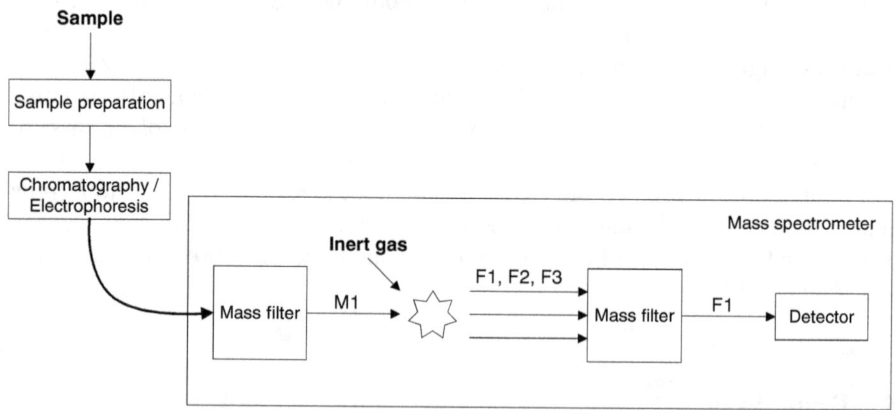

Fig. 1 Principle of liquid or gas chromatography with tandem mass spectrometry detection. The sample is cleaned up for chromatographic separation of drugs and metabolites from matrix components. After chromatography or electrophoresis, the effluent enters the mass spectrometer. After selection of molecules of a specific molecular weight (M1) by the first mass filter, the molecules are fragmented with an inert gas. The resulting fragments (F1, F2, and F3) are sent through the second filter in which one individual fragment is selected to be quantified at the detector

simultaneous quantification of different analytes in a single run by rapidly changing the mass filter settings (Marzo and Bo 2007; Vogeser 2003). Another separation method, which can be used in combination with mass spectrometric detection with small sample volumes (especially for different drug enantiomers), is capillary electrophoresis (CE-MS) (Chen and Chen 1999; Sung and Chen 2006), but due to wide experience and superior sensitivity, LC-MS and GC-MS remain the cornerstones of drug microassays. Whereas urine and serum or plasma are the main biofluids in experimental pharmacology, some biochemical markers and compounds can also be quantified in extracts from dried blood spots. This poses additional requirements on the assay method and its validation, drug or metabolite stability, and the availability of reference values for drugs concentrations in whole blood (see Spooner et al. 2009; Edelbroek et al. 2009). Nevertheless, the logistical advantages are appealing. Dried bloodspot collection allows sampling at remote locations, if necessary even by patients or parents themselves. Once dry, the blood spots can be sent via regular mail services to a central laboratory, without many additional measures to minimize biohazard. Even samples from large multinational studies can then be processed at a single laboratory, which greatly improves efficiency regarding method validation at different study sites, refrigeration or freezing during sample storage and transport, reliability of assay results due to increased experience with the assay, and reduction of interlaboratory variability, etc. Re-assay, however, is usually not possible, since most methods require the entire dried drop of blood to be processed. So far, there are few published assay methods with dried blood spots, but their number seems to be increasing; examples include the quantification of topiramate (la Marca et al. 2008), everolimus (van der Heijden et al. 2008), tacrolimus (Hoogtanders et al. 2007), metformin (Aburuz et al. 2006), and antiretroviral drugs (Koal et al. 2005).

5.2   Sample Preparation

Exogenous and endogenous components in the biological matrix can interfere with sample preparation or quantification, which compromises accuracy and precision. The mechanisms of these so-called matrix effects are not fully understood, but have been linked to coelution of different compounds (including inorganic ions and plasma phospholipids) that can interfere with analyte ionization (Taylor 2005; Careri and Mangia 2006). The degree of signal enhancement or suppression could therefore vary from individual to individual, but also within individuals upon changes in physiological constitution, either due to disease progression or growth and maturation. This implies that validation of the assays should include an evaluation of matrix effects in biological specimens ("blank matrix") from the intended patient population. The US Food and Drug Administration has issued guidelines on the validation requirements for bioanalytical chromatographic methods (Anonymous 2001b) without mentioning a specific method to assess matrix effects; current reports on new LC-MS and GC-MS assays often contain a qualitative visual assessment or a quantitative calculation based on work by Matuszewski et al. (Matuszewski et al. 2003; Matuszewski 2006).

Samples are cleaned up via solid phase extraction (SPE) or liquid–liquid extraction (LLE) to separate analytes from interfering components and, if possible, to concentrate the analyte in a smaller volume to increase sensitivity (Hyotylainen 2009; Hernandez-Borges et al. 2007). In pediatric and neonatal studies in particular, sample volumes are small. When volumes become too small to reliably be transferred from one vial to another, sample preparation can be a challenge, and preassay concentration in a smaller volume is impossible. Therefore, microassays often contain minimal sample preparation (i.e., protein precipitation or direct injection, also called "dilute-and-shoot") and rely heavily on the chromatographic prowess of LC-MS or GC-MS equipment to maintain accuracy and precision without matrix effects. When extensive cleanup cannot be avoided, it is possible to use LLE with minimal amounts of organic solvents or sophisticated and expensive microtechniques such as 96-well SPE (Saito and Jinno 2003; Shen et al. 2006; Ahsman et al. 2010).

5.3 Multiple Drug Assays

The efficiency of pharmacological studies can sometimes be increased by quantifying multiple analytes in a single sample, since it requires less biological material per patient while reducing the total analytical workload. Multiple-analyte assays have been developed for drugs and their main metabolites (Witjes et al. 2009; Liang et al. 2009; Patel et al. 2009) and for drugs from different therapeutic classes that are often coprescribed in specific patient populations (Ahsman et al. 2009; de Velde et al. 2009; Gomes et al. 2008). Especially for biobanked samples, these assays can be used to maximize scientific output from limited sample volumes. This requires careful selection of sampling times in relation to the expected dose regimens to allow reliable estimation of pharmacokinetic parameters.

5.4 Alternative Drug Matrices

For studies on fetal drug or pollutant exposure, compounds are assayed in unusual biological matrices such as meconium, hair, or cord blood. For these biofluids, it may be even more difficult to find suitable blank material. For meconium in particular, special sample preparation methods may be necessary to prepare solutions that are suitable for LC-MS or GC-MS analysis. See Gray et al. (2009), Rigourd et al. (2008), Frison et al. (2008), Kacinko et al. (2008), and Yeh et al. (2009) for examples of analytical methods that were developed specifically for these matrices.

6 Conclusion

In summary, pharmacological studies in children are possible, but require careful selection of an appropriate sampling method and sample volume. An assay method should be developed and validated, with special attention to the required sensitivity level, matrix effects, and sample preparation. See Table 1 for a checklist with the main points that should be addressed when designing a pediatric study.

Table 1 Items to be considered before engaging in a pediatric study involving sample collection and drug quantification

Sample collection

What are the maximum allowed sample volumes per occasion and per study period?

Which sampling times are informative (based on population PK study design) and practical?

Is blood the preferred biological specimen or can alternatives be used?

How much sample is required, taking into account the intended assay requirements and potential future studies into different analytes with leftover material?

Which sampling methods are suitable?

Can these methods be implemented as part of routine clinical procedures and/or do involved staff need extra training?

Biobanking and leftover samples

Have patients or their guardians given permission for biobanking and use of leftover samples?

Is there a separate long-term storage facility with temperature control, compliant with GCP guidelines available?

How are patient data being recorded; is the database suitable for (anonymized) long-term storage and extraction?

Who decides whether to grant individual researchers access to samples and data, and is there a system that allows tracking of individual samples and researchers that use them?

Which departments or individuals are responsible for maintenance, logging access rights to samples, etc?

Shipping and storage

How stable are the biofluid specimens and analytes at standard storage conditions: ambient temperature (20–25°C), refrigerated (4–7°C), frozen (−20°C), and deep-frozen (−80°C)?

What are the average and worst-case shipping conditions and time?

Is privacy of study participants guaranteed during storage and shipping?

What arrangements have been made to allow sampling, storage, and processing outside standard working hours, in weekends, and on holidays?

Have roles and responsibilities been agreed upon by the clinical department, logistical services, and the laboratory?

Have standard operating procedures (SOP) containing contact details, storage conditions, etc., been agreed upon by and made available to the involved staff?

Assay

How much sample is required for the assay, taking into account reassay in case of instrument failure?

Are the expected concentrations within the assay's calibration range?

Has the assay been validated for this specific type of sample and analyte?

Have matrix effects been evaluated in appropriate batches of blank matrix? (preferably from patients of the intended age, comedication, and disease state)

References

Aburuz S, Millership J, McElnay J (2006) Dried blood spot liquid chromatography assay for therapeutic drug monitoring of metformin. J Chromatogr B Analyt Technol Biomed Life Sci 832:202–207

Ahsman MJ, Wildschut ED, Tibboel D, Mathot RA (2009) Microanalysis of beta-lactam antibiotics and vancomycin in plasma for pharmacokinetic studies in neonates. Antimicrob Agents Chemother 53:75–80

Ahsman MJ, Van der Nagel BC, Mathot RA (2010) Quantification of midazolam, morphine and metabolites in plasma using 96-well solid-phase extraction and ultra-performance liquid chromatography-tandem mass spectrometry. Biomed Chromatogr 24(9):969–976

Allegaert K, Rayyan M, de Hoon J, Tibboel D, Verbesselt R, Naulaers G, Van den Anker JN, Devlieger H (2006) Contribution of glucuronidation to tramadol disposition in early neonatal life. Basic Clin Pharmacol Toxicol 98:110–112

Anonymous (2000) E11: Guidance for industry – clinical investigation of medicinal products in the pediatric population. US Food and Drug Administration, Center for Drug Evaluation and Research, Rockville, MD

Anonymous (2001a) Clinical investigation of medicinal products in the paediatric population, vol E11. European Medicines Agency, London

Anonymous (2001b) Guidance for industry – bioanalytical method validation. Biopharmaceutics Coordinating Committee, Center for Drug Evaluation and Research, US Food and Drug Administration, Rockville, MD

Anonymous (2004) The Hospital for Sick Children (SickKids) Research Ethics Board Blood Sampling Guidelines. Toronto

Anonymous (2008) E11: Ethical considerations for clinical trials on medicinal products with the paediatric population. Guidelines for Directive 2001/20/EC. European Commission, Brussels

Anonymous (2009) Good Clinical Laboratory Practice (GCLP). World Health Organization Special Programme for Research and Training in Tropical Disease. WHO, Geneva

Burke N (1995) Alternative methods for newborn urine sample collection. Pediatr Nurs 21:546–549

Careri M, Mangia A (2006) Validation and qualification: the fitness for purpose of mass spectrometry-based analytical methods and analytical systems. Anal Bioanal Chem 386:38–45

Chen SH, Chen YH (1999) Pharmacokinetic applications of capillary electrophoresis. Electrophoresis 20:3259–3268

de Paula M, Saiz LC, Gonzalez-Revalderia J, Pascual T, Alberola C, Miravalles E (1998) Rifampicin causes false-positive immunoassay results for urine opiates. Clin Chem Lab Med 36:241–243

de Velde F, Alffenaar JW, Wessels AM, Greijdanus B, Uges DR (2009) Simultaneous determination of clarithromycin, rifampicin and their main metabolites in human plasma by liquid chromatography-tandem mass spectrometry. J Chromatogr B Analyt Technol Biomed Life Sci 877:1771–1777

de Wildt SN, Knibbe CA (2009) Knowledge of developmental pharmacology and modeling approaches should be used to avoid useless trials in children. Eur J Clin Pharmacol 65:849–850, author reply 851–842

de Wildt SN, Kerkvliet KT, Wezenberg MG, Ottink S, Hop WC, Vulto AG, van Den Anker JN (2001) Use of saliva in therapeutic drug monitoring of caffeine in preterm infants. Ther Drug Monit 23:250–254

de Wildt SN, Berns MJ, van den Anker JN (2007) 13C-erythromycin breath test as a noninvasive measure of CYP3A activity in newborn infants: a pilot study. Ther Drug Monit 29:225–230

Drummer OH (2006) Drug testing in oral fluid. Clin Biochem Rev 27:147–159

Edelbroek PM, van der Heijden J, Stolk LM (2009) Dried blood spot methods in therapeutic drug monitoring: methods, assays, and pitfalls. Ther Drug Monit 31:327–336

Elliott P, Peakman TC (2008) The UK Biobank sample handling and storage protocol for the collection, processing and archiving of human blood and urine. Int J Epidemiol 37:234–244

Ezzelle J, Rodriguez-Chavez IR, Darden JM, Stirewalt M, Kunwar N, Hitchcock R, Walter T, D'Souza MP (2008) Guidelines on good clinical laboratory practice: bridging operations between research and clinical research laboratories. J Pharm Biomed Anal 46:18–29

Farin D, Kitzes-Cohen R, Piva G, Gozlan I (1999) High performance liquid chromatography method for the determination of meropenem in human plasma. Chromatographia 49:253–255

Fell JM, Thakkar H, Newman DJ, Price CP (1997) Measurement of albumin and low molecular weight proteins in the urine of newborn infants using a cotton wool ball collection method. Acta Paediatr 86:518–522

Frison G, Favretto D, Vogliardi S, Terranova C, Ferrara SD (2008) Quantification of citalopram or escitalopram and their demethylated metabolites in neonatal hair samples by liquid chromatography-tandem mass spectrometry. Ther Drug Monit 30:467–473

Gallardo E, Queiroz JA (2008) The role of alternative specimens in toxicological analysis. Biomed Chromatogr 22:795–821

Gomes NA, Vaidya VV, Pudage A, Joshi SS, Parekh SA (2008) Liquid chromatography-tandem mass spectrometry (LC-MS/MS) method for simultaneous determination of tenofovir and emtricitabine in human plasma and its application to a bioequivalence study. J Pharm Biomed Anal 48:918–926

Gray TR, Shakleya DM, Huestis MA (2009) A liquid chromatography tandem mass spectrometry method for the simultaneous quantification of 20 drugs of abuse and metabolites in human meconium. Anal Bioanal Chem 393:1977–1990

Hawcutt DB, Rose AC, Nunn T, Turner MA (2008) NIHR Medicines for Children Research Network (MCRN): points to consider when planning the collection of blood samples in clinical trials of investigational medicinal products. MCRN Guide. NIHR, London

Helgesson G, Dillner J, Carlson J, Bartram CR, Hansson MG (2007) Ethical framework for previously collected biobank samples. Nat Biotechnol 25:973–976

Hernandez-Borges J, Borges-Miquel TM, Rodriguez-Delgado MA, Cifuentes A (2007) Sample treatments prior to capillary electrophoresis-mass spectrometry. J Chromatogr A 1153:214–226

Hoeyer K, Olofsson BO, Mjorndal T, Lynoe N (2005) The ethics of research using biobanks: reason to question the importance attributed to informed consent. Arch Intern Med 165:97–100

Hoogtanders K, van der Heijden J, Christiaans M, Edelbroek P, van Hooff JP, Stolk LM (2007) Therapeutic drug monitoring of tacrolimus with the dried blood spot method. J Pharm Biomed Anal 44:658–664

Hyotylainen T (2009) Critical evaluation of sample pretreatment techniques. Anal Bioanal Chem 394:743–758

Ince I, de Wildt SN, Tibboel D, Danhof M, Knibbe CA (2009) Tailor-made drug treatment for children: creation of an infrastructure for data-sharing and population PK-PD modeling. Drug Discov Today 14:316–320

Kacinko SL, Shakleya DM, Huestis MA (2008) Validation and application of a method for the determination of buprenorphine, norbuprenorphine, and their glucuronide conjugates in human meconium. Anal Chem 80:246–252

Koal T, Burhenne H, Romling R, Svoboda M, Resch K, Kaever V (2005) Quantification of antiretroviral drugs in dried blood spot samples by means of liquid chromatography/tandem mass spectrometry. Rapid Commun Mass Spectrom 19:2995–3001

la Marca G, Malvagia S, Filippi L, Fiorini P, Innocenti M, Luceri F, Pieraccini G, Moneti G, Francese S, Dani FR, Guerrini R (2008) Rapid assay of topiramate in dried blood spots by a new liquid chromatography-tandem mass spectrometric method. J Pharm Biomed Anal 48:1392–1396

Liang X, Li Y, Barfield M, Ji QC (2009) Study of dried blood spots technique for the determination of dextromethorphan and its metabolite dextrorphan in human whole blood by LC-MS/MS. J Chromatogr B Analyt Technol Biomed Life Sci 877:799–806

Marzo A, Bo LD (2007) Tandem mass spectrometry (LC-MS-MS): a predominant role in bioassays for pharmacokinetic studies. Arzneimittelforschung 57:122–128

Matuszewski BK (2006) Standard line slopes as a measure of a relative matrix effect in quantitative HPLC-MS bioanalysis. J Chromatogr B Analyt Technol Biomed Life Sci 830:293–300

Matuszewski BK, Constanzer ML, Chavez-Eng CM (2003) Strategies for the assessment of matrix effect in quantitative bioanalytical methods based on HPLC-MS/MS. Anal Chem 75:3019–3030

Mehta AC (1989) Preanalytical considerations in drug assays in clinical pharmacokinetic studies. J Clin Pharm Ther 14:285–295

Moyer TP, Johnson P, Faynor SM, Sterioff S (1986) Cyclosporine: a review of drug monitoring problems and presentation of a simple, accurate liquid chromatographic procedure that solves these problems. Clin Biochem 19:83–89

Paine MF, Wagner DA, Hoffmaster KA, Watkins PB (2002) Cytochrome P450 3A4 and P-glycoprotein mediate the interaction between an oral erythromycin breath test and rifampin. Clin Pharmacol Ther 72:524–535

Patel BN, Sharma N, Sanyal M, Shrivastav PS (2009) An accurate, rapid and sensitive determination of tramadol and its active metabolite O-desmethyltramadol in human plasma by LC-MS/MS. J Pharm Biomed Anal 49:354–366

Peakman TC, Elliott P (2008) The UK Biobank sample handling and storage validation studies. Int J Epidemiol 37(Suppl 1):i2–i6

Pons G, Blais JC, Rey E, Plissonnier M, Richard MO, Carrier O, d'Athis P, Moran C, Badoual J, Olive G (1988) Maturation of caffeine N-demethylation in infancy: a study using the 13CO$_2$ breath test. Pediatr Res 23:632–636

Premaud A, Rousseau A, Picard N, Marquet P (2006) Determination of mycophenolic acid plasma levels in renal transplant recipients co-administered sirolimus: comparison of an enzyme multiplied immunoassay technique (EMIT) and liquid chromatography-tandem mass spectrometry. Ther Drug Monit 28:274–277

Rigourd V, Amirouche A, Tasseau A, Kintz P, Serreau R (2008) Retrospective diagnosis of an adverse drug reaction in a breastfed neonate: liquid chromatography-tandem mass spectrometry quantification of dextropropoxyphene and norpropoxyphene in newborn and maternal hair. J Anal Toxicol 39:787–789

Saito Y, Jinno K (2003) Miniaturized sample preparation combined with liquid phase separations. J Chromatogr A 1000:53–67

Shen JX, Tama CI, Hayes RN (2006) Evaluation of automated micro solid phase extraction tips (micro-SPE) for the validation of a LC-MS/MS bioanalytical method. J Chromatogr B Analyt Technol Biomed Life Sci 843:275–282

Spooner N, Lad R, Barfield M (2009) Dried blood spots as a sample collection technique for the determination of pharmacokinetics in clinical studies: considerations for the validation of a quantitative bioanalytical method. Anal Chem 81:1557–1563

Strazdins L, Meyerkort S, Brent V, D'Souza RM, Broom DH, Kyd JM (2005) Impact of saliva collection methods on sIgA and cortisol assays and acceptability to participants. J Immunol Methods 307:167–171

Streetman DS, Kashuba AD, Bertino JS Jr, Kulawy R, Rocci ML Jr, Nafziger AN (2001) Use of midazolam urinary metabolic ratios for cytochrome P450 3A (CYP3A) phenotyping. Pharmacogenetics 11:349–355

Sung WC, Chen SH (2006) Pharmacokinetic applications of capillary electrophoresis: a review on recent progress. Electrophoresis 27:257–265

Tate J, Ward G (2004) Interferences in immunoassay. Clin Biochem Rev 25:105–120

Taylor PJ (2005) Matrix effects: the Achilles heel of quantitative high-performance liquid chromatography-electrospray-tandem mass spectrometry. Clin Biochem 38:328–334

Tribut O, Gaulier JM, Allain H, Bentue-Ferrer D (2005) Major discrepancy between digoxin immunoassay results in a context of acute overdose: a case report. Clin Chim Acta 354:201–203

Tucker GT, Rostami-Hodjegan A, Jackson PR (1998) Determination of drug-metabolizing enzyme activity in vivo: pharmacokinetic and statistical issues. Xenobiotica 28:1255–1273

van der Heijden J, de Beer Y, Hoogtanders K, Christiaans M, de Jong GJ, Neef C, Stolk L (2008) Therapeutic drug monitoring of everolimus using the dried blood spot method in combination with liquid chromatography-mass spectrometry. J Pharm Biomed Anal 50(4):664–670

van der Schoor SR, de Koning BA, Wattimena DL, Tibboel D, van Goudoever JB (2004) Validation of the direct nasopharyngeal sampling method for collection of expired air in preterm neonates. Pediatr Res 55:50–54

Vaught JB (2006) Blood collection, shipment, processing, and storage. Cancer Epidemiol Biomark Prev 15:1582–1584

Vogeser M (2003) Liquid chromatography-tandem mass spectrometry – application in the clinical laboratory. Clin Chem Lab Med 41:117–126

Witjes BC, Ahsman MJ, van der Nagel BC, Tibboel D, Mathot RA (2009) Simultaneous assay of sildenafil and desmethylsildenafil in neonatal plasma by ultra-performance liquid chromatography-tandem mass spectrometry. Biomed Chromatogr 24(2):180–185

Yeh RF, Rezk NL, Kashuba AD, Dumond JB, Tappouni HL, Tien HC, Chen YC, Vourvahis M, Horton AL, Fiscus SA, Patterson KB (2009) Genital tract, cord blood, and amniotic fluid exposures of seven antiretroviral drugs during and after pregnancy in human immunodeficiency virus type 1-infected women. Antimicrob Agents Chemother 53:2367–2374

Ethical Considerations in Conducting Pediatric Research

Michelle Roth-Cline, Jason Gerson, Patricia Bright, Catherine S. Lee, and Robert M. Nelson

Contents

Abstract The critical need for pediatric research on drugs and biological products underscores the responsibility to ensure that children are enrolled in clinical research that is both scientifically necessary and ethically sound. In this chapter, we review key ethical considerations concerning the participation of children in clinical research. We propose a basic ethical framework to guide pediatric research, and suggest how this framework might be operationalized in linking science and

M. Roth-Cline • J. Gerson • P. Bright • C.S. Lee • R.M. Nelson (✉)
U.S. Department of Health and Human Services, Food and Drug Administration, Office of the Commissioner, Office of Pediatric Therapeutics, Silver Spring, MD 2011, USA
e-mail: Robert.Nelson@fda.hhs.gov

H.W. Seyberth et al. (eds.), *Pediatric Clinical Pharmacology*,
Handbook of Experimental Pharmacology 205,
DOI 10.1007/978-3-642-20195-0_11, © Springer-Verlag Berlin Heidelberg 2011

ethics. Topics examined include: the status of children as a vulnerable population; the appropriate balance of risk and potential benefit in research; ethical considerations underlying study design, including clinical equipoise, placebo controls, and non-inferiority designs; the use of data monitoring committees; compensation; and parental permission and child assent to participate in research. We incorporate selected national (USA) and international guidelines, as well as regulatory approaches to pediatric studies that have been adopted in the USA, Canada, and Europe.

Keywords Ethics • Pediatrics • Children • Subpart D • International guidelines • Extrapolation • Component analysis • Equipoise • Risk assessment • Choice of control group • Placebo • Minor increase • Scientific necessity • Minimal risk • Direct benefit • Parental permission • Child assent

1   Children as Research Subjects

Historically, children were viewed as vulnerable subjects who should be protected from the risks of research. The result was a paucity of safety and effectiveness data that made the use of therapeutic agents a virtual uncontrolled experiment whenever they were prescribed for children (American Academy of Pediatrics 1977). Tens of thousands of children were harmed by therapies that were assumed in the absence of research to be safe and effective (Fost 1998). More recently, pediatric research has come to be seen as a moral imperative (Shaddy and Denne 2010). Additionally, some disorders primarily affect children, necessitating studies to develop therapeutics in these populations.

The vulnerability of children stems from a number of factors (Kipnis 2003). Children commonly lack mature decision-making capacity; they are subject to the authority of others; they may defer in ways that can mask underlying dissent; and their rights and interests may be socially undervalued. As with adults, children may have acute medical conditions requiring immediate decisions without adequate time for education and deliberation; they may have serious medical conditions that cannot be effectively treated; and they may lack important socially distributed goods that would be provided as a consequence of research participation. Kipnis suggests that parental permission and child assent procedures alone cannot mitigate these vulnerabilities. Rather, studies in the pediatric population must be designed to minimize risk and maximize the possibility of therapeutic benefit (Kipnis 2003).

Recognition of this vulnerability has led many countries to develop regulations or guidelines specific to research with children. In 1973, the US Department of Health, Education and Welfare published its first proposals to develop regulations providing additional protections for vulnerable populations that had "limited capacities to consent" (Department of Health Education and Welfare 1973). The problem of regulating research on children was also assessed by the National Commission (Department of Health Education and Welfare 1978b). The US Food and Drug Administration (FDA) proposed establishing regulations for the protection of human subjects in 1979, including protections pertaining to clinical investigations involving children (Department of Health Education and Welfare 1979). In 1981, FDA regulations were promulgated regarding informed consent (21 CFR Part 50, 2011) and institutional review board (IRB) review of research (21 CFR Part 56, 2011). Based on recommendations made by the National Commission, regulations were promulgated in 1983 that governed research on children conducted or funded by the Department of Health and Human Services (Department of Health Education and Welfare 1983). In 2001, similar protections were extended to research regulated by FDA (2001).

Specific guidelines on pediatric research within the European Union were promulgated in 2001. Directive 2001/20/EC required Member States to develop laws, regulations, and administrative provisions for the implementation of good clinical practice in the conduct of clinical trials (European Parliament and the Council 2001). Specific protections were to be implemented to ensure adequate protections for minors, including parental permission and assent of able children, assurance of direct benefit for the child or for the group of patients with the particular condition, minimization of risk, and scientific necessity of the research. An ad hoc group responsible for guideline development made further recommendations for implementation of this Directive (2008).

The additional protections for children to be enrolled in a clinical investigation can be divided into four "nested" domains with each protection building on an adequate response to the prior protection. The enrollment of children in a clinical investigation must be considered scientifically necessary before the evaluation of whether the research interventions or procedures present an appropriate balance of risk and potential benefit. A clinical investigation must be found to have an appropriate balance of risk and potential benefit before considering the role of parental permission and child assent. This chapter will address these four nested protections.

2 The Principle of Scientific Necessity

A fundamental pillar of pediatric research is the ethical principle of "scientific necessity." This principle holds that children should not be enrolled in a clinical investigation unless necessary to achieve an important scientific and/or public health objective concerning the health and welfare of children. An "important scientific question" may be one that generates information that is necessary and timely for establishing the appropriate pediatric use of investigational therapeutics. A corollary is that children should not be enrolled in studies that are duplicative or unlikely to yield important knowledge applicable to children about the product or condition under investigation. These principles are grounded in regulations and/or guidelines governing human subject protections worldwide. FDA regulations require that risks to subjects are minimized by eliminating unnecessary procedures

(21 CFR 56.111(a)(1) 2011), and that the selection of subjects must be equitable (21 CFR 56.111(b) 2011).

Consistent with the recommendations of the National Commission, equitable selection requires that subjects who are capable of informed consent (i.e., competent adults) should be enrolled prior to subjects who cannot consent (e.g., children) (Department of Health Education and Welfare 1978b). There is broad international agreement on this approach, assuming there are no significant scientific reasons to enroll younger children preferentially to older children and/or adults. EMA regulations (2001), International Conference on Harmonisation (ICH) guidelines E6 (1996) and E11 (2000), and the Declaration of Helsinki (World Medical 2008) all state explicitly that vulnerable populations such as children should not be enrolled in a clinical investigation unless their involvement is essential to answer a scientific objective relevant to the health and welfare of that vulnerable population.

The ethical principle of "scientific necessity" has been operationalized in the scientific principle of "extrapolation." As described in the Pediatric Research Equity Act of 2007 "if the course of the disease and the effects of the drug are sufficiently similar in adults and pediatric patients, the Secretary may conclude that pediatric effectiveness can be extrapolated from adequate and well-controlled studies in adults, usually supplemented with other information obtained in pediatric patients, such as pharmacokinetic studies" (Food and Drug Administration Amendments Act of 2007). The principle of extrapolation also can be found in the International Conference on Harmonization guidance on pediatric research (ICH 2000). The need for pediatric studies is assessed by asking a series of questions about the similarity of the adult and pediatric disease, response to treatment, drug-exposure response, and pharmacokinetic and pharmacodynamic measurements that could be used to predict efficacy (see Fig. 1).

3   Appropriate Balance of Risk and Potential Benefit

The additional safeguards for children enrolled in research are based on two ethical principles. First, the risks to which children would be exposed must be low if there is no prospect of direct therapeutic benefit (PDB) to the enrolled children. Second, children should not be placed at a disadvantage by being enrolled in a clinical trial, either through exposure to excessive risks or by failing to get necessary health care. Consequently, the data necessary to initiate a pediatric investigation must demonstrate *either* an acceptably low risk of the experimental intervention *or* a sufficient PDB to justify the risks of the intervention. A major challenge facing the development of a new product for the treatment of a pediatric disorder or condition is bridging this "risk gap" between (a) research involving procedures and/or interventions that present only a low risk given the absence of sufficient data to establish the PDB, and (b) the conduct of either "proof of concept" or pivotal trials for dosing, safety and/or efficacy that offer a sufficient PDB to the enrolled children to justify exposure to interventions that present greater than low risk.

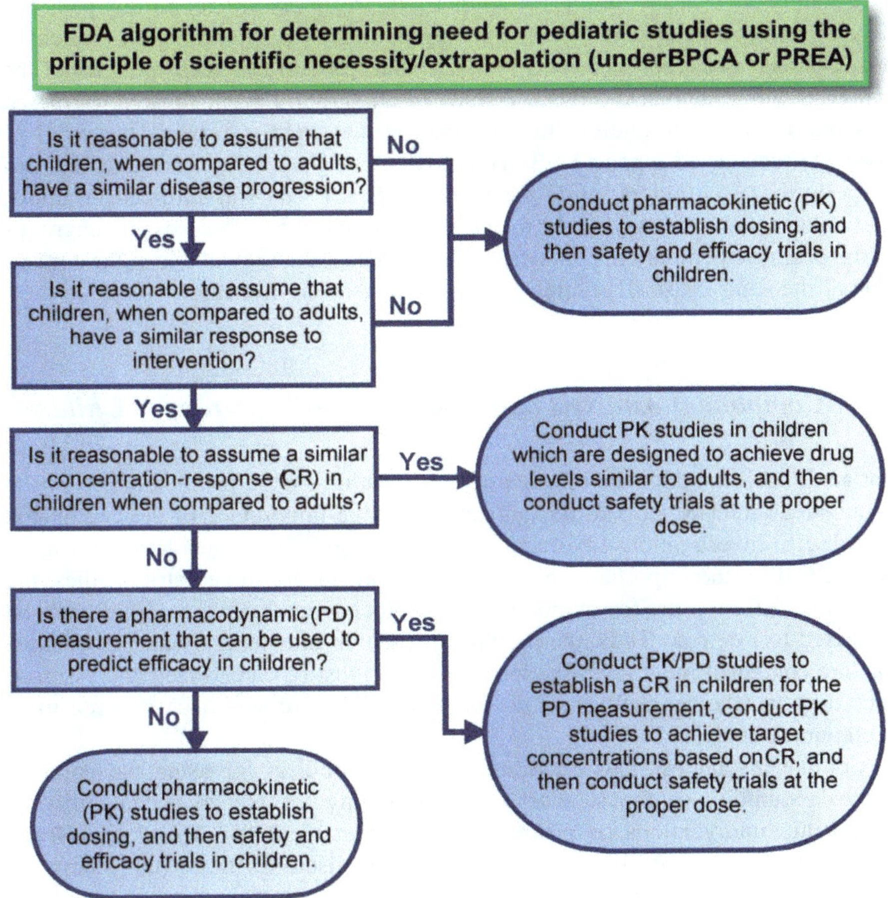

Fig. 1 FDA algorithm for determining need for pediatric studies using the principle of scientific necessity/extrapolation

There are several pathways to pediatric licensure of investigational products. If the product is being developed for a pediatric indication alone (if no comparable adult indication exists), sufficient preclinical data must be developed to support the initiation of pediatric clinical trials. In this case, a major hurdle is establishing a sufficient PDB using a preclinical animal model. If the product is being developed for an indication that occurs in both children and adults, the goal should be concurrent licensure unless there are safety concerns that would delay or even preclude pediatric studies. Adult and pediatric development may proceed either sequentially or concurrently, depending on the product and factors such as the anticipated risks to children and availability of alternate treatments. However, concurrent development still requires sufficient information about PDB in children to support initiating pediatric trials.

If safety or efficacy results of adult trials are necessary to inform pediatric development, sequential development may be necessary. Importantly, sequential development does not necessarily mean that concurrent licensure cannot be achieved. For example, if a phase 2 study of an antiviral agent showed decreased viral burden in adult studies, this information may help to provide the proof of concept necessary to support PDB in children. Dosing and safety studies could then be performed in children while the pivotal efficacy trial was initiated in adults. Particularly if the efficacy of the agent was extrapolated to some or all subgroups of the pediatric population, sufficient pediatric data may be available at the conclusion of the adult phase III studies to support concurrent licensure.

3.1 Component Analysis and Additional Safeguards for Children

For adult subjects, the risks of research participation can be justified *either* by the anticipated direct benefits to the subjects *or* by the importance of the anticipated knowledge. Investigations involving children that pose more than low risk cannot be justified by the importance of anticipated knowledge. In pediatric studies, the allowable risk exposure for an intervention or procedure not offering a PDB must be restricted to low risk. Thus, the individual research interventions and procedures that are contained in an investigational protocol must be categorized and assessed according to whether they do or do not offer PDB – an approach referred to as "component analysis."

Component analysis has come under recent criticism for using the norm of clinical equipoise as the standard for determining the ethical acceptability of therapeutic interventions or procedures (Miller et al. 2003; Miller and Brody 2007). The concept of clinical equipoise will be discussed more fully below. A related (albeit unconvincing) criticism of component analysis is directed toward the manner in which the distinction between therapeutic and non-therapeutic procedures is made (Wendler and Miller 2007). Wendler and Miller (2007) argue that the consequences of the intervention are what matters to the determination of the PDB, rather than the intent of the investigator or the design of the individual intervention. All parties to the debate agree on the need to avoid the term "therapeutic research" which may justify (or offset) the risks of non-beneficial procedures through the inclusion of unrelated beneficial procedures in the same protocol (i.e., the fallacy of the "package deal") (Department of Health Education and Welfare 1978b; Institute of Medicine 2004; Medical Research Council 2004). Otherwise a non-beneficial research intervention that presents considerable risk could be justified by adding unrelated therapeutic components to the protocol, such as free health care.

The analysis of a proposed clinical investigation can be approached either (1) by assessing whether or not each intervention or procedure does or does not offer the PDB, followed by an assessment of the risks of each component, or (2) by assessing the risks of each intervention and procedure, followed by an assessment of the PDB for those components that present greater than minimal risk. An intervention or procedure that presents no more than minimal risk may or may not offer a PDB. We will discuss the "minimal risk" category under the heading of interventions or procedures that do not offer the PDB.

3.2 Interventions or Procedures that Do Not Offer the PDB

There is general international consensus that a child's exposure to risk in pediatric research must be minimal/low in the absence of direct therapeutic benefit to that child. Although there are differences in terminology (minimal risk, minor increase over minimal, low risk, minimal burden, etc.), international regulations share the ethical commitment to limit a child's exposure to non-therapeutic risk. General guidance from European directives is supplemented below by a more detailed review of the US Code of Federal Regulations (CFR) – exploring the categories of "minimal risk" and "minor increase over minimal" in the context of no direct benefit for the individual pediatric participant.

3.2.1 Minimal/Low Risk: No Direct Benefit

For research on non-consenting subjects that does not offer direct therapeutic benefit, the ICH (1996) E6 Guidelines specify that "the foreseeable risks to the subjects are low" and that "the negative impact on the subjects' well-being is minimized and low." FDA regulations use the term "minimal risk" (21 CFR 50.51, 2011) and define it as "the probability and magnitude of harm or discomfort anticipated in the research are not greater in and of themselves than those ordinarily encountered in daily life or during the performance of routine physical or psychological examinations or tests" (21 CFR 50.3(k) 2011). This definition appears to allow for a "relativistic interpretation" indexed to the research participants' own experiences as well as provides two comparators for assessing minimal risk (a) ordinary daily life, and (b) routine physical or psychological examinations or tests (Institute of Medicine 2004). There is well-documented variability in the interpretation and application of "minimal risk" (Shah et al. 2004; Institute of Medicine 2004; Kopelman 2000).

Three US-based advisory panels – the Institute of Medicine (IOM), The Secretary's Advisory Committee on Human Research Protections (SACHRP), and The National Human Research Protections Advisory Committee – recommend the international use of a uniform standard for minimal risk (Fisher et al. 2007). Grounded in the ethical principle of justice as fairness (Institute of Medicine 2004), this approach indexes minimal risk to the normal experiences of average, healthy children rather than to risk levels routinely experienced by the research participants. According to this standard, research interventions and procedures should not involve potential harm or discomfort beyond that which average, healthy, normal children may encounter in their daily lives or in routine physical or psychological examinations or tests (Institute of Medicine 2004). This protects children with a disorder or condition or children who are at increased risk due, for example, to poor socioeconomic status from research unrelated to their condition that is considered greater than minimal risk for a healthy child.

The US-based National Commission listed "routine immunization, modest changes in diet or schedule, physical examination, obtaining blood and urine specimens . . .developmental assessments. . . most questionnaires, observational techniques, noninvasive physiological monitoring, [and] psychological tests and puzzles" as minimal risk (Department of Health Education and Welfare 1978b). While not specified here, "obtaining blood" has been understood to mean venipuncture in many settings in the USA. Other examples include "obtaining stool samples, administering electroencephalograms, . . . [and] a taste test of an excipient or tests of devices involving temperature readings orally or in the ear" (Food and Drug Administration 2001). SACHRP lists a number of physical (e.g., measurement of height, weight, and head circumference; assessment of obesity with skin fold calipers; hearing and vision tests; testing of fine and gross motor development; non-invasive physiological monitoring) and psychological (e.g., child and adolescent intelligence tests; infant mental and motor scales; educational tests; reading and math ability tests; social development assessment; family and peer relationship assessments; emotional regulation scales; scales to detect feelings of sadness or hopelessness) examinations or tests as being no more than minimal risk (Office for Human Research Protections 2005). Finally, some limited exposure to radiation from diagnostic procedures may be viewed as minimal risk (Nelson 2006). However, some of the above procedures may be considered greater than minimal risk depending on the context of the research and the specific population to be enrolled (Office for Human Research Protections 2005).

In assessing for minimal risk, harm or discomfort should be interpreted in relation to the ages (and developmental status) of the children to be studied (Institute of Medicine 2004; Department of Health Education and Welfare 1978a). The duration, cumulative risks, and reversibility of harm also impact on the overall level of risk (Fisher et al. 2007). The use of background risk associated with daily life as a standard for minimal risk has been the subject of debate (Nelson 2007; Wendler 2009; Wendler and Glantz 2007; Wendler and Miller 2007). Data about the risks of "daily life" or "routine examinations or tests" contribute to an informed evaluation of minimal risk, but they alone are not sufficient. The moral acceptability of the risks of research reflects the obligation of a scrupulous parent to evaluate and weigh research risks. These risks should be evaluated against the risks of daily life or routine examinations of a healthy child who is supervised by a *prudent* parent (Nelson 2007; Nelson and Ross 2005). Some general risks that healthy children experience in daily life as part of their growth and development may be deemed excessive if the risk is introduced only for the purpose of producing generalizable knowledge (Fisher et al. 2007).

3.2.2 Minor Increase over Minimal Risk: No Direct Benefit

FDA regulations also include a classification of "minor increase over minimal risk" (21 CFR 50.53, 2011). An intervention or procedure approved under this category must also involve "experiences to subjects that are reasonably commensurate with those inherent in their actual or expected... situations" and be "likely to yield generalizable knowledge about the subjects' disorder or condition that is of vital importance for the understanding or amelioration of the subjects' disorder or condition." This category has been the most controversial, garnering two dissenting votes from members of the US National Commission (Department of Health Education and Welfare 1978b). The justification for this classification has included that the increased risk is warranted due to scientific necessity (CIOMS 2002; Institute of Medicine 2004), scrupulous parents can be entrusted with the authority to evaluate such non-beneficial risk exposures (Nelson and Ross 2005), and that the absolute difference in risk exposure is meant to be "slight" (Department of Health Education and Welfare 1978a). The regulations do not, however, define "disorder or condition," "vital importance," "reasonably commensurate," and "minor increase over minimal risk." These concepts are explored below.

The IOM defined "disorder or condition" as a set of "specific physical, psychological, neurodevelopmental, or social characteristics" that scientific evidence or clinical knowledge has shown to compromise the child's health or "to increase risk of developing a health problem in the future" (Institute of Medicine 2004). Therefore, a child could be healthy, but "at risk" for the condition that is the object of the research based on scientific and/or clinical evidence. Consistent with international guidelines, this definition excludes the use of healthy not-at-risk children from greater than minimal risk research without a PDB (CIOMS 2002; European Parliament and the Council 2001; ICH 1996). The IOM also understood the requirement for "vital importance" to be consistent with the principle of scientific necessity and thus closely tied to the child's "disorder or condition" (Institute of Medicine 2004). The overall plan for pediatric product development should be taken into consideration since information gained from the specific protocol under consideration may be an important yet intermediate step leading to further investigations.

The National Commission uses "commensurate" to describe research activities that are reasonably similar (but need not be identical) to procedures that prospective research participants may ordinarily experience. The IOM elaborated on this approach, noting that "although a child might not have experienced a particular research procedure...the procedure could still be described to the child as potentially presenting levels of pain, immobility, anxiety, time away from home, or other effects that would be similar to those produced by procedures that they have experienced" (Institute of Medicine 2004). The goal is to make the research procedures tangible for the child and parents, thereby improving child assent and parental permission (CIOMS 2002; Department of Health Education and Welfare 1978b).

In assessing whether an intervention or procedure presents no more than a minor increase over minimal risk, there must be sufficient data that any research-related pain, discomfort or stress will not be severe and that any potential harms will be transient and reversible (Fisher et al. 2007). Even if the average risk associated with an intervention or procedure is thought to be low, if the risk estimate is unknown, reflects a large degree of variability, or has not been adequately characterized, then the risks of an intervention or procedure cannot be considered only a minor increase over minimal risk.

For example, single-dose pharmacokinetic (PK) studies of cough and cold medicines in children may qualify as presenting only a "minor increase over minimal risk," depending on the associated data. PK studies may be necessary to establish the correct dose to be used in subsequent efficacy studies. However, the single-dose of a product is unlikely to offer a direct benefit to the child (unless symptomatic) and is associated with a small, but higher than minimal risk (based on prior data). Therefore, to be enrolled, children must have a disorder (symptoms) or a condition (asymptomatic, but at risk based on empiric criteria). A child may be considered "asymptomatic, but at risk" using a combination of three criteria: (frequency) >6 infections per year for children 2 to <6, >4 infections per year for children aged 6 to <12; (crowding) four or more persons living in a home or three or more people sleeping in one bedroom; and (exposure) another ill family member in the home or a child in the family who is attending preschool or school with six or more children per group (Nelson 2010).

Procedures that may present a minor increase over minimal risk (depending on the research context, the specific population of children and the skill of the investigator) have included: lumbar puncture, bone marrow aspirate with appropriate procedural sedation (CIOMS 2002; Institute of Medicine 2004), placement of a blood-drawing peripheral intravenous line for a limited time period, selected approaches to procedural sedation (Institute of Medicine 2004) and perhaps limited radiation exposure (Nelson 2006). The risk of a single-dose PK study depends on both the approach to blood sampling and on the risks of the drug that is being administered.

Although FDA regulations include this classification of "minor increase over minimal risk," EU pediatric regulations do not include such a category of research. Instead, EU guidance documents refer to research which offers potential direct benefits to *individual* research participants and/or to *the group* (i.e., children affected by the same disease, or a disease which shares similar features and for which the product could be of benefit) (European Parliament and the Council 2001). European regulations that specify direct benefit to the individual are closely aligned with US regulations that require direct benefit, discussed in the next section. The "direct benefit to the group" category allows studies to proceed in Europe that would be approved in the USA under the "minor increase over minimal risk" category. Thus, while differences in nomenclature exist, the USA and European approaches are essentially aligned in practice.

In summary, although the ethical importance of restricting risk exposure in pediatric studies in the absence of direct benefit to the child is widely appreciated, implementing associated regulations can be challenging and experts have debated their interpretation. FDA regulations may allow for assessing minimal risk based on the participants' routine experiences, however, there are persuasive ethical arguments for implementing a uniform standard for minimal risk – drawing on normal experiences of average, healthy children, tempered by the child's age, risk duration, cumulative risks, and reversibility of harm. The risks of daily life can also factor into (rather than determine) the scrupulous parent's assessment of minimal risk. In addition, FDA regulation offers the category of "minor increase over minimal risk" and, with clarification of key concepts, provides guidance for more challenging evaluations of risk acceptability when there is no direct benefit to pediatric participants.

3.3   *Interventions or Procedures that Offer the PDB*

Children should not be placed at a disadvantage by being enrolled in a clinical trial, either through exposure to excessive risks or by failing to get necessary health care. Thus, research guidelines worldwide stipulate that persons who cannot provide informed consent – including children – should be enrolled in clinical trials only when the risks are low or the research offers a compensating potential for direct benefit that is comparable to available alternatives (ICH 1996; CIOMS 2002). Similarly, FDA regulations permit pediatric research involving an intervention or procedure that presents more than a minor increase over minimal risk only if it "holds out the PDB for the individual subject" or "is likely to contribute to the subject's well-being." Such interventions or procedures must meet two conditions (1) "the risk is justified by the anticipated benefit to the subjects"; and (2) "the relation of the anticipated benefit to the risk is at least as favorable to the subjects as that presented by available alternative approaches" (21 CFR 50.52, 2011). Research that offers a PDB includes several key concepts that require interpretation: PDB/contribution to well-being, justification of risk, and available alternative approaches.

3.3.1   PDB/Contribution to Wellbeing

Current regulatory frameworks or national and international clinical research guidelines do not explicitly define "direct" benefits, and the literature offers varying views on which benefits are direct. King (2000) provided an influential account of research-related benefits in which she distinguishes between direct (clinical benefits arising from receiving the experimental intervention), collateral (arising from other aspects of the protocol, e.g., medical care), and aspirational (social value of scientific knowledge) benefits. Direct benefit must accrue to the individual research participant, and result from the specific research intervention or procedure, not from ancillary benefits such as health care that may be provided in the trial. The consequences of an intervention cannot be determined a priori, and thus cannot serve as the basis for an assessment of direct benefit that Wendler and Miller (2007) suggest. The determination of the "prospect of direct benefit" is based on the design of the intervention (i.e., choice of dose, duration, method of administration, and so forth) given the available evidence, and not the investigator's state-of-mind or belief in the therapeutic value. The evidence in support of the PDB is generally based on mechanistic and in vivo studies of the intervention in animal models or studies in adult humans.

This account does not squarely address the status of diagnostic or monitoring procedures that are needed to help answer the scientific questions posed by the study (e.g., additional scans, blood draws, or biopsies). As noted earlier, an appropriate balance of risk and potential benefit is required for *each* of the interventions and procedures included in the trial. Monitoring procedures may not per se offer a PDB, yet may be critical in evaluating the safety of other interventions that do offer a PDB. More recent accounts of direct benefit have explicitly considered these procedures (Friedman et al. 2010; Nelson et al. 2010; Miller et al. 2003).

Under current US regulations, there are two ways that the risks of such a monitoring procedure could be evaluated. If the monitoring procedure is made necessary by the administration of the investigational product, the risks of the monitoring procedure may be justified by the PDB of the experimental intervention. Using this approach, the administration of the investigational product *and* the monitoring made necessary by that administration could both be considered under 21 CFR 50.52 (greater than minimal risk with PDB). Alternatively, the monitoring procedure may be viewed as not offering a PDB, and thus considered under either 21 CFR 50.51 (minimal risk) or 21 CFR 50.53 (minor increase over minimal risk). In addition, monitoring procedures that may impact on clinical care may offer PDB. For example, if clinical monitoring of blood levels in order to adjust drug dosing were necessary, the risks of venipuncture would be justified because the blood levels obtained in this way may affect clinical management.

3.3.2 Justification of Risk

Whether the risks of an experimental intervention are justified by the potential direct benefits is a complex evaluation, involving a mix of quantitative and qualitative judgments similar to those made in clinical practice (Department of Health Education and Welfare 1978b; National Commission 1979; CIOMS 2002). There should be empirical evidence of sufficient direct benefit [i.e., "scientifically sound" expectation of success (Department of Health Education and Welfare 1978b)] to justify exposure to the risks. Consistent with component analysis, the risks of an intervention or procedure can only be justified by the benefits to be expected from that same intervention or procedure (Department of Health Education and Welfare 1978b). The justification of risk can include: the possibility of avoiding greater harm from the disease; the provision of important anticipated benefit to the individual exposed to risk; the severity of the disease (e.g., degree of disability, life-threatening); and the availability of alternative treatments.

3.3.3 Available Alternative Approaches

The underlying ethical reason for considering "available alternative approaches" is the view that a child's health or welfare should not be placed at a disadvantage by being enrolled in a clinical investigation (Institute of Medicine 2004). The application of this general principle hinges to a large extent on the interpretation of "available." Some have argued that the other approaches that need to be taken into consideration include "any other course of action (or non-action)" (Department of Health Education and Welfare 1978b). However, the modification of "alternative" by "available" raises the question whether *all* alternatives need to be considered, or only those that are "available" to the subjects to be enrolled in the clinical investigation (Wendler 2008). In other words, should the range of available alternatives against which the risks and potential benefits of the experimental intervention are compared be all those that are "universally" available, or should the alternatives be limited to those that are "locally" available (Lie et al. 2004; Macklin 2001; London 2000)?

To help address this question, we turn now to selected ethical issues in the design and conduct of pediatric clinical trials. The topic of clinical equipoise is followed by a discussion of the choice of an appropriate control group, including the use of a placebo control in pediatric clinical trials. The alternative of an actively controlled trial is explored, with special attention to issues of randomized withdrawal and non-inferiority (NI) designs in the pediatric population. Finally, we pursue the question of when to initiate first-in-human (FIH) studies in the pediatric population, followed by two issues related to the conduct of trials: optimal safety-monitoring practices and compensation in pediatric research.

4 Selected Ethical Issues in the Design and Conduct of Pediatric Research

4.1 Clinical Equipoise

Clinical equipoise is commonly defined as "genuine uncertainty on the part of the expert medical community about the comparative therapeutic merits of each arm of a clinical trial." Advocates of clinical equipoise argue that it "provides a clear moral foundation to the requirement that the health care of subjects not be disadvantaged by research participation" (Canadian Institutes of Health Research 1998; with 2000, 2002 and 2005 amendments; Medical Research Council 2004).

The concept of equipoise combines two separate principles (Miller and Brody 2007). The first principle is the scientific principle of "uncertainty" (i.e., the null hypothesis between the investigational product and the comparator or control group). However, this principle is a requirement of *all* ethical research, and the specification and application of this principle of "uncertainty" is complex (Veatch 2007). The uncertainty of the individual clinician is not decisive, but rather the uncertainty of the relevant community. The morally problematic area is where sufficient data have been developed such that clinical equipoise is disturbed, but insufficient data exist to justify a scientific (or policy) conclusion (Veatch 2007; Gifford 2007).

The second principle contained within the concept of equipoise is the ethical norm that no one enrolled in a trial should receive an inferior treatment (i.e., known effective treatment should be provided). Here clinical equipoise is seen as a specification of the "duty of care" (Miller and Brody 2007). From this perspective, the dispute about the role of equipoise is primarily about whether the "duty of care" (carried over from the clinical setting based on the fiduciary duty of a physician to act in a patient's best interest) should be the ethical framework for clinical research (Institute of Medicine 2004). Proponents of equipoise may argue in favor of actively-controlled comparator trials, as such trials may provide more useful clinical information. However, this approach does not solve the tension between having enough information to make an "individual patient decision" and enough to "warrant making a policy decision" (Gifford 2007).

All parties to the debate over equipoise as a guiding principle of clinical research accept the need for a demarcation between interventions or procedures that either offer or do not offer a PDB. The regulations of many countries are grounded on this distinction. The view that no child should be disadvantaged by participation in a clinical trial bears some resemblance to clinical equipoise. However, an affirmation of the child-patient's right to competent medical care and to protection from undue risk of harm when participating in a clinical investigation does not require nor entail the principle of clinical equipoise. The patient-subject's right to competent medical care should be operationalized in the structure of the investigational protocol (London 2007). The nature of the scientific uncertainty to be resolved by the study design should be specified, and the comparability of alternatives – namely, the ethical and scientific argument in favor of the chosen control group – should be justified.

4.2 Choice of Control Group and Placebo Controls

The choice of an appropriate control group for a clinical investigation should be approached from two perspectives – scientific and ethical. From a scientific perspective, what is the appropriate comparator to use in order to demonstrate the safety and/or efficacy of the intervention? The primary focus is on designing the clinical investigation so that any uncertainty about the research objective(s) is resolved. From an ethical perspective, does enrollment in a clinical investigation place subjects at an unreasonable risk (i.e., one that is not compensated by a sufficient PDB)? Are individuals enrolled in the clinical investigation not receiving a treatment that they should otherwise receive as part of competent medical care? Importantly, the enrollment of a subject in the placebo group does not offer that subject a PDB. No direct medical benefit will be available from the placebo itself, and the avoidance of exposure to an unknown risk of the experimental intervention cannot be considered a direct medical benefit. As noted earlier, direct benefits are limited to desirable clinical effects arising from receipt of the experimental intervention.

The ethics of the choice of control group has been the subject of much debate, focused on either the use of placebo controls or on the choice of a local standard (which may or may not be a placebo) as the control group. The starting point of this debate is often the Declaration of Helsinki, which currently states that "a placebo-controlled trial may be ethically acceptable, even if proven therapy is available, under the following circumstances (1) where no current proven intervention exists; *or* (2) where for compelling and scientifically sound methodological reasons the use of placebo is necessary to determine the efficacy or safety of an intervention and the patients who receive placebo or no treatment will not be subject to any risk of serious or irreversible harm" (World Medical Association 2008). The ICH E-10 Choice of Control Group guidance argues that a placebo-controlled trial may be ethically justified when there would be "no serious harm" from withholding known effective treatment (2001). Even if there would be a good scientific reason to withhold a known effective treatment in order to demonstrate the efficacy of a new treatment, ICH and CIOMS make it clear that withholding proven therapy would *only* be ethically acceptable if the use of placebo would not add any risk of serious or irreversible harm to the subjects, even if the use of an active comparator would undermine the ability of the clinical investigation to produce scientifically sound results (ICH 2001; CIOMS 2002).

Arguably, the clarification of when a placebo control may be used in place of proven effective treatment remains consistent with clinical equipoise. From this perspective, a placebo is acceptable when "patients have provided an informed refusal of standard therapy for a minor condition for which patients commonly refuse treatment and when withholding such therapy will not lead to undue suffering or the possibility of irreversible harm of any magnitude" (Canadian Institutes of Health Research 1998; with 2000, 2002 and 2005 amendments). However, whether or not subjects would commonly refuse standard therapy for a minor condition is not relevant to the ethical justification of the use of a placebo in the absence of "any risk of serious or irreversible harm to the subjects." The withholding of a known effective treatment from children enrolled in a clinical investigation may appear to violate the principle of clinical equipoise. Nevertheless, such a violation may be ethically justified if the risk exposure is limited to low risk (Institute of Medicine 2004). In effect, the risk exposure must be limited to that same level of risk that would be acceptable for an intervention or procedure that does not offer a PDB. Thus, the risk related to withholding a known effective treatment from children enrolled in the placebo arm of a study, for example, must be limited to no more than a minor increase over minimal risk because the placebo arm of a study does not offer a PDB.

A variant of the discussion about placebo (or no treatment) controls concerns the use of "local" versus "universal" standards to determine the appropriate control group. In other words, should "proven effective therapy" only refer to treatments that are actually available in the location where the clinical investigation is being conducted? Some argue that the purpose of a clinical investigation is to alter clinical practice. Thus, "it is crucial... to take the study context into account when designing and conducting such studies." Simply, the appropriate control group (or comparator) should be drawn from actual clinical practice in that setting (Weijer and Miller 2004). However, others argue that the withholding of known effective treatment based on the underlying inequities in the distribution of medical care is unjust and exploits those less fortunate (Shaddy and Denne 2010). A middle ground in this debate requires that the proposed study provide valuable and timely information about a health care need important to the local population, such that there is a reasonable likelihood that the local population could benefit from the research (World Medical Association 2008).

4.3 Alternatives to Placebo Controlled Trials

If a classical placebo-controlled trial is not ethical or practical, there are several alternatives that may reduce or eliminate the exposure to placebo. In a randomized withdrawal trial, all eligible patients with a particular disease are initially treated with the experimental drug. Patients that have a successful initial response are then randomized in a double-blind fashion to remain on the drug or be switched to placebo (or lower doses). The primary study endpoint is time to relapse, usually defined as the duration of time before which clinical signs and/or symptoms of the disease recur. These designs are useful when a trial of medication withdrawal or change in therapy may be clinically indicated, particularly if the experimental drug is similar to those already marketed (Balfour-Lynn et al. 2006). Any child that relapses may immediately be provided with "rescue" medication to reduce the harm or discomfort to no more than a minor increase over minimal risk.

If any exposure to placebo is unacceptable, actively controlled trials may be an alternative. These trials can be designed to test either superiority or non-inferiority (NI) of the experimental intervention relative to the control. Superiority trials generally pose few ethical or interpretational difficulties, provided that the dose of the control product is not artificially low. However, NI designs can pose ethical dilemmas under certain circumstances and deserve further comment.

Non-inferiority trials are intended to show that the effect of a new treatment is not worse than that of an active control by more than a specified margin (Snapinn 2000). The design and interpretation of NI trials is not straightforward. For the NI trial to be valid, one must have historical studies that provide reliable and precise estimates of the effect of the active control regimen relative to placebo (ICH 2001). Further, NI trials do not assure that the experimental agent is "at least as effective" as the active regimen unless superiority of the experimental agent is demonstrated. An experimental intervention may be inferior to the active control and still demonstrate non-inferiority.

Therefore, the primary ethical question is whether it is appropriate to use an NI design for pediatric trials where the inferior performance of the experimental intervention may be associated with serious morbidity or mortality in children. For example, suppose a new antibiotic were tested for life-threatening infections. Even if the experimental drug were shown to be non-inferior, more children may still be at risk of dying due to inferiority of the experimental drug. The ethical acceptability of this design depends on a variety of factors. There may be times when the new treatment offers a potential benefit in lower toxicity or improved usability that may justify using the new treatment in a given population even if it were shown to be slightly inferior to standard care. However, the burden of proof should be on the advocates of the NI study to present convincing evidence that the benefits of the new product outweigh the potential inferiority such that the trial should be allowed to proceed.

4.4 Special Concerns in FIH Pediatric Clinical Trials

An FIH trial is a clinical investigation in which a therapeutic intervention, previously developed and assessed through in vitro or animal testing, or through mathematical modeling, is tested on human subjects for the first time. FIH studies are heterogeneous in design, ranging from dose escalation studies testing conventional oncology drugs to gene transfer trials or monoclonal antibodies that target newly discovered biological pathways. A major ethical question concerning the conduct of FIH trials is whether or not an FIH experimental intervention offers a PDB to the enrolled child. Some take the view that such research *can* offer a PDB, contending that it should be seen as "therapeutic research" (Ackerman 1995) or arguing for a "relativistic understanding of prospect of benefit" (Kodish 2003). Others believe that the objective of FIH is not to produce clinical benefits, and that promoting PDB to participants fosters a therapeutic misconception (Ross 2006; Sankar 2004; Miller 2000). A middle ground requires the recognition that a key ethical dilemma concerning FIH trials is not simply about whether or not they offer a PDB, but whether the PDB is of sufficient likelihood, magnitude, and type to justify the anticipated risks of the experimental intervention (King 2000). Understanding PDB as an empirical matter laden with uncertainty places the focus on assessing the strength of evidence – particularly nonclinical evidence – that provides the scientific rationale for undertaking an FIH trial. There is no consensus, however, on the quantity or quality of nonclinical or adult human evidence necessary to justify a pediatric FIH study.

We propose a "sliding threshold" evidentiary approach, arguing that data (whether animal or adult human) necessary to establish sufficient PDB to justify the risks of the experimental intervention varies with the severity of the disease and the adequacy of alternate treatments. The sliding threshold is hierarchical in character: evidence about *structure* (design) is considered weaker than evidence about *function* (mechanism of action, e.g., molecular targets, biomarkers, physiologic pathways), which in turn is considered weaker than evidence related to a *clinical disease model* (surrogate or clinical endpoints). Kimmelman's principle of "modest translational distance" similarly tries to establish an evidentiary basis for PDB in FIH studies through a critical examination of the assumptions linking nonclinical and clinical models (2009, 2010).

A critical issue in the design of many FIH trials is the question of starting dose. Currently the estimation of a maximum recommended starting dose (MRSD) in an FIH study often is based on the "no observed adverse effect level" (NOAEL), as determined in toxicity studies in relevant animal species. The starting dose for human intervention is then reduced by a substantial safety margin. While this approach may be acceptable in adults, using a very low dose in children may eliminate any PDB from the intervention. Dosing studies in animal models using an appropriate biomarker or physiologic endpoint may therefore be particularly important for establishing a dose in children that is likely to have some biological effect.

4.5   Data and Safety Monitoring in Pediatric Clinical Trials

Data Monitoring Committees (DMC) are advisory to the sponsor, and charged with conducting periodic reviews of accumulated data from ongoing clinical trials to assess for substantial evidence of benefit, harm, or futility of collecting additional data (U.S. Department of Health and Human Services FDA 2006). While all pediatric clinical trials require careful safety monitoring, they do not uniformly require a formal DMC. The only mandatory use of a DMC in US regulations is for research studies in emergency settings in which the informed consent requirement has been waived [21 CFR 50.24(a)(7)(iv) 2011].

However, a DMC is recommended in additional circumstances: large, multi-center studies of long duration; strong a priori safety concerns, potential serious toxicity related to study product use; and populations at elevated risk of death/serious morbidity or in populations deemed potentially fragile (U.S. Department of Health and Human Services FDA 2006). Current guidance from the American Academy of Pediatrics recommends DMCs for all pediatric trials (Shaddy and Denne 2010). In practice, however, DMCs may not be warranted in trials with few or well-characterized risks or at early stages of product development when studies have few participants and are not blinded.

4.6   Compensation for Pediatric Research

Compensation for participation in research is a common practice for research studies that involve both children and adults. A number of different types of compensation are used in clinical studies, including material or monetary compensation such as reimbursement for travel, parking, or inconvenience. The amount paid to study subjects can vary from site to site as well as study to study, even at the same institution for similar tasks (Shaddy and Denne 2010). The American Academy of Pediatrics recommends the giving of gifts instead of money to children as a token of appreciation after the child has completed (or withdrawn from) the trial (1995). While this model may be appropriate for younger children, remuneration using a wage model based on time or effort (e.g., a percentage of trial visits or procedures that have been completed) may be appropriate for older adolescents (Bagley et al. 2007).

Offering payment in studies that enroll children requires parents, investigators, and IRBs to weigh the importance of several competing values (Bagley et al. 2007). Incentive payments may be essential to the recruitment and retention of pediatric study subjects. The obligation to treat all patients fairly might include compensating them for their time, effort, and discomfort and for their contribution to the social good. However, payments to parents for their child's research participation could potentially influence parents to decide in favor of participation without regard for the child's wishes, because there is no personal risk to them (Shaddy and Denne 2010). Some foreign countries prohibit inducements in pediatric trials, either for the parents, legal representatives or children (Federal Agency for Medicines and Health Products (Belgium) 2004). In other instances, parents/legal representatives can only be compensated for their time and expenses (European Union 2008). These concerns must be carefully weighed to ensure that pediatric research can continue without unduly influencing a parent to enroll a child in a research protocol that is not consistent with the best interests of the individual child (Bagley et al. 2007; Institute of Medicine 2004). The exposure of children to excessive risk due to undue influence may be avoided if pediatric trials are designed with an appropriate balance of risk and potential direct benefit.

We now consider a final protection for children in research: parental permission and the assent of children. We also explore conditions under which parental permission may no longer be needed under the applicable law of the jurisdiction in which research is being conducted.

5   Child Assent and Parental Permission

5.1   The Assent Requirement

The requirement for child assent emerged in a 1978 report by The National Commission (1978b). William Bartholome defined four fundamental elements of child assent (1) a developmentally appropriate understanding of the nature of the condition; (2) disclosure of the nature of the proposed intervention and what it will involve; (3) an assessment of the child's understanding of the information provided and the influences that impact on the child's evaluation of the situation; and (4) a solicitation of the child's expression of willingness to accept the intervention (Bartholome 1996). Considerable disagreement among experts remains about many fundamental components of assent, including: the definition of assent, the age at which investigators should solicit assent from children; who should be involved in the assent process; how to resolve disputes between children and their parents; the relationship between assent and consent; the quantity and quality of information to disclose to children and their families; how much and what information children desire and need, the necessity and methods for assessing both children's understanding of disclosed information and of the assent process itself; and what constitutes an effective, practical, and realistically applicable decision-making model (Unguru et al. 2008; Carroll and Gutmann 2010; National Commission 1979).

Children must affirmatively agree to participate in research unless the assent requirement is waived. The absence of dissent does not qualify as assent (21 CFR 50.3(n) 2011). US regulations allow the assent requirement to be waived only when the research holds out the possibility of direct benefit that is available only in the research context, or if the child is judged incapable of assent (Department of Health Education and Welfare 1983). Evaluating the capacity of a child to assent to research participation presupposes an understanding of what the giving of assent means. If we expect the child to make an adult-like judgment of the risks and possible benefits of the research, such a capacity may not develop until mid-adolescence. However, if a child simply needs to agree based on their own perspective on the acceptability of the experience (e.g., the pain of having a blood test), a younger child would be capable of assent. While not specifying the elements of assent as Bartholome did (1996), The National Commission opined that children as young as 7 years of age are capable of assent (Department of Health Education and Welfare 1978b).

The criteria are found in US regulations are similar to those in international regulations on child assent and participation in research. For example, the EU Directive 2001/20/EC states that the following conditions must be met for any pediatric clinical trial: "(a) consent must represent the minor's presumed will and may be revoked at any time, without detriment to the minor; (b) the minor has received information according to its capacity of understanding regarding the trial, the risks and the benefits; and (c) the explicit wish of a minor who is capable of forming an opinion and assessing this information to refuse participation or to be withdrawn from the clinical trial at any time is considered by the investigator" (European Parliament and the Council 2001). Specific guidance on age requirements and assent procedures is again not included.

5.2   Parental Permission

Since children are unable to provide informed consent, pediatric research relies on parental permission to authorize the enrollment of children in research. There is wide international agreement on this requirement of surrogate (usually parental) consent. A parent is generally defined as a child's biological or adoptive parent, and a guardian is defined as an individual who is authorized under applicable state or local law to consent on behalf of a child to general medical care. The parental permission requirement is intended to protect the child from assuming unreasonable risks (Rossi et al. 2003).

However, the feasibility of obtaining parental permission may be a problem in certain circumstances. For example, great distances, lack of communication infrastructure, social dislocation, or high parental mortality (e.g., HIV affected populations) may serve to make parents unreachable. US regulations governing Health and Human Services-funded research at (45 CFR 46.408(c) 2011) allow for a waiver of the requirement for parental or guardian permission if a research ethics committee determines that the requirement is unreasonable. However, FDA regulations for the protection of children (21 CFR 50, Subpart D 2011) do not include this waiver. Thus, for the majority of FDA-regulated research, parental permission is required for the enrollment of children. The exception from informed consent allowed under (21 CFR 50.24, 2011) for research conducted in emergency settings applies to children as well as adults.

5.3   The Definition of a Child

Children are defined in FDA regulations as "persons who have not attained the legal age for consent to treatments or procedures involved in clinical investigations, under the applicable law of the jurisdiction in which the clinical investigation will be conducted" (21 CFR 50.3(o) 2011). In effect, whether or not an individual subject is considered a child for the purposes of the application of Subpart D depends on how the age of majority is defined by state law. State law also defines certain conditions under which a child who is younger than the age of majority may be considered emancipated (i.e. not under the control of a parent or guardian) and thus effectively an adult. These conditions generally include marriage, military service, or a court order, but vary considerably from state to state. FDA regulations would allow a minor who meets one of these conditions to be considered an adult for the purposes of research. In addition, state law may allow a minor to consent for certain interventions and procedures such as treatment for sexually transmitted diseases and drug abuse. If the clinical investigation involves one of these conditions, a minor may be considered an adult for the purposes of obtaining informed consent (absent parental permission). Such a determination would be made by the local research ethics committee in consultation with legal counsel.

International regulations do not define the pediatric population according to the age of consent to specific interventions or procedures. For instance, both the European Commission (2008), and ICH E11 (2000) refer to the pediatric population as birth to 18 years. The policy of using local judicial or legal procedures to either appoint a guardian or establish that an adolescent is legally able to consent to the interventions and procedures included in the research is more defensible than relying on the interpretation of particular permission guidelines by individual research ethics committees. The use of established, transparent, and fair judicial procedures to establish the right of an adolescent to consent to research participation under the applicable laws of the appropriate jurisdiction respects the differing moral and legal views of local communities while affirming a liberty interest of parents to raise their children as they see fit (Nelson et al. 2010).

6 Summary

In recognition of the benefits of pediatric research, research ethics has evolved from a position of excluding children to one of cautious advocacy – acknowledging the critical role of pediatric research, but accompanied by careful consideration of the scientific context, evaluation of risks and benefits, and protection to participants. Many countries have adopted regulations or guidelines to protect children in research. Typically, this requires a careful analysis of the risk associated with each intervention and/or procedure, an evaluation of potential benefits, provisions for child assent, and ensuring adequate parent/guardian permission. The regulatory agencies overseeing pediatric research need to make a careful ethical assessment weighing sometimes complex trade-offs so as to protect children's welfare and prevent undue risk of harm while generating scientifically valuable information to answer important questions concerning the health and welfare of children.

References

21 CFR 50, Subpart D. http://www.accessdata.fda.gov/scripts/cdrh/cfdocs/cfcfr/CFRSearch.cfm?CFRPart=50&showFR=1&subpartNode=21:1.0.1.1.19.4. Accessed 3 Jan 2011

21 CFR 50.3(k). http://www.accessdata.fda.gov/scripts/cdrh/cfdocs/cfcfr/CFRSearch.cfm?fr=50.3. Accessed 3 Jan 2011

21 CFR 50.3(n). http://www.accessdata.fda.gov/scripts/cdrh/cfdocs/cfcfr/CFRSearch.cfm?fr=50.3. Accessed 3 Jan 2011

21 CFR 50.3(o). http://www.accessdata.fda.gov/scripts/cdrh/cfdocs/cfcfr/CFRSearch.cfm?fr=50.3. Accessed 3 Jan 2011

21 CFR 50.24. http://www.accessdata.fda.gov/scripts/cdrh/cfdocs/cfcfr/CFRSearch.cfm?fr=50.24. Accessed 3 Jan 2011

21 CFR 50.24(a)(7)(iv). http://www.accessdata.fda.gov/scripts/cdrh/cfdocs/cfcfr/CFRSearch.cfm?fr=50.24. Accessed 3 Jan 2011

21 CFR 50.51. http://www.accessdata.fda.gov/scripts/cdrh/cfdocs/cfcfr/CFRSearch.cfm?fr=50.51. Accessed 3 Jan 2011

21 CFR 50.52. http://www.accessdata.fda.gov/scripts/cdrh/cfdocs/cfcfr/CFRSearch.cfm?fr=50.52. Accessed 3 Jan 2011

21 CFR 50.53. http://www.accessdata.fda.gov/scripts/cdrh/cfdocs/cfcfr/CFRSearch.cfm?fr=50.53. Accessed 3 Jan 2011

21 CFR 56.111(a)(1). http://www.accessdata.fda.gov/scripts/cdrh/cfdocs/cfcfr/CFRSearch.cfm?fr=56.111. Accessed 3 Jan 2011

21 CFR 56.111(b). http://www.accessdata.fda.gov/scripts/cdrh/cfdocs/cfcfr/CFRSearch.cfm?fr=56.111. Accessed 3 Jan 2011

21 CFR Part 50. http://www.accessdata.fda.gov/scripts/cdrh/cfdocs/cfcfr/CFRsearch.cfm?CFRPart=50. Accessed 3 Jan 2011

21 CFR Part 56. http://www.accessdata.fda.gov/scripts/cdrh/cfdocs/cfcfr/cfrsearch.cfm?cfrpart=56. Accessed 3 Jan 2011

45 CFR 46.408(c). http://www.hhs.gov/ohrp/humansubjects/guidance/45cfr46.htm#46.408. Accessed 3 Jan 2011

Ackerman TF (1995) Phase I pediatric oncology trials. J Pediatr Oncol Nurs 12(3):143–145

Ad hoc group for the development of implementing guidelines for Directive 2001/20/EC (2008) Ethical considerations for clinical trials on medicinal products with the paediatric population. Ad hoc group for the development of implementing guidelines for Directive 2001/20/EC relating to good clinical practice in the conduct of clinical trials on medicinal products for human use. http://ec.europa.eu/health/files/eudralex/vol-10/ethical_considerations_en.pdf. Accessed 10 Dec 2010

American Academy of Pediatrics (1977) Committee on drugs. Guidelines for the ethical conduct of studies to evaluate drugs in pediatric populations. Pediatrics 60(1):91–101

American Academy of Pediatrics (1995) Committee on drugs. Guidelines for the ethical conduct of studies to evaluate drugs in pediatric populations. Pediatrics 95(2):286–294

Bagley SJ, Reynolds WW, Nelson RM (2007) Is a "wage-payment" model for research participation appropriate for children? Pediatrics 119(1):46–51. doi:10.1542/peds.2006-1813

Balfour-Lynn IM, Lees B, Hall P, Phillips G, Khan M, Flather M, Elborn JS (2006) Multicenter randomized controlled trial of withdrawal of inhaled corticosteroids in cystic fibrosis. Am J Respir Crit Care Med 173(12):1356–1362. doi:200511-1808OC [pii] 10.1164/rccm.200511-1808OC

Bartholome W (1996) Ethical issues in pediatric research. In: Vanderpool HY (ed) The ethics of research involving human subjects. University Publishing Group, Fredrick, MD

Canadian Institutes of Health Research (1998; with 2000, 2002 and 2005 amendments) Tri-council policy statement: ethical conduct for research involving humans. Canadian Institutes of Health Research – Natural Sciences and Engineering Research Council of Canada and Social Sciences and Humanities Research Council of Canada. http://www.pre.ethics.gc.ca/english/policystatement/introduction.cfm. Accessed 10 Dec 2010

Carroll TW, Gutmann MP (2010) The limits of autonomy: the Belmont report and the history of childhood. J Hist Med Allied Sci 60(1):82–115. doi:10.1093/jhmas/jrq021

CIOMS (2002) International ethical guidelines for biomedical research involving human subjects. Council for International Organizations of Medical Sciences (CIOMS) in collaboration with the World Health Organization (WHO). http://www.cioms.ch/publications/layout_guide2002.pdf. Accessed 10 Dec 2010

Department of Health Education and Welfare (1973) Protection of human subjects: policies and procedures. Fed Regist 38(221):31738–31749

Department of Health Education and Welfare (1978a) Notice of proposed rule-making: subpart D – additional protections for children. Fed Regist 43:31785

Department of Health Education and Welfare (1978b) Research involving children: report and recommendations of the national commission for the protection of human subjects of biomedical and behavioral research. Fed Regist 43(9):2083–2114

Department of Health Education and Welfare (1979) Protection of human subjects; proposed establishment of regulations. Fed Regist 44(80):24106–24111

Department of Health Education and Welfare (1983) Subpart D: additional protections for children involved as subjects in research. Fed Regist 48:9818–9820

European Parliament and the Council (2001) Directive 2001/20/EC of the European Parliament and the Council on the approximation of the laws, regulations, and administrative provisions of the Member States relating to the implementation of good clinical practice in the conduct of clinical trials on medicinal products for human use. Off J Eur Commun 121:34

European Union (2008) Ethical considerations for clinical trials on medicinal products conducted with the paediatric population. Eur J Health Law 15(2):223–250

Federal Agency for Medicines and Health Products (Belgium) (2004) Law of May 7th 2004: unofficial consolidated version. http://www.fagg-afmps.be/en/human_use/medicines/Medicines/research_development/clinical_trials/index.jsp. Accessed 10 Dec 2010

Fisher CB, Kornetsky SZ, Prentice ED (2007) Determining risk in pediatric research with no prospect of direct benefit: time for a national consensus on the interpretation of federal regulations. Am J Bioeth 7(3):5–10. doi:10.1080/15265160601171572

Food and Drug Administration (2001) Additional safeguards for children in clinical research. Fed Regist 66(79):20589–20600

Food and Drug Administration (2007) Food and Drug Administration Amendments Act of 2007 – Pediatric Research Equity Act (reauthorization), 110th Congress ed: H.R. 3580, Public Law 110-85

Food and Drug Administration Amendments Act of 2007. Title VI: Pediatric Research Equity Act of 2007. Pub. L. no. 110-85, 121 Stat 823 (2007)

Fost N (1998) Ethical dilemmas in medical innovation and research: distinguishing experimentation from practice. Semin Perinatol 22(3):223–232

Friedman A, Robbins E, Wendler D (2010) Which benefits of research participation count as 'Direct'? Bioethics. doi:BIOT1825 [pii] 10.1111/j.1467-8519.2010.01825.x

Gifford F (2007) So-called "clinical equipoise" and the argument from design. J Med Philos 32(2):135–150. doi:777158743 [pii] 10.1080/03605310701255743

ICH (1996) International Conference on Harmonisation E6(R1): guideline for good clinical practice. http://www.ich.org/LOB/media/MEDIA482.pdf. Accessed 10 Dec 2010

ICH (2000) International Conference on Harmonisation Guidance on E11 clinical investigation of medicinal products in the pediatric population. Available via HSR. http://www.fda.gov/downloads/RegulatoryInformation/Guidances/ucm129477.pdf. Accessed 10 Dec 2010

ICH (2001) International Conference on Harmonisation E10: choice of control group and related issues in clinical trials available via HSR. http://www.fda.gov/RegulatoryInformation/Guidances/ucm125802.htm. Accessed 10 Dec 2010

Institute of Medicine (2004) IOM committee on clinical research involving children: ethical conduct of clinical research involving children. National Academies Press, Washington, DC, 2010/07/30 edn

Kimmelman J (2009) Ethics of cancer gene transfer clinical research. Methods Mol Biol 542:423–445

Kimmelman J (2010) Gene transfer and the ethics of first-in-human research: lost in translation, 1st edn. Cambridge University Press, Cambridge, UK

King NM (2000) Defining and describing benefit appropriately in clinical trials. J Law Med Ethics 28(4):332–343

Kipnis K (2003) Seven vulnerabilities in the pediatric research subject. Theor Med Bioeth 24(2):107–120

Kodish E (2003) Pediatric ethics and early-phase childhood cancer research: conflicted goals and the prospect of benefit. Account Res 10(1):17–25

Kopelman LM (2000) Children as research subjects: a dilemma. J Med Philos 25(6):745–764

Lie RK, Emanuel E, Grady C, Wendler D (2004) The standard of care debate: the Declaration of Helsinki versus the international consensus opinion. J Med Ethics 30(2):190–193

London AJ (2000) The ambiguity and the exigency: clarifying 'standard of care' arguments in international research. J Med Philos 25(4):379–397

London AJ (2007) Two dogmas of research ethics and the integrative approach to human-subjects research. J Med Philos 32(2):99–116. doi:10.1080/03605310701255727

Macklin R (2001) After Helsinki: unresolved issues in international research. Kennedy Inst Ethics J 11(1):17–36

Medical Research Council (2004) Medical research involving children. Medical Research Council, London

Miller FG, Brody H (2007) Clinical equipoise and the incoherence of research ethics. J Med Philos 32(2):151–165. doi:777158978 [pii] 10.1080/03605310701255750

Miller FG, Wendler D, Wilfond B (2003) When do the federal regulations allow placebo-controlled trials in children? J Pediatr 142(2):102–107. doi:S0022-3476(02)40245-4 [pii] 10.1067/mpd.2003.43

Miller M (2000) Phase I cancer trials. A collusion of misunderstanding. Hastings Cent Rep 30(4):34–43

National Commission (1979) The Belmont Report: ethical principles and guidelines for the protection of human subjects of research from the National Commission for the Protection of Human Subjects of Biomedical and Behavioral Research. National Commission, Washington, DC

Nelson R (2006) Issues in the Institutional Review Board Review of PET scan protocols. In: Charron M (ed) Practical pediatric PET imaging. Springer, New York

Nelson RM (2007) Minimal risk, yet again. J Pediatr 150(6):570–572. doi:10.1016/j. jpeds.2007.03.040

Nelson RM (2010) The scientific and ethical path forward in pediatric product development. http://www.bioethics.nih.gov/hsrc/slides/Nelson%20-%20NIH%20HSP%20Course%2010-20-2010.pdf. Accessed 10 Dec 2010

Nelson RM, Lewis LL, Struble K, Wood SF (2010) Ethical and regulatory considerations for the inclusion of adolescents in HIV biomedical prevention research. J Acquir Immune Defic Syndr 54(Suppl 1):S18–S24. doi:10.1097/QAI.0b013e3181e2012e

Nelson RM, Ross LF (2005) In defense of a single standard of research risk for all children. J Pediatr 147(5):565–566. doi:10.1016/j.jpeds.2005.08.051

Office for Human Research Protections (2005) Appendix B: Secretary's Advisory Committee on Human Research Protections (SACHRP) – Chair Letter to HHS Secretary Regarding Recommendations. http://www.hhs.gov/ohrp/sachrp/sachrpltrtohhssecApdB.html. Accessed 10 Dec 2010

Ross L (2006) Phase I research and the meaning of direct benefit. J Pediatr 149(1 Suppl):S20–S24. doi:S0022-3476(06)00372-6 [pii] 10.1016/j.jpeds.2006.04.046

Rossi WC, Reynolds W, Nelson RM (2003) Child assent and parental permission in pediatric research. Theor Med Bioeth 24(2):131–148

Sankar P (2004) Communication and miscommunication in informed consent to research. Med Anthropol Q 18(4):429–446

Shaddy RE, Denne SC (2010) Clinical report – guidelines for the ethical conduct of studies to evaluate drugs in pediatric populations. Pediatrics 125(4):850–860. doi:peds.2010-0082 [pii] 10.1542/peds.2010-0082

Shah S, Whittle A, Wilfond B, Gensler G, Wendler D (2004) How do institutional review boards apply the federal risk and benefit standards for pediatric research? JAMA 291(4):476–482. doi:10.1001/jama.291.4.476

Snapinn SM (2000) Noninferiority trials. Curr Control Trials Cardiovasc Med 1(1):19–21

U.S. Department of Health and Human Services FDA (2006) Guidance for clinical trial sponsors: establishment and operation of clinical trial data monitoring committees. http://www.fda.gov/downloads/RegulatoryInformation/Guidances/ucm127073.pdf. Accessed 10 Dec 2010

Unguru Y, Coppes MJ, Kamani N (2008) Rethinking pediatric assent: from requirement to ideal. Pediatr Clin North Am 55(1):211–222. doi:10.1016/j.pcl.2007.10.016, xii

Veatch RM (2007) The irrelevance of equipoise. J Med Philos 32(2):167–183. doi:777159077 [pii] 10.1080/03605310701255776

Weijer C, Miller PB (2004) When are research risks reasonable in relation to anticipated benefits? Nat Med 10(6):570–573. doi:10.1038/nm0604-570

Wendler D (2008) Is it possible to protect pediatric research subjects without blocking appropriate research? J Pediatr 152(4):467–470. doi:S0022-3476(07)00887-6 [pii] 10.1016/j.jpeds.2007.09.027

Wendler D (2009) Minimal risk in pediatric research as a function of age. Arch Pediatr Adolesc Med 163(2):115–118. doi:10.1001/archpediatrics.2008.524

Wendler D, Glantz L (2007) A standard for assessing the risks of pediatric research: pro and con. J Pediatr 150(6):579–582. doi:10.1016/j.jpeds.2007.02.018

Wendler D, Miller FG (2007) Assessing research risks systematically: the net risks test. J Med Ethics 33(8):481–486. doi:10.1136/jme.2005.014043

World Medical Association (2008) Declaration of Helsinki – ethical principles for medical research involving human subjects. http://www.wma.net/en/30publications/10policies/b3/index.html. Accessed 10 Dec 2010

Pediatric Regulatory Initiatives

Steven Hirschfeld and Agnes Saint-Raymond

Contents

S. Hirschfeld (✉)
National Children's Study Eunice Kennedy Shriver, National Institute of Child Health and Human
Development, 31 Center Drive, Room 2A03, MSC 2425, Bethesda, MD 20892, USA
e-mail: hirschfs@mail.nih.gov

A. Saint-Raymond
Scientific Advice, Paediatrics, and Orphan Drug Sector, European Medicines Agency, 7 Westferry
Circus, Canary Wharf, London E14 4HB, United Kingdom

H.W. Seyberth et al. (eds.), *Pediatric Clinical Pharmacology,*
Handbook of Experimental Pharmacology 205,
DOI 10.1007/978-3-642-20195-0_12, © Springer-Verlag Berlin Heidelberg 2011

Abstract A series of government actions have evolved since the 1990s to facilitate the development of medicinal products for pediatric use using a combination of incentives and mandates. The initiatives have been successful in stimulating activity and interest in products developed for pediatric use. The initiatives continue to evolve as experience accumulates and regulatory agencies develop robust cooperative programs. A multidimensional program is necessary to achieve the necessary goal of aligning pediatric therapeutics with adult therapeutics and providing children the most favorable opportunity to benefit and minimize risk to vulnerable populations.

Keywords Pediatric medicines • Therapeutic orphans • ICH E11 guidelines • United States Federal Pediatric Initiatives • European Pediatric Regulation • Written request • Pediatric rules • Pediatric investigation plan • Waivers • Deferrals

1 Regulatory Part 1: United States Federal Pediatric Initiatives

1.1 Introduction

A quotation from Vice President Hubert Humphrey, who trained as a pharmacist, is inscribed in wall of the lobby of the building named after him in Washington, DC, which is the headquarters of the United States Department of Health and Human Services. The inscription reads "The moral test of a government is how it treats those who are at the dawn of life, the children; those who are in the twilight of life, the aged; and those who are in the shadow of life, the sick, the needy, and the handicapped (1976)."

Protections for animals have existed since the nineteenth century, but legal protections and rights for human children have been a twentieth century development. The early part of the twentieth century saw the emergence of specialists in the diseases of children and the establishment of professional societies.

The United States is governed by a federal system where each of the individual states govern, regulate, and license commerce and other services within their own border, and a federal government governs and regulates commerce only between states and establishes national standards. The foundation of United States law is the Constitution and its amendments. The Federal government has three branches – one to generate law (Legislative Branch with two houses of Congress), one to enact and enforce law (Executive Branch with the President and the Departments and agencies), and one to judge the law based on the principles in the Constitution (Judicial Branch or the Supreme Court). When a law is passed by both Houses of the Congress and signed by the President, it becomes effective. The term "Law" is synonymous with the term "Act." Once a law is in effect it becomes part of the United States Code. The Executive Branch has the authority to issue Regulations (or Rules) to further clarify the law. Regulations are not voted on but are vetted for public comment before they become finalized. A Final Rule or Regulation is published in the Code of Federal Regulations. Regulations are enforceable, but can be challenged in a Federal court.

1.2 Brief Regulatory History

The general regulation of biologics and medicines in the United States began in the early twentieth century with a series of laws triggered by several widely publicized events involving the administration of tainted products causing the deaths of children. The establishment of laws to regulate the medicinal products began in 1902 when the use of an equine tetanus antitoxin that was not properly purified and resulted in fatalities among those who received it was widely circulated as a news story. The United States Congress passed the Biologics Control Act in 1902 to regulate the purity and safety of serums, vaccines, and other biologics. In 1906, deaths among infants given a colic syrup containing morphine contributed to the passage of the Food and Drug Act that required the ingredients of products to be listed. The authority of the federal government to regulate interstate commerce for medicinal products was challenged in the courts and upheld in 1912. A subsequent amendment to the Food and Drug Act known as the Sherley Amendment confirmed the federal government's authority.

Over 100 deaths due to a preparation of the antibiotic sulfanilamide containing diethylene glycol in 1937 triggered debate that led to the Food Drug and Cosmetic Act of 1938, establishing a legal requirement to demonstrate safety of regulated medicinal products prior to marketing. The law was amended in 1962 following deaths and malformations associated with the use of thalidomide to include a requirement for establishing effectiveness through investigations. Subsequent regulations clarified the intent to state that the investigations must be adequate and controlled studies with descriptions of the characteristics of such studies.

The last major principle to be enacted into law was the authority of the federal government to grant incentives for certain classes of products through the Orphan Drug Act of 1983. Support for the law came from reports of children with rare diseases unable to find any available therapy in the United States and traveling to other countries to seek treatment.

Due to different legal definitions for different types of products, the Food and Drug Administration (FDA) operates under the authority of many laws and regulations. Administratively the FDA is organized into different centers based on the type of product. For example, the Center for Biologics Evaluation and Research, the Center for Devices and Radiological Health, and the Center for Drug Evaluation and Research each operate under and apply different sets of laws and regulations, and other FDA Centers each have their own specific legal framework and responsibilities. The entire agency is under the direction of a Commissioner. A license for marketing authorization for the use of product that is classified as a drug is termed a New Drug Application (NDA) and the corresponding license for a product classified as a biological is a Biologics License Application (BLA).

Research programs directed to children began to emerge following World War II, particularly in the field of pediatric leukemia but also to study infectious diseases, effects of radiation, and nutrition. While some studies were initiated and supported by the federal government, others were not. Public media reports and the academic medical literature began to describe inconsistencies and harm to participants, particularly children, in research studies. Consequently, a National Commission was established by the United States Congress through the National Research Act of 1974 to examine human research practices and make recommendations. The general principles, as summarized in the Belmont Report published in 1979, are that research should be conducted with respect for person, beneficence, and justice. Regulations to protect research participants were published in the late 1970s. The legal inability of children to formally consent to participate in research and recognition of the need for specific oversight resulted in an additional section of the regulations, Title 45 Code of Federal Regulations, Part 46 Subpart D, published in 1983, that specifically outlines the expectation and responsibilities for research enrolling children. The regulations apply to research that is funded by the U.S. federal government. The regulations were revised for consistency and adopted by a total of 16 federal agencies in 1991.

1.3   Early Efforts to Address Pediatric Therapeutics

The term "therapeutic orphan" was invented in 1968 to describe the status of sick children who lacked appropriate medications. The American Academy of Pediatrics published a White Paper in 1974 outlining expectations for research enrolling infants and children. Concurrently awareness of the need for adequate information to treat children with medicinal products led to several analyses of product package inserts of FDA-approved products that showed 78% had no information pertaining to pediatric use other than, in some cases, a disclaimer that the product is not for use in children.

The FDA began to specifically address the needs of children with a regulation establishing a Pediatric Use section for the product package insert, also known as the product label, in 1979. The FDA subsequently encouraged voluntary development of products for pediatric use through the potential use of extrapolation of adult efficacy under certain conditions in a regulation known as the Pediatric Rule of 1994. The result of the initiative, despite a new regulation and FDA staff writing hundreds of letters to companies and promoting the opportunity, was that the most common response was a statement that a product is not intended for use in children.

1.4   First Generation of Coordinated Federal Pediatric Initiatives

The enactment of the Prescription Drug User's Fee Act of 1992 provided the FDA with additional resources and the Food and Drug Administration Modernization Act of 1997 (FDAMA) followed with FDA review performance standards and a section (Section 111) that introduced an incentive for pediatric use of medicinal products. The principle of providing an incentive that first appeared in the Orphan Drug Act was now extended not just to products intended to treat diseases or conditions that met the definition of a rare disease, but to most medicinal products classified as drugs, with a few exceptions, independent of intended use. Biologics and some antibiotics were not included in the program. The intent was to enhance a voluntary program with a financial incentive.

The specific incentive was a 6-month extension of patent life or marketing exclusivity for all indications, doses, and dosage forms of a product from a sponsor that use the same chemical moiety as its active ingredient. A patent in the United States is issued by the Patent and Trademark Office of the Department of Commerce to protect intellectual property. Marketing exclusivity is a license granted by the FDA in the form of an NDA to provide product innovators with a period of time without competition in the market place to sell a product for its claimed use. The initial standard exclusivity period is 5 years and exclusivity for Supplements (known in other regions of the world as Variations) is for 3 years. A product approved for an orphan indication receives 7 years of exclusivity. The result of receiving a 6-month exclusivity extension for a product was 5½ years of exclusivity for a new product, 3½ years for a Supplement, and 7½ years for a product with orphan designation.

When marketing exclusivity expires, other manufacturers may sell a similar product if they either have intellectual property rights under license from an active patent holder or the patent has expired, in which case no license is required. The new manufacturer must make the product within legal specifications as determined by federal regulations and register the product through an Abbreviated New Drug Applications (ANDA) with the FDA in order to market it. A 6-month extension blocks other manufacturers from entering the market place until the extension expires. The general expectation is that when marketing exclusivity expires, the price of a product will decrease due to competition from other manufacturers. The potential economic impact of a delay caused by an exclusivity extension on the US health care system costs as well as the potential economic benefit to a product innovator was considered in the selection of the 6-month time frame.

The incentive process is initiated by a formal pediatric Written Request from the FDA. The rationale for requiring a pediatric Written Request from the FDA to perform studies that could qualify for an incentive was to ensure that the studies were of sufficient quality, design and public health need to justify the potential risks to children, and avoid the perception of exploitation of a vulnerable population for financial gain.

The specific model was that the FDA would issue a Written Request to the product sponsor stating a general framework for the type of pediatric information expected and an outline of the types of studies, both nonclinical and clinical, to be performed and a due date. The types of studies could include dose finding studies in various pediatric populations, safety studies, pharmacokinetic, or pharmacodynamic studies in various pediatric populations, or a demonstration of clinical benefit. The specific diseases or conditions and the relevant pediatric populations were independent of whatever use the product may have for adults and determined by the public health needs. The due date was determined by a reasonable estimate of the time and resources needed to generate the requested information and was not influenced by expiration dates for a marketing license or patent.

The deliverable from a pediatric Written Request was a report describing how the sponsor responded to the terms of the Written Request by the due date.

A sponsor or a third party could send to the FDA a Proposed Pediatric Study Request outlining a proposal. The FDA then had the option to utilize or modify the proposal in developing a formal Written Request. The FDA also had the option to issue a Written Request without an external proposal.

Proposed Pediatric Study Requests and the study reports in response to a pediatric Written Request were reviewed in the various review divisions within the Center for Drug Evaluation and Research to provide the most specific subject matter expertise. The review divisions would then submit the draft Written Requests to a centralized multidisciplinary Pediatric Implementation Team to provide consistency and additional expertise. Following secondary review and discussion by the Pediatric Implementation Team, the Written Request would be issued by the appropriate FDA Office Director.

The study reports in response to a Written Request were submitted to the issuing FDA review division for initial review. Subsequently, the review division would present a summary and recommendations as to the adequacy of the response to a multidisciplinary Pediatric Exclusivity Board. The adequacy of the response was evaluated on the basis of the data quality, information content, and adequacy to inform pediatric use. It was not based on whether the requested studies demonstrated efficacy or suggested effectiveness in children. The major principle was to obtain high-quality information to guide pediatric use, regardless of the potential for clinical benefit. The knowledge that a product is not effective in a particular population has value in avoiding risk and unnecessary exposure. The Pediatric Exclusivity Board then made a determination that was subsequently communicated to the sponsor. The establishment of the Pediatric Implementation Team and the Pediatric Review Board provided a uniform framework for pediatric needs and product assessment.

The entire pediatric incentive program was developed on a time-limited basis of 5 years after inception and scheduled to expire in the year 2002. The rationale was that if the program were successful, it could be renewed and even improved, and if it were not successful, other approaches would have to be developed.

In 1998, the FDA published a regulation known as the Pediatric Rule of 1998 that was intended to be a mandate to complement the incentive program in the FDAMA. The Pediatric Rule targeted products where the disease or condition that the product was intended to be used for in adults also existed in a pediatric population. All products with a new active ingredient, new indication, new dosage form, new dosing regimen, or new route of administration that were likely to be used in children either due to their potential meaningful therapeutic benefit that would be considered an advance over currently existing therapy in a limited population or the product had the potential for widespread use in the pediatric population were included. Widespread use was calculated use by greater than 50,000 children using the assumption that the threshold for an orphan indication was a prevalence of less than 200,000 in the United States and that children are about one quarter of the population; therefore, an adjusted threshold could be used. In contrast to the incentive program that only applied to medicinal drugs, the mandate program applied to both drugs and biologics. It did not, however, apply to products with orphan designation for the orphan indication. The contemplated penalty for noncompliance was that a product could be considered to be misbranded, meaning that the product had a use that was intended but not included in the language of the product package insert or label. A product that is misbranded can be subject to injunction (legal blockage of production or distribution) and product seizure.

The 1998 Pediatric Rule had provisions for waivers of the requirement for some or all pediatric subpopulations on the basis that the disease or condition did not exist in children or that pediatric studies would not be practical. In addition, sponsors could request a deferral for compliance so that licensing and marketing a product for adult use would not be compromised if the pediatric data were not yet available. Waivers and deferrals had to be requested from the FDA, and deferrals would be granted with a due date for when the pediatric data would be submitted for review to the FDA. A full waiver referred to all children and a partial waiver would refer to only a pediatric subpopulation, usually defined on the basis of age.

The incentive program and the mandate were intended as complementary regulatory tools in a comprehensive program to advance the need for adequate information to manage the risks and provide the benefits that medicinal products can provide to children. As early as 1998, discussions on the pediatric initiatives between the FDA and other regulatory authorities began, built partially on the successful experience of developing orphan drug programs in other regions based on the experience of the US Orphan Product program. In December 2000 under the French presidency of the European Union, with the FDA consulting on the preparation of documents, the European Council of Health Ministers adopted a resolution requesting the European Commission to develop a program for pediatric therapeutics. Further details and elaboration are given in the next section on the European Regulation.

1.5 Second Generation of Pediatric Initiatives

The initial experience with the FDAMA incentive program was favorable, so in January 2002, the pediatric incentive program was renewed for another 5 years when the Best Pharmaceuticals for Children Act (BPCA) became law and included some new provisions including the study of off-patent medications in partnership with the National Institutes of Health (NIH), establishment of pediatric specific FDA advisory committees, enhanced safety reviews, and publication of FDA clinical and pharmacology reviews on the FDA Web site.

The 1998 Pediatric Rule was challenged in court under the premise that if a sponsor did not intend to market a product for a particular use, the federal government lacked authority to force a sponsor to develop a product for an unintended use. In October 2002, a federal court in Washington, DC, heard the case and ruled against the 1998 Pediatric Rule partially on the basis that the US Congress did not intend to give the FDA the authority to compel a manufacturer to study medicinal products in children. The court opinion was based in part on the recent renewal of the pediatric incentive program in BPCA using the argument that Congress had an opportunity to contemplate pediatric therapeutics and chose an incentive mechanism.

Rather than challenge the court decision, the Department of Health and Human Services waited until 2003 when the Pediatric Research Equity Act (PREA) became law and gave the FDA the authority to enforce the development of therapeutic products for children under the same conditions as in the 1998 Pediatric Rule – when the disease or condition was similar in adults and children and when the product was either a meaningful therapeutic advance or would be widely used. As in the original 1998 Rule, options to request waivers and deferrals were included and orphan products were excluded.

The PREA required that products develop a Pediatric Assessment and Plan. The specific language is that all applications (or supplements to an application) submitted under section 505 of the Act (21 U.S.C. 355) or section 351 of the Public Health Service Act (PHSA) (42 U.S.C. 262) for a new active ingredient, new indication, new dosage form, new dosing regimen, or new route of administration to contain a pediatric assessment unless the applicant has obtained a waiver or deferral (section 505B(a) of the Act). It also authorizes FDA to require holders of approved NDAs and Biologic Licensing Applications for marketed drugs and biological products to conduct pediatric studies under certain circumstances (section 505B (b) of the Act). The PREA applied to all products that received marketing authorization since April 1, 1999, because that was the date the 1998 Pediatric Rule became effective.

If a product did not meet the criteria for compliance with the need for pediatric studies, then the Pediatric Assessment and Plan would be to request a waiver. Nonetheless, the potential use of a product in children must be contemplated by every sponsor wishing to file a product use claim for marketing authorization.

Waivers are considered for three general circumstances:

- Studies are not practical due, for example, to the rarity of the disease or condition in children.
- The product is likely to be unsafe or ineffective in children.

- The product is considered neither a meaningful therapeutic advance nor is likely to have widespread use.

Generic products that are licensed under ANDA are generally exempt, but ANDAs submitted under an approved suitability petition under section 505(j)(2)(C) of the PHSA for changes in dosage form, route of administration, or new active ingredient in combination products are subject to the pediatric assessment requirements that PREA imposes. If clinical studies are required under PREA for a product submitted under an approved suitability petition and a waiver is not granted, that application is no longer eligible for approval under an ANDA.

PREA requires development of age-appropriate pediatric formulations with a waiver possible if the applicant can demonstrate that reasonable attempts to produce a pediatric formulation necessary for that age group have failed.

The off-patent program in partnership between the FDA and the NIH was guided by a process to determine priorities for products to study based on chemical entities that were ranked on the basis of discussion at public meetings by subject matter experts. The results of the prioritization process were published annually in the Federal Register.

1.6 Use of Extrapolation

The FDA organized a pediatric extrapolation working group that presented a framework in 2003 for using nonpediatric data in supporting pediatric efficacy. In order to define the nature of the evidence used to extrapolate adult clinical data to a pediatric population, applications from 34 drugs in 23 indications that were granted Pediatric Exclusivity under the 1997 FDAMA were reviewed for the approaches used to relate diseases or conditions found in both adult and pediatric populations. Multiple sources of data were used. Clinical indications approved for adults for each drug were analyzed with respect to pathophysiology, nonclinical data, pharmacokinetics, exposure–response relationships, clinical signs and symptoms, laboratory and surrogate measures, natural history and response to therapy, and then compared to the pediatric condition. Components important in determining relationships between adult and pediatric conditions were identified and classified into four categories: (1) nonclinical data, (2) pathophysiology, (3) natural history, or (4) response to therapy. Analysis showed that similarity of pathophysiology was the most common basis for supporting extrapolation, followed by similar response to therapy.

An algorithm on the use of extrapolation was published in an FDA Guidance Document on "Exposure–Response Relationships – Study Design, Data Analysis and Regulatory Applications" (2003) that outlined the need for pediatric studies using available data. http://www.fda.gov/downloads/Drugs/GuidanceCompliance RegulatoryInformation/Guidances/UCM072109.pdf

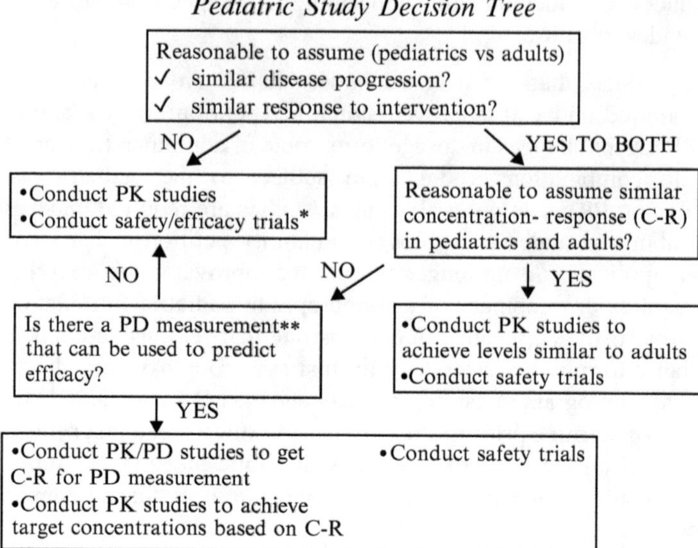

The FDA continues to refine the use of extrapolation through a multidisciplinary extrapolation working team.

1.7   Comparison and Interaction of the Pediatric Regulatory Initiatives

A comparison of the pediatric mandate and incentive programs is outlined in Table 1.

With both the incentive and the mandate for pediatric product research in law, the interaction between the opportunity to qualify for an incentive and the need to comply with the mandate required clarification. The FDA issued a draft Guidance

Table 1 Comparison of major features of US Pediatric Initiative Programs

US Pediatric Mandate Program (PREA)	US Pediatric Incentive Program (BPCA)
Applies to all drugs and biologicals except orphan designation	Biologicals and some drugs excluded but includes orphan designation
Only applies to the drug product and indication under review	Applies to all products with same active moiety
Only applies if an approved or pending indication occurs in adults and children	Eligible indications for study must occur in pediatric populations
Only applies if there is a meaningful therapeutic advance or widespread use	Only applies when there is underlying patent or exclusivity protection
May be used as often as public health need arises	May only be used once in a product lifetime
Mandatory – compliance expected	Voluntary – no compliance expected

document in 2005 to address the question. A Guidance document is a nonbinding public statement from a regulatory agency that reflects current thinking and represents a framework for discussion and interaction.

The FDA Guidance notes that the FDA cannot issue a Written Request for studies that have already been submitted to the agency. Thus, a sponsor that wishes to qualify for the incentive must obtain a Written Request under BPCA prior to submitting studies that are mandated under PREA. Studies performed to address PREA requirements may not be adequate to address a BPCA Written Request because the Written Request can have a broader scope. PREA is limited to conditions where the adult and pediatric diseases are considered similar, while a Written Request is based on public health needs that could extend to any potential pediatric use, including diseases or conditions that are not found in adults.

The opportunity for a sponsor to address the mandate and qualify for the incentive is therefore time limited and context dependent. In addition, the timing of the receipt of a Written Request and the submission of pediatric study data are critical. The interaction between the incentive and the mandate when the two are separate programs under separate laws has been approached by the European pediatric initiatives in a combined program.

1.8   Extension of Human Research Subject Protections

The US regulations in the Code of Federal Regulations Title 45 Part 46 that pertain to human research protection developed during the 1970s and 1980s and revised in the 1990s apply to research that is funded by the federal government. Research not funded by the federal government but regulated by the FDA is covered under regulations in Title 21 Part 50. In 1996, the FDA published the International Conference on Harmonization of Technical Requirements for Registration of Pharmaceuticals for Human Use (ICH) E6 Guidelines, also known as the Good Clinical Practice Guidelines as a Guidance Document. In 2000, the FDA published ICH E11 on Clinical Investigation of Medicinal Products in the Pediatric Population as a Guidance Document. Guidance documents, however, are not legally binding, so in order to provide the same level of protection to children who participate in nonfederal government funded research as provided to children who participate in federally funded research, the FDA adapted the provisions in Title 45 Part 46 Subpart D that pertain to children to Title 21 Part 50 in 2003.

1.9   Interim Results of the Pediatric Regulatory Initiatives

The BPCA and the PREA were scheduled to expire in 2007. By the end of March 2007, under the incentive programs in FDAMA and BPCA, the FDA had issued about 340 Written Requests, granted the incentive for 136 products representing

129 active chemical moieties, and revised 118 product package inserts with new pediatric information. The total number of submissions for an incentive was 149, so the favorable determination rate was about 91%. Under the mandate program for PREA, the FDA revised 55 product package inserts with new pediatric information. The total for both programs was 173 products with new pediatric information.

Of products that received the incentive, 73 had FDA medical or pharmacology reviews or both posted on the FDA Web site by March 2007.

An analysis of these reviews showed that there were 195 individual pediatric studies across 33 drug classes in 12 disease categories. The average number of studies per product was about 3 with a range from 1 to 9 and the average number of patients per product was about 360 with a range from 11 to 1,550. The total number of pediatric patients enrolled for all products was about 25,000.

Studies could be classified into four types – pharmacokinetic only (19%), pharmacokinetic and pharmacodynamic (17%), pharmacodynamic only (conventionally referred to as proof of concept or Phase 2 studies) (32%), and efficacy studies (32%). An efficacy study was defined as a study with a clinically relevant outcome measure and with adequate statistical power to formally establish efficacy. All studies were considered to varying degrees to be safety studies. About one third of all studies had a formal pharmacokinetic component, underlying the importance of dose determination in different pediatric subpopulations. A common theme in many of the studies was the need for dose adjustments in 3- to 5-year-old children.

1.10   Third Generation of Pediatric Initiatives

The Food and Drug Administration Amendments Act of 2007 (FDAAA) renewed the BPCA as Title V of FDAAA with some modifications and the PREA for an additional 5 years. The major modifications in the BPCA are as follows:

- Listing of off-patent drug prioritization process.
- Prioritization of off-patent products to be studied framed by public health needs based on diseases and conditions rather, as in the prior version of the BPCA, based on specific products.
- Flexibility in funding mechanisms that the NIH may use for pediatric studies related to either off-patent drugs or on-patent drugs in the case of the sponsor declining a Written Request.
- Enhanced program for training in pediatric pharmacology.
- Description of the role and responsibilities of the Pediatric Committee (PeRCO) at the FDA to review Written Requests, review pediatric study reports, and track and make public pediatric activity.

The PREA was renewed as Title IV of FDAAA and a new law, Title III – The Pediatric Medical Device Safety and Improvement Act, was added. The Pediatric Medical Device Safety and Improvement Act has provisions for:

1. Requirement to perform pediatric studies in relevant populations for medical devices that are either under development or will be licensed for marketing.
2. Applicability of the law to "patients" who "suffer from" a disease or condition.
3. Definition of a "pediatric patient" as "patients who are 21 years of age or younger at the time of the diagnosis or treatment."
4. Specific safety monitoring requirements.
5. Funding of demonstration projects.
6. Development of a federal pediatric medical device plan.
7. Designation of a pediatric medical device point of contact at the NIH.

The demonstration projects for pediatric medical device development have been funded in 2009 and are under the direction of the FDA Office of Orphan Products with scientific input from the NIH and consist of a consortium of three university-based centers in different geographic regions of the United States.

As of mid-2009, about 370 drugs had been issued Written Requests under the pediatric incentive, about 160 drugs had been granted an incentive based on pediatric data, and about 160 product package inserts had been changed. The pediatric mandate resulted in about 80 product package insert changes for a total of about 240 products with new pediatric information as a result of the pediatric initiatives.

1.11   International Harmonization and Other Trends

The near term future of the US pediatric initiatives includes the harmonization and coordination of a fragmented and diverse clinical research infrastructure. The NIH are supporting several programs designed to augment current clinical research efforts and transform the culture of research to one of stability, cooperation, and collaboration. The most comprehensive is the Clinical and Translational Science Awards Consortium administered by the National Center for Research Resources to build a national infrastructure for translational and clinical research with a man-dated pediatric component. Additional programs from other institutes and centers are coordinating with the Clinical and Translational Science Awards program as they evolve their own programs.

A major operational principle of all the efforts is the concept of interoperability – the capacity to integrate technical and scientific functions on multiple levels. Examples include standards for data acquisition, data transmission and data archiv-ing, agreement on terminology and harmonization of definitions, and assessments of outcome measures. The technical and scientific alignment in several domains has been a priority for the pharmaceutical and biotech industries for over a decade and is actively supported by and has participation of the FDA.

In the United States, most pediatric patients enrolled in clinical research studies are referred and evaluated by academic investigators. A series of workshops and meetings over the last decade have addressed the expectations of commercial sponsors and regulatory authorities with academic investigators to facilitate the operations and compliance of pediatric clinical research. As a consequence of the federal pediatric initiatives, many pharmaceutical companies now have pediatric investigators and pharmacologists on staff. The interactions between pediatric investigators in the regulated industry and academic pediatric investigators are a basis to facilitate pediatric product development.

The FDA has been engaged in formal interactions with international partners for the past 20 years and with attention to pediatric issues for the past decade. Structured and scheduled interactions occur monthly between the FDA and the European Medicines Agency and less frequent, but substantive interactions occur between other international partners and the FDA and other US agencies.

In combination with the European pediatric initiatives, a culture change has occurred in medicinal product development that has extended from the heads of companies to the lecture halls and clinics where specialists are trained to anticipate and plan for a pediatric component in all development plans.

Co-funding between public and private sources for pediatric projects had its origins in the Orphan Drug program and became formalized with the BPCA. Federal funding agencies now work routinely with foundations and other nonprofit partners as well as commercial partners and have dedicated staff and a legal framework to function in. As an example, a public–private partnership to develop biomarkers, The Biomarkers Consortium, has the FDA, the NIH, and other Federal partners along with academic and industry partners and an expectation to examine the pediatric implications for each project the Consortium supports. Other examples of public–private partnerships that involve the FDA are the Critical Path Institute and the Reagan-Udall Foundation.

Coordination of technical and harmonization efforts at the interface of pediatric clinical research, medicinal product development, and regulatory practice has begun with information sharing and future efforts will address resource sharing along with specific technical standards in terminology, outcome assessments, data standards, data sharing, registries, and analyses. Related and parallel international activities to harmonize human research subject protections and ethical and regulatory review are also in progress.

The integrated effect of these initiatives will bring the global community into alignment with the goals and principles described by Hubert Humphrey in 1976.

2　Regulatory Part 2: The European Regulation and Pediatric Medicines

As presented in the first section of this chapter on US initiatives, European pediatricians and authorities also identified the lack of appropriate medicines for children and relevant data. Although most catastrophes with medicines affected children, they led to changes in regulatory requirements for the development of medicines intended for adults.

The adoption of legislation took more time in Europe than in the USA. Despite European publications and active lobbying by pediatricians as early as the 1980s, the first initiative was in 1997 with the organization of a roundtable by the European Commission; the need for legislation was identified, but more time elapsed before the legislative initiative.

In the meantime, Europe with the USA and Japan adopted a guideline on the development of pediatric medicines through the ICH process. This guideline was a follower to the 1997 European guideline. This new guideline, named Clinical Investigations of Medicinal Products in the Pediatric Population, ICH E11, became effective in 2000 in the European Union (EU).

2.1   European Legislation and Pharmaceutical Regulation

Made of six countries in 1957, the European Union includes an expanding number of countries. These Member States have over the years signed various successive Treaties creating a specific supranational environment of free circulation of citizens, goods, and capital. The Union has progressively accumulated laws to harmonize the internal market. To date, the EU includes 27 Member States: Austria, Belgium, Bulgaria, Cyprus, Czech Republic, Estonia, Finland, Denmark, France, Germany, Greece, Hungary, Ireland, Italy, Latvia, Lithuania, Luxembourg, Malta, Poland, Portugal, Romania, Slovakia, Slovenia, Spain, Sweden, The Netherlands, and the UK. Several countries are candidate to accession (Croatia, Former Yugoslavian Republic of Macedonia, Turkey, and Iceland). Three more countries from the European Economic Area/European Free Trade Area are associated with the work of the European Union without having formally joined: Norway, Liechtenstein, and Iceland (which has now requested accession). They apply the same regulation of medicinal products and participate in the work of the European Agency. The EU has currently 23 official languages (not including Norwegian and Icelandic) among 60 regional or minority languages. All approval decisions concerning medicines are issued in all official languages.

The European Parliament, representing the people of Europe, in consultation with the European Council of Ministers, representing governments, usually adopt European legislation through a co-decision procedure, but a legislative initiative is under the sole responsibility of the European Commission. Two sets of laws can be adopted in the European Union: Regulations and Directives. A Regulation is a law directly applicable to Member States; a Directive is a more flexible framework, which requires to be transposed into national law in a given timeframe. A Regulation has clearly a different meaning in the USA and in the EU.

Since 1965, the EU issued various Directives regulating the authorization and pharmacovigilance of medicines (i.e., medicinal products encompassing biologicals, vaccines, and chemicals), medical devices, and clinical trials. In 1993, a Regulation created a European Medicines Evaluation Agency (EMEA), since 2004 the European Medicines Agency (EMA), and established a Community procedure of authorization valid across the EU. In 2004, a codification exercise of all pharmaceutical legislation consolidated the various texts and took account of innovation in this area.

Two major laws are framing the regulation of medicinal products in the EU, Regulation (EC) No 726/2004, which covers the Community procedures and the Agency, and Directive 2001/83/EC, which covers the marketing authorization of medicinal products, the content of an application, and "decentralized" (or national) and referral procedures. Both laws have already been amended several times and complemented by the Regulation on medicinal products for paediatric use in 2006[1] (Regulation (EC) No 1901/2006, hereafter the Pediatric Regulation) and the Regulation on Advanced Therapies (Regulation (EC) No 1394/2007).

Additionally, a Directive (2001/20/EC) sets the framework for interventional clinical trials using medicinal products, and several Directives cover the supervision of medical devices. The European Medicines Agency is coordinating activities relating to authorization and supervision of medicinal products in collaboration with National Medicines Authorities, but both the authorization of clinical trials and that of medical devices remain activities of national authorities.

The European Commission is the decision-making body for Community procedures once the Agency has given a positive scientific opinion on the quality, safety, and efficacy of the product through its Committees. National Authorities grant authorizations for national marketing authorization procedures only. The choice of using the Community instead of a national procedure depends on the nature of the medicine or its intended indication. Biologicals, orphan medicines, and medicines intended for the treatment of cancer, diabetes, HIV, neurodegenerative diseases, viral diseases, and autoimmune diseases must go through the Community procedure. The Community procedure is optional for other medicines, but in practice all new medicines are now using the Community procedure, whereas many generics use the national procedures. Once authorized, a medicinal product is protected by 10 years of data protection, during which no generic can be authorized. Since the implementation of the Regulation on orphan medicinal products in 2000, designated orphan medicines receive 10 years of market exclusivity protecting not only against generic competition, but also against similar medicines, therefore receiving wider protection. In Europe, similar to the Pediatric Exclusivity of the US BPCA, medicines developed for children can receive 6 months of extension of the patent [under the form of an extension of the Supplementary Protection Certificate (SPC)], provided they meet all necessary requirements.

Scientific opinions to support various regulatory activities on medicines are given by the Scientific Committees of the European Medicines Agency. These committees include experts from all Member States, and in most Committees also include patients' representatives as full members. The Agency has six permanent Committees, generally referred to by their acronym: the approval Committee

---

[1]Please note that American English spelling is used except where specific terms are referred to, as British English spelling is generally used in Europe.

(Committee for Medicinal Products for Human Use, CHMP), the Committee for Orphan Medicinal Products (COMP), the Committee on Advanced Therapies (CAT), the Committee on Herbal Medicinal Products (HMPC), and the Paediatric Committee PDCO. The sixth one is a Committee on veterinary medicines (CVMP). Most Committees have set up and delegated preparatory work (e.g., guidelines) to expert groups, the Working Parties. One is of particular relevance for the pediatric development of medicines, the Scientific Advice Working Party, which advises companies on their proposed development. For orphan and pediatric medicines, the Agency staff has a direct complementary role in the evaluation. For other procedures, the Agency has only a coordination role, as the evaluation is performed by experts and regulators working in the Member States and finalized by the relevant Committee.

Following the receipt of an Agency opinion, the European Commission takes all administrative decisions (e.g., orphan designation) except on Paediatric Investigation Plans (PIP), which are signed into Decisions by the Executive Director of the Agency.

2.2   The European Pediatric Regulation: A Concise History

The French Presidency of the EU of 2000 submitted a memorandum to the European Council of Ministers on the need for pediatric medicines. As a consequence, the Council adopted unanimously a resolution urging the Commission to initiate legislation on medicines for children. Between 2000 and 2004, the European Commission went through a long exercise of consultation of stakeholders, of drafting proposals, and analyzing the potential impact of such legislation. The existing US model was scrutinized to take account of its successes and limitations. In September 2004, a first draft of a Regulation was submitted to the European Parliament and to the Council. The Pediatric Regulation was adopted by the end of 2006 (Regulation (EC) 2006) after two readings and substantial amendments. The most significant amendment introduced by the Parliament was the transparency of pediatric clinical trials.

The Regulation took effect on 26 January 2007, but some obligations were deferred; this was intended to give time to the pharmaceutical industry to prepare to what is a dramatic and sweeping change of the regulatory framework for medicines, affecting not just Europe. At the difference of the US Acts described in the first section of this chapter, this legislation does not have a sunset clause, but the Commission must report on its impact after 6 and 10 years of operation.

2.3   Major Aspects of the Pediatric Regulation

The Pediatric Regulation is extremely complex and affects many other regulatory procedures. It creates not only rewards or incentives, but also obligations for pharmaceutical companies developing medicinal products. The development of medicines for children becomes the rule rather than the exception. An expert Committee, the PDCO at the Agency, must agree the pediatric development presented in a PIP, including for national authorization procedures, or when the medicine was intended for an adult indication only. The Agency Decision on a PIP is binding for the company, and compliance with its content is necessary for the submission of applications at Agency or national level. The main other measures of the Regulation include strengthened measures for pediatric pharmacovigilance, transparency measures, the creation of a network of pediatric research, and the funding of off-patent medicines.

2.4   The Paediatric Committee

The PDCO consists of one expert member per Member State, including five holding simultaneous membership of the approval Committee (CHMP). In addition, there are three patients' representatives and three health professionals; Norway and Iceland are represented (Liechtenstein has no representative). Each member has an alternate, so currently the full Committee includes 33 members, plus the 2 Norwegian and Icelandic members, and 35 alternates. The scope of expertise of the Committee members is defined by the Regulation. The Committee was established in July 2007 with a Chair elected for 3 years (renewable once). The Committee meets once a month for 4 days and its main activity is to issue scientific opinions on PIP and compliance; it can also provide pediatric expertise to the other Committees of the Agency, or to the Member States.

2.5   The Paediatric Investigation Plan

A PIP or a request for a Waiver must be proposed at an early stage by any company intending to apply for marketing authorization, i.e., around the end of phase 1 in adults, and must be agreed by the PDCO. The development must aim at a full pediatric indication including an age-appropriate formulation and timelines, and cover all pediatric age groups, i.e., from birth to 17 years inclusive. The least studied subset of the pediatric population, the neonate, should always be included in the development where relevant. The scope relates to the potential pediatric use generally close to the condition developed for adults, or the proposed pediatric indication when adults are not affected. This is mandatory for new medicines (biologicals, vaccines, and chemicals are all regulated by the same laws in the EU), and when the company applies for a new indication, new route of administration, and/or a new pharmaceutical form for an active substance covered by a SPC or by a patent, which qualifies for an SPC. The SPC is a European extension of the patent to compensate for the unusually long development phase of medicinal products compared to other industrial products; it is variable in length, up to 5 years maximum.

Orphan medicines must also submit a PIP; however, generics, biosimilars, traditional herbal, and homeopathic medicines are excluded. Off-patent medicines can follow a voluntary procedure to be developed according to an agreed PIP, and, if successful, approved via a specific authorization covering exclusively the pediatric indication(s), the so-called Paediatric Use Marketing Authorization (PUMA)

PIPs are submitted to the Agency in electronic format (xml file) and entered directly into an administrative and scientific database, which will determine and monitor timelines, generate a number of documents automatically, and allow tracking the scientific content of applications. The Agency pediatric staff and two members (or alternates) of the PDCO assess sequentially but independently the plan over 60 days. The outcome is discussed by the PDCO, which can require modifications from the company. The PIP assessment is then completed over a second period of 60 days followed by a month (or less) of decision-making. The Decision is issued in English and, on request, in the official language of the applicant. The procedure is free of charge. The PIP Decision specifies the key elements (e.g., design, end points, and comparator timelines) of each study, trial, and/or pediatric formulation required by the PDCO. This is close to a Written Request. However, an agreed PIP or a Waiver is required to validate the marketing authorization application. A company can apply for Modifications of an agreed PIP if and when they encounter difficulties to perform the plan, or there is a change in the state of the art; this procedure takes a maximum of 60 days.

Decisions on PIP or Waivers and Modifications and Opinions on compliance are available on the Agency pediatric webpage (Decisions on PIP or Waivers 2010).

2.6 Waivers and Deferrals of the Pediatric Development

Similar to the USA, waivers can be obtained where pediatric development is not necessary, but the legal basis is not identical. In the EU, the pediatric development can be waived if the disease does not occur in children, if the product is likely to be unsafe or ineffective in children, and/or if the product does not bring significant therapeutic benefit, which means that the medicine would not meet an unmet pediatric need. Development in rare conditions is not waived (unless a study would not be feasible). In addition, systematic waivers can be issued by the PDCO to avoid repeated administrative procedures; these are published on the Agency pediatric webpage and can be referred to without applying to the PDCO (Class waivers).

Although the PIP must be agreed early, the performance of studies and trials in children can be deferred until it is safe to do so, consistent with the ICH E11 guideline.

2.7   Characteristics of the European Pediatric Initiative

Main elements of the Regulation

- Paediatric Committee
- Pediatric Development (PIP) or Waiver to be agreed with the Committee
- Applies to all medicinal products (chemicals, vaccines, and biologicals, orphan medicines)
- Early submission of PIP
- All subsets from birth to 18 years to be covered by PIP
- Waiver of the pediatric development if the condition only occurs in adults, if the product is likely to be ineffective or unsafe, or if product does not represent significant therapeutic benefit
- Obligations continue to apply once reward has been obtained
- Reward can be obtained only once
- Transparency of clinical trials
- Transparency of PIP Decisions
- Network of pediatric research networks
- Community funding for priority research into off-patent medicines

2.8   Further Research on Pediatric Development

The PDCO has issued or contributed to several guidelines on drug development, including one in neonates. Working groups were set up to ensure consistency and to progress the scientific knowledge on specific aspects of pediatric development such as pediatric formulations, juvenile animal studies, and the extrapolation of efficacy. Limiting unnecessary investigations in the vulnerable pediatric population is an ethical duty, but little is known on how or when extrapolation of efficacy is legitimate, and, for example, what could be "similar" conditions in adults and children, or in different pediatric subsets. Gaps in knowledge, once identified by the PDCO, are discussed with the relevant learned pediatric societies with a view to stimulating further research.

During the legislative discussion, the European Parliament requested to set up the ethical framework for the protection of children involved in clinical trials, based on the legal principles of Directive 2001/20/EC on good clinical practice for clinical trials. This led to the publication of Ethical Considerations for clinical trials with the paediatric population.

As pediatric development is complementary to adult development and to avoid divergences between different Committees, collaboration between the PDCO, the CHMP, and the Scientific Advice Working Party is ensured. Scientific Advice for pediatric issues is free of charge at the Agency (in contrast to adult development requests).

As of December 2009, after less than 2.5 years of operation more than 620 applications for PIP or a Waiver covering more than 960 conditions have been received by the Agency. The Committee has finalized more than 200 PIP opinions and the pediatric development has been completed for 14 medicines. The product information for these medicines is being updated after assessment, and the first companies can now claim the patent extension.

2.9   International Collaboration

The vast majority of pharmaceutical companies develop medicines at the global level; it is therefore important to consider not just EU but other regions' expectations or plans for pediatric development as well. As mentioned in the first section of this chapter, under the umbrella of the Confidentiality Arrangements (in place since 2003 between EU and the US), monthly teleconferences are held between the Agency and the FDA; the Japanese authorities have recently joined as observers; PIP's and Written Requests are extensively discussed to understand any differences and avoid unnecessary duplication. Since August 2007, more than 170 products (on average five per teleconference) and 14 topics of relevance for pediatric development have been discussed in depth.

Other initiatives are ongoing through the World Health Organization (WHO) to stimulate pediatric development of medicines (in particular formulations) for other regions of the world, especially developing and emerging countries. This is particularly important from the ethical perspective as many pediatric trials will take place in less developed countries and children should not be used as commodities by developed countries.

2.10   Rewards and Incentives

In the EU, an extension by 6 months of the SPC (patent extension) can be granted to a marketing authorization holder who has not only completed the pediatric development in conformity with the agreed PIP, but also included all results in the Product information and obtained a marketing authorization in all Member States of the EU. The reward can be obtained even when the results show that the product is unsafe or ineffective in children. It can be obtained only once despite the fact that several PIPs might still be required.

Provided the same requirements for information and authorization are met, pediatric development of orphan medicines is rewarded by two supplemental years of market exclusivity, in addition to the 10 years granted for medicines intended for rare diseases in the EU.

The voluntary procedure of PUMA attracts incentives of reduced application fees and 10-year data protection for the pediatric indication and formulation.

2.11   Transparency Measures

The Pediatric Regulation has introduced a number of breakthrough measures giving clear precedence to public health over commercial (competitive) interests.

PIP Opinions and Decisions are required to be made public; therefore, development plans and timelines will be disclosed, which previously were considered commercially confidential, including for currently unapproved products.

The Pediatric Regulation also requires that any clinical trial or study involving subjects between birth and 18 years of age be registered into the existing European database of clinical trials (EudraCT) if at least one investigation site is in the European Economic Area, or wherever the study takes place if the study is mentioned in a PIP. The EudraCT database, created in 2004, used to include only information related to the trial authorization and the database access was limited to the National Authorities, the Commission, and the Agency. Public access will now be given to the protocol and to the trial results that have to be submitted within 6 or 12 months of completion. The European Parliament introduced this measure during the co-decision procedure, on request from pediatric academics and patients' organizations; this is of high ethical value. The database is currently under modification to accommodate this requirement and public access should be implemented in 2010. In parallel, international collaboration is taking place to ensure convergence of information requirements with clinicaltrials.gov (NIH) and the WHO portal.

Some existing pediatric study results were never submitted to the European Authorities. This was all the more obvious when studies included in Written Requests and submitted to the FDA did not reach European Authorities. To avoid repeating unnecessarily studies, the Pediatric Regulation mandates companies to submit all existing pediatric studies completed before the entry into force of the Regulation and, within 6 months of completion, the results of new pediatric studies performed with EU-authorized medicines. Existing studies for more than 1,000 active substances, authorized at national level mostly, were submitted and are undergoing evaluation by National Agencies in a work-sharing exercise. These studies and their assessments will also be made public through the EudraCT database.

2.12   Pharmacovigilance and Long-Term Safety Monitoring

In the EU, adverse reactions occurring with medicinal products authorized or studied in clinical trials must be reported regularly or on an ad hoc basis. In addition, since 2004, the so-called Risk Management Plans introduce regulatory measures to prevent and minimize the risks of medicines. These requirements are strengthened for pediatric medicines and Risk Management Plans are normally part of submissions for pediatric approval. Long-term safety or efficacy monitoring can similarly be required by the Agency.

2.13 The Network of Pediatric Research

As the Pediatric Regulation introduces requirements to study medicines in high-quality ethical research, it also includes provisions to encourage collaboration between pediatric research centers, investigators, and networks. The Agency is establishing a network of networks to facilitate the performance of sufficiently powered studies, to facilitate access to relevant expertise, and to speed up recruitment. This network will also contribute to capacity building in pediatric research.

2.14 Priority for and Funding of Pediatric Development of Off-Patent Medicines

The Pediatric Regulation provides for specific funding of off-patent medicines through Community research programs (the Community Framework Programmes, currently the seventh, spanning 2007–2013) managed by the Commission. To this effect, a first priority list of about 60 off-patent medicines established in 2004 was updated and renewed annually since the implementation of the Regulation. The prioritization was based on public health considerations, using a simple combination of priority criteria for the conditions to be treated, and for the medicines based on available data with a view to selecting those likely to be effective and safe in children. Various learned societies were involved or consulted and the process of prioritization was efficient. Funding is available each year and twelve projects (e.g., morphine in neonates and pediatric oral formulations of methotrexate) have been funded since 2007. The first results are expected in the next years. This exercise is now a collaborative effort with the United States National Institutes of Health.

2.15 Survey of all Pediatric Uses of Medicines

As requested by the Regulation and based on data provided by each Member State on all pediatric uses of medicines, the Agency is preparing a report on pediatric use of medicines to the European Commission, who will make it available to the public. This report will contribute to the identification of pediatric needs that the PDCO has to consider when assessing a PIP.

2.16 Reporting on benefits and infringements

In addition to the impact reports due after 6 and 10 years of operation of the Pediatric Regulation prepared by the European Commission, the European Medicines Agency should report every year on companies and products, which have benefited from incentives and rewards, and on those which fail to comply with the Regulation. This information will be made public and can be considered as part of a "naming and praising" or "naming and shaming" process to encourage compliance. Additionally, financial penalties could be imposed by the Commission on companies failing to comply, but to date the legislation on penalties has not been updated to take account of pediatric obligations; thus, this possibility remains quite theoretical.

2.17 Conclusions

Several years after the USA, the European Union adopted a complex law aimed at improving the available information on medicines for pediatric use through ethical high-quality research and increasing the overall number of medicines specifically authorized for children. Through a stringent system of obligations compensated by economic rewards, a dramatic change in the way medicines are developed is taking place. This effort is placed under the sign of international collaboration with the USA and with other regions including developing countries. These new measures are implemented within an ethical framework to obtain evidence-based information while protecting the children involved in research.

References

Class waivers. http://www.ema.europa.eu/htms/human/paediatrics/classwaivers.htm. Accessed 11 Jan 2010

Decisions on PIP or Waivers. http://www.ema.europa.eu/htms/human/paediatrics/decisions.htm. Accessed 11 Jan 2010

European Medicines Agency pediatric webpage http://www.ema.europa.eu/htms/human/paediatrics/introduction.htm. Accessed 11 Jan 2010

Network of pediatric research. http://www.ema.europa.eu/htms/human/paediatrics/network.htm. Accessed 11 Jan 2010

Paediatric Committee http://www.ema.europa.eu/htms/general/contacts/PDCO/PDCO.html. Accessed 11 Jan 2010

Regulation (EC) No 1901/2006 of the European Parliament and of the Council of 12 December 2006 on medicinal products for paediatric use, and amending Regulation (EEC) No 1768/92, Directive 2001/20/EC Directive 2001/83/EC and Regulation (EC) No 726/2004 (as amended). http://ec.europa.eu/enterprise/sectors/pharmaceuticals/files/eudralex/vol-1/reg_2006_1901/reg_2006_1901_en.pdf. Accessed 11 Jan 2010

Part III
Specific Pediatric Pharmacology

Fetal Medicine and Treatment

Magnus Westgren

Contents

Abstract Fetal medicine covers a broad spectrum of conditions that can be diagnosed before birth. Different disorders will require different treatment strategies and there is often an important ontogenetic aspect on how and when treatment can be implemented. Due to the limited availability there is a general lack of knowledge on how pharmacotherapy can be provided in the most efficient way. Until recently most knowledge about how different drugs are transferred and metabolized in the human fetus is based on very limited observational studies on concentrations of drugs in fetal blood and other fetal compartments. It might be that the rapid development of other non-invasive methods for fetal diagnostics such as isolation of fetal DNA and RNA in maternal serum, NMR imaging and other techniques could in the future be explored in fetal pharmacotherapy.

M. Westgren
Division of Obstetrics and Gynecology, Department of Clinical Science, Intervention and Technology, Centre for Fetal Medicine, Karolinska University Hospital, Karolinska Institutet, S-141 86 Stockholm, Sweden
e-mail: magnus.westgren@ki.se

H.W. Seyberth et al. (eds.), *Pediatric Clinical Pharmacology*,
Handbook of Experimental Pharmacology 205,
DOI 10.1007/978-3-642-20195-0_13, © Springer-Verlag Berlin Heidelberg 2011

Introduction of new treatment strategies are often based on extrapolation from experience in neonates and adults. However some fetal conditions are very specific for this time period in life. This especially entails disturbances in development as malformations, early growth restriction and several congenital disorders. Here it might be required to introduce new treatment strategies without any previous experience in humans. Example of this ethical dilemma is gene therapy for lung growth in severe cases of diaphragmatic hernia and early growth restriction. The risk–benefit issues need to be discussed in all these alternatives. However, it is likely that the concept of the human fetus as a potential patient is still in its infancy and with an improved understanding about fetal patho-physiology there will be a continued need for better knowledge of pharmacotherapy during this crucial time period in life.

Keywords Fetal therapy • Fetal medicine • Congenital anomalies • Fetal analgesia • Gene therapy • Stem cell therapy

1 Introduction

During the last decades fetal medicine has evolved from traditional obstetrics. Cornerstones in this process have been the development of effective fetal diagnostic means such as advanced ultrasound techniques, cytogenetics, and more recently molecular genetics. Improved knowledge about fetal conditions has formed the diagnostic foundation for different fetal treatment strategies.

The pioneering work within this new field was made by physicians and scientists from New Zealand. Liley, frustrated by severely hydropic fetuses in rhesus immunized mothers and a devastating high stillborn rate among these patients, introduced intrauterine transfusions in 1959 (Liley 1963). He showed that it was possible to rescue severely ill fetuses, and his contribution is not only that he developed effective treatment but also that the human fetuses could be regarded as a patient accessible for diagnosis and therapy.

Effective non-invasive fetal therapy was introduced by his countryman Liggins (Liggins 1969; Liggins and Howie 1972). He reported on the effectiveness of transplacental steroid treatment to the mother in preventing respiratory stress syndrome. Intrauterine transfusion and corticosteroids are still by far the most common modalities for fetal therapy. There are continuous attempts to introduce new treatment strategies, and the present chapter will give a brief review on this topic.

2 Basic Principles for Placental transfer of Drugs and Fetal Pharmacokinetics

Most drugs move across the placenta by simple diffusion and the degree of diffusion depends on the chemical properties and concentration of the unbound drug (Boreus 1967; Yaffe 1980). Drugs with a molecular weight less than 1,000 are lipid soluble and these drugs penetrate the trophoblast barrier easily and can reach the fetal circulation readily (Juchau and Dyer 1972). With advancing gestational age, drug transfer is increasing. Any drug in maternal blood will cross the placenta, especially if maternal effective drug concentrations have been maintained under extended periods (Leeder 2009). Different pathological conditions affecting the placenta such as preeclampsia, preterm premature rupture of membranes, etc. can affect the placental blood flow and thus placental transfer. Some drugs will be metabolized and biotransformed in the placenta as occurs in liver. Drugs may also induce or inhibit placental enzymes necessary for metabolic conversion of exogenous substances.

For most drugs that cross the placenta fetal concentration will be 50–100% of the mother concentration. When steady state is reached, the fetal concentration can be higher than in the mother. The complete exposure of the drug and its metabolites are more important than the rate of placental transportation. In the human fetus proportionally more blood is directed to the brain, and the blood–brain permeability is greater in the fetus than in the adult (Myllynen et al. 2009). Consequently, the developing brain is more vulnerable to circulating drug levels. Despite preferential circulation to the brain, the distribution eventually becomes diffuse. Plasma protein concentration and protein binding capacity is lower in the fetus than in the mother leading to higher unbound drug concentration. Thus, conclusions about drug disposition in the fetus based on maternal and fetal serum concentrations may not accurately reflect true fetal pharmacokinetics.

Receptor and the strength of the receptor response for different drugs may differ with advancing gestational age. Several fetal organs are capable of substantial metabolic activity, but drug metabolism does preferentially take place in the liver. Human fetal liver microsomes have significant P-450 levels and NADPH cytochrome c reductase (Yaffe 1980). Oxidation and reduction reaction have been observed already from the first trimester but are probably less than in the adult. Therefore direct effects of drugs can be more prolonged in the fetus than in the mother. The excretion in the fetus is slower than in the mother. Primary routes for excretion are placenta and amniotic fluid. The placental transfer of the drugs from the fetus to the mother is the primary route in early pregnancy while drug elimination in late pregnancy depends on the immature fetal kidneys.

The transplacental route is the standard means of administrating drugs to the fetus. Exceptions are if the drug crosses the placenta poorly, or if the disease of the fetus affects the placental transfer, the fetus is moribund requiring fast intervention, or if severe maternal side effect can be anticipated. Direct administration to the fetus can be performed in several ways; intraamniotically, intravascularly, intramuscularly, and finally intraperitoneally (Table 1). There is limited information on how the route for direct administration affects the pharmacokinetics of different drugs.

Table 1 Principal routes for drug administration in human fetuses

Route	Example in clinical practice
Maternal	Digoxin
	Sotalol
	Flecainide
Intraamniotic	Thyroxin
Intravenously (fetus)	Alfentanil
	Digoxin
	Plasma products
Intramuscular (fetus)	Curare
	Alfentanil
Intraperitoneal	Curare
	Alfentanil

3 Different Fetal Treatment Strategies

3.1 Fetal Transfusions

Fetal transfusions were introduced in the 1960s. From the beginning, blood was transfused into the intraperitoneal cavity, but later intravascular transfusions were introduced. In 1984, Rodeck published a report on fetoscopically guided intravascular transfusions (Rodeck et al. 1981). Later Bang introduced ultrasound-guided fetal transfusions, and this technique is considered common practice fetal medicine today (Bang et al. 1982). The most common sites for intravascular transfusions are the umbilical vein close to the placental insertion, umbilical vein in a free lope, and the intrahepatic part of the umbilical vein. The free lope approach is associated with a higher rate of complications; i.e., bleedings into the amniotic cavity. Puncturing of the umbilical vein is associated with certain risks, and the procedure-related complication rate is about 3%. The most common reason for fetal transfusions is severe erythrocyte immunization. Another well-known indication is fetal anemia due to parvovirus infection.

Patients at risk of fetal anemia are monitored non-invasively with Doppler flow recordings of the cerebral arteries. In case of signs of anemia (increased velocities), the patient will undergo cordocentesis with direct measurement of fetal hemoglobin concentration. If the fetus is anemic, a blood transfusion will be carried out. Mostly O negative blood with high hematocrit will be used and the amount of blood required will be calculated from the initial hemoglobin value and the size of the fetus. Usually, repeated transfusions are required and typically a patient will undergo treatment every second week. Most centers for fetal medicine today prefer to perform transfusions until the 33rd–34th week. Intravascular transfusions can be commenced as early in the 18th–19th week of gestation, and such a patient will require 7–8 transfusions until she can be safely delivered. Depending on the degree of anemia and if the fetus has developed hydrops survival rate differ, but most units report survival rates in the range of 80–95% (Westgren et al. 1988; Weiner et al

1991). Long-term outcome of children treated in utero for fetal anemia is favorable, and it is amazing how the human fetus can withstand very severe anemia.

Other blood products have been transfused for other fetal disorders. Platelets have been administrated in cases of fetal alloimmune thrombocytopenia. The risk for bleedings in increased in such cases, and today most fetal medicine units avoid cordocentesis in this condition. In cases of non-immune hydrops of unknown origin, plasma and albumin have been given to the fetus. However, this is highly experimental and is practiced in very few centers.

3.2 Fetal Stem Cell Therapy

The fetus and its environment are unique in many ways. This has led to the assumption that the fetus is a potential suitable candidate for stem cell transplantations (Touraine et al 1989; Flake and Zanjani 1999). The arguments for fetal transplantations are the following: In some disorders the fetus is severely affected already during fetal life. An example of such a condition is homozygous alpha-thalassemia, almost always lethal before birth. Furthermore, from experience with bone marrow transplantation in cases of metabolic disorders or hemoglobinopathies, it is quite clear that the earlier in life a transplantation is carried out the better the prognosis. Thus, there are many arguments favoring early stem cell transplantation. The immunological naivety in the early gestation fetus has given rise to the concept of fetal tolerance, i.e., the inability to raise an immunological response against foreign antigens. During fetal life, the developing immune system is educated to distinguish between autologous and foreign antigens. However, if introduced early enough, foreign antigens can be recognized as self and not rejected. Consequently, in theory it should be possible to carry out fetal stem cell transplantations without chemotherapy and myoablation and across HLA barriers. Furthermore, during normal fetal life, naturally occurring stem cells expand and migrate and seed different anatomical compartments. An example of this relationship is the development of hematopoietic stem cells that originally are located in the dorsal aorta, from the 5th week in the liver and from week 12 in the bone marrow. These different compartments provide a potential and specialized supportive environment for engraftment, proliferation, and differentiation of stem cells. Exogenous administrated stem cells could possibly take advantage of these favorable conditions. Other arguments are that the intrauterine environment is sterile and very protective and the small size of the fetus ensures a much larger cell dose on a per kilogram basis than can be achieved after birth.

In-utero stem cell transplantation has been studied in several different animal models, most extensively in mouse, sheep, canine, and primates (Zanjani et al. 1992; Harrison et al. 1989; Blakemore et al. 2004). With few exceptions mixed chimerism of different percentage (0.5–30%) is achieved in these models. Thus it seems possible to perform intrauterine transplantation if it is done early during fetal life.

In humans the experience with fetal stem cell transplantation is limited, and we know about 50 cases reported so far. Most of these cases have been reported adequately in previous reviews on this topic (Tiblad and Westgren 2008; Westgren 2009). The most successful group of patients transplanted in utero are those with immunodeficiencies. Engraftment has been reported in 8 of 12 cases, and several of these children have had a benign clinical course. In comparison with postnatal transplantation, in-utero transplantation is associated with several advantages. It is less expensive and the recipient does not need any chemotherapy or radiation. Furthermore, it might reduce the risk for graft-versus-host disease, a problem associated with SCID, and it has an obvious psychological advantage before postnatal transplantations (Flake et al. 1996; Westgren et al. 2002).

In quite a number of cases with hemoglobinopathies and storage disorders, intrauterine transplantation has convincingly failed (Westgren et al. 1996). In a few of these cases engraftment has occurred but the phenotype has not been changed. The reason why intrauterine transplantation has failed in these cases is unclear but it seems that the human fetal immunological system is more mature than has been anticipated and failure of transplant could also be considered. In recent years, there are some reports on successful transplantation of mesenchymal stem cells (MSC) for osteogenesis imperfecta (Le Blanc et al. 2005). Interestingly, some of these transplantations have been performed across HLA barriers and rather late during gestation. It seems that MSC have unique immunological properties and if these results will be confirmed in larger studies MSC could be used for transplantation between mismatched individuals.

In conclusion, intrauterine transplantation is a highly experimental type of fetal treatment. Widespread clinical application is premature based on the limited success that has been achieved so far.

3.3　Fetal Analgesia

Invasive therapeutic options have drawn attention to the need of fetal analgesia. Currently no defined evidence-based fetal anesthesia or analgesia protocol exists for these procedures. Whether the fetus can respond to noxious stimulus with pain is based on our current knowledge on neurodevelopment of anatomical pathways as well as observational studies on fetal behavior at pain exposition in utero.

It has been claimed that an intact spinothalamic connection exists as early as in the seventh week of gestation (Lagercrantz and Changeux 2009; Derbyshire 2006). At this stage, no laminal structure is present connecting thalamus to cortex, and without thalamic projection to the cortex the neuronal cells cannot process noxious information from the periphery. The first projections from thalamus to cortex appear at 12th–16th week. However, not until the 23rd–25th week afferent neurons penetrate and form synapses to the cortex. Theoretically, the spinothalamic projections into the cortex may provide the necessary anatomical foundation for pain experience in the human fetus. That the human fetus is capable to experience pain from late second trimester is also supported by several observational studies.

Withdraw reflexes at needling procedures as a sign of nociceptial reaction can be observed from the 19th week. Fisk et al. showed from their experience on puncturing the human fetus with a needle an increase in cortisol, beta-endorphin, and noradrenalin in cord blood from the 20th week (Giannakoulopoulos et al. 1994; Fisk et al. 2001; Teixeira et al. 1999). In preterm children, face reactions similar to that seen in adults experiencing pain can be observed from the 28th week (Van de Velde et al. 2006).

Thus, there is evidence suggesting that analgesia to blunt nociceptive responses in utero should be used from the 20th–23rd week of gestation. However, although most centers performing invasive fetal procedures are using analgesia, there is a general lack of information on how it may be safely and effectively administrated. Opioid agonists have been widely used and have been given directly intravenously to fetuses before open surgery. Direct administration into the intravascular space of the fetus is known to be associated with certain risks. Direct intravenous administration has later in most centers been replaced by intramuscular administration, but due to slower absorption this will prolong the procedure and might require multiple injections of the fetus (Van de Velde et al. 2006). In our center, we have since more than a decade used intraperitoneal administration for administration of different pharmacological agents at invasive procedures (cisatracurare 0.30 mg/kg, alfentanil 0.015 mg/kg) after the 20th week of gestation. The intraperitoneal cavity is easy to puncture and rapid absorption enables us to perform fetal procedures within 5 min after administration without any sign of fetal distress. Other routes to consider is intra amniotic where it was recently shown that intra-amniotic sufentanil is easily absorbed by the sheep fetus and it was suggested that this route might provide a simple and fast method for fetal analgesia (Van de Velde et al. 2005; Strumper et al. 2003).

Different fetal procedures may require a different type of analgesia. In open fetal surgery, inhalation agents to the mother provide effective maternal and fetal analgesia and anesthesia. In addition, uterine relaxation is often obtained by these agents. Most endoscopic procedures are performed under regional or local maternal analgesia. If analgesia and paralysis of the fetus are required, this is usually obtained by injection of opioids and/or muscle relaxants. If only immobilization of the fetus is wanted during the procedure, maternally administrated remifentanil resulted in effective maternal sedation and fetal immobilization.

The potential benefit of the fetus with analgesia and anesthesia needs to be balanced against the risk for the mother. In such equation it is important to consider the old obstetric dictum that the mother's life should always be at highest priority. Finally, we are lacking information on long-term outcome of fetuses exposed for in-utero procedures. In this context pain experience during fetal life is an area of concern that requires much more attention in the future.

3.4   Fetal Medical Treatment Due to Fetal Heart Arrhythmias

The most common reason for medical treatment is fetal tachycardias. It is defined as a tachycardia of non-sinus origin with a heart frequency exceeding 180–200 beats per minute. There are several variants with different electrophysiological background and prognosis. The most common is an atrioventricular re-entry tachycardia caused by the presence of an accessory pathway between the atrium and the ventricle. Another type is the one with atrium flatter with re-entry in the atrium wall. Altogether these two types represent approximately 95% of all cases of fetal tachycardias (Simpson and Sharland 1998; Carvalho et al. 2007; Krapp et al. 2003).

Usually the mother will not experience any symptoms and the high fetal heart rate is picked up at a routine antenatal check-up in weeks 28–34. In some cases, the fetus has developed signs of heart failure with polyhydramniosis and/or reduced fetal movements. Ultrasound examination will in a third of these cases reveal increased amount of fluid in the fetus or in more severe cases full blown hydrops. The reason for the heart failure is an impaired diastolic filling of the ventricules when the heart rate increases. Consequently, cardiac output decreases and the intraatrial and central vein pressure increases. The increased pressure in the atria predisposes for atrial flatter.

Management of fetal tachycardia requires knowledge about the electrophysiological background and the hemodynamic situation of the fetus. The degree of heart failure or hydrops will be in most cases an important denominator for prediction of the prognosis. Other issues to consider are if the tachycardia is continuous or intermittent, frequency of the ventricles, relationship between atrial and ventricular systolic phase, heart malformations, and finally the gestational age. If the fetus has no hemodynamic signs of heart failure, different options can be considered. Maternal medication and treatment across the placenta, direct therapy to the fetus, delivery and treatment of the newborn, or if tachycardia is intermittent just to observe. To deliver a fetus with heart failure is usually a worse alternative than treating the fetus in utero.

In absence of hydrops, first line drug is digoxin. In many cases digoxin needs to be combined with sotalol or flecainide (Oudijk et al. 2000; Jaeggi et al. 2004). Approximately 85% of the cases will convert to normal heart rate on this treatment, and these children will do well. In fetuses with hydrops there is poor transplacental passage of digoxin, and in these cases sotalol is to be recommended. Another option is to treat the fetus with direct dixoxin administration.

Fetal bradycardia is defined as a heart rate less than 100 bpm. Short episodes of bradycardia is a common phenomenon and of no significance. In cases of continued ventricular arrhythmia, treatment with beta blockers could be considered. A severe form of bradycardia is due to a complete A–V block. In approximately 50% of these cases, it is combined with heart malformations. In cases with no malformations, the condition is usually caused by anti-Ro and Anti-L antibodies (Bergman et al. 2009; Strandberg et al. 2008). Transplacental treatment with digoxin for improvement of ventricular contractions, beta stimulator for increasing the heart rate and dexamethasone for anti-inflammation could be considered in these cases.

3.5 Corticosteroids for Accelerated Fetal Lung Maturation

Respiratory distress syndrome (RDS) is a serious consequence of preterm delivery and causes significant mortality and morbidity. Liggins when investigating dexamethasone and preterm labor in lambs found evidence of accelerated lung maturation (Liggins 1969). Later Liggins and Howie performed the first prospective randomized study on the value of antenatal corticosteroids and were able to demonstrate prevention of RDS (Liggins and Howie 1972). Since then a large number of prospective randomized trials have been carried out and confirmed Liggin's original observation and hypothesis. An extensive Cochrane review and meta-analysis was published in 2006 on the use of antenatal steroids (Dalziel 2008). Treatment with antenatal corticosteroids reduces the risk of neonatal death, RDS, cerebroventricular hemorrhages, necrotising enterocolitis, infectious morbidity, and need of respiratory support and neonatal intensive care. There is evidence on benefit from 24 to 34 weeks. There is also evidence on beneficial effect in cases of premature rupture of membranes and in hypertensive disorders.

It seems that this beneficial effect is achieved by single-dose antenatal corticosteroids. Thus, corticosteroids are by far the most common used drugs for fetal therapy. It seems safe for the fetus and mother, but long-term follow-up of the children to adulthood after corticosteroid exposition in utero are still needed to ensure the long-term safety of this treatment.

3.6 Medical Treatment for Intrauterine Fetal Virus Infections

Intrauterine cytomegalovirus (CMV) infection is a serious condition with far-reaching consequences for the fetus. Infection during pregnancy occurs in 1% of nonimmune and 5% of immune pregnant women, with a vertical transmission of 30% and 0.2–8%, respectively. Intrauterine infection is associated with severe growth restriction, microcephaly, jaundice, hepatosplenomegaly, and severe thrombocytopenia. Approximately 30% of the fetuses with symptoms will die, and of the remainder, a substantial number will develop neurological handicaps (Lazzarotto et al. 2000; Lanari et al. 2006). Recently there are also reports on an association between CMV infections and neuroblastomas later during infancy (Söderberg-Nauclér 2008). Thus congenital CMV infection represents a major medical challenge in fetal medicine. Jacquemard et al. treated affected cases with maternal oral administration of valaciclovir (VACV) (Jacquemard et al. 2007). They could demonstrate that they achieved therapeutic concentrations in maternal and fetal blood. The viral load decreased significantly after 1–12 days of treatment. They could not prove the therapeutic effect which needs to be addressed in a prospective randomized study.

There is limited information on pharmacokinetics of VACV. VACV is an orally administrated prodrug of acyclovir with improved oral bioavailability and pharmacokinetic properties. A substantial number of fetuses have been exposed for acyclovir with no teratogenic effects. Therefore acyclovir has been given in serious maternal complications such as pneumonia and herpes encephalitis, etc. (Frenkel et al. 1991; Stone et al. 2004). There are no data on VACV and the risk for the fetus, but based on the outcome from acyclovir exposition, the risk seems low. Another option treatment strategy for CMV infection is to provide CMV hyperimmune globulin. Promising results have been published but these studies needs to be confirmed in controlled trials (Nigro et al. 2005; Adler and Nigro 2009).

3.7 Medical Treatment for Fetal Goiter

Fetal goiter may be associated with hypo- or hyperthyroidism. With high resolution ultrasound the thyroid gland can easily be visualized and consequently most cases of fetal goiter are diagnosed in utero (Ballabio et al. 1989). Congenital hypothyroidism is rare and is mostly caused by thyroid dysgenesis. Transient fetal hypothyroidism is usually caused by maternal antithyroid drug intake, commonly carbimazole or propylthiouracil due to Grave's disease. Fetal hyperthyroidism is usually caused by maternal Grave's disease. Some of these mothers have thyroid-stimulating immunoglobulins, and sometimes these stimulating immunoglobulins cross the placenta and may activate fetal TSH receptors (Mitsuda et al. 1992).

Timely diagnosis and treatment are important in cases of fetal thyroid disturbances. The diagnosis of fetal goiter is usually quite straightforward. It warrants a thorough evaluation of other thyroid-associated manifestations such as tachycardia, polyhydramniosis, and growth restriction.

Fetal thyroid status can be assessed by cordiocentesis and direct blood sampling. If the fetal goiter is found in an euthyroid mother, it is usually possible to treat the mother with antithyroid drugs and get a good response in the fetus. However, the mother usually needs T4 supplementation during the treatment. If the fetal goiter is diagnosed in a mother with Grave's disease it is necessary to evaluate if the goiter is a result from transplacental passage of thyroid-stimulating antibodies. At concomitant fetal hyperthyroidism, the mother usually requires higher doses of antithyroid drugs. In cases of need for T4 supplementation to the fetus, direct administration of thyroid hormones can be carried out by intra-amniotic, intravascular or intramuscular routes. Since the fetus in this situation often requires repeated injections the intra-amniotic route is preferable. Adequate fetal thyroid replacement therapy can be achieved by intra-amniotic administration of 250–500 mg T4 at 7–10 days intervals.

References

Adler SP, Nigro G (2009) Findings and conclusions from CMV hyperimmune globulin treatment trials. J Clin Virol 46(Suppl 4):S54–S57

Ballabio M, Nicolini U, Jowette T, Ruiz de Elvira MC, Ekins RP, Rodeck CH (1989) Maturation of thyroid function in normal human foetuses. Clin Endocrinol 31(5):565–571

Bang J, Bock JE, Trolle D (1982) Ultrasound guided fetal intravenous transfusion for severe rhesus haemolytic disease. Br Med J 284:373–374

Bergman G, Eliasson H, Bremme K, Wahren-Herlenius M, Sonesson SE (2009) Anti-Ro52/SSA antibody-exposed fetuses with prolonged atrioventricular time intervals show signs of decreased cardiac performance. Ultrasound Obstet Gynecol 34(5):543–549

Blakemore K, Hattenburg C, Stetten G et al (2004) In utero hematopoietic stem cell transplantation with haploidentical donor adult bone marrow in a canine model. Am J Obstet Gynecol 190:960–973

Boreus LO (1967) Pharmacology of the human fetus: dose-effect relationship for acetylcholine during ontogenesis. Biol Neonat 11:328–337

Carvalho JS, Prefumo F, Ciardelli V et al (2007) Evaluation of fetal arrhythmias from simultaneous pulsed wave Doppler in pulmonary artery and vein. Heart 93:1448–1453

Dalziel RD (2008) Antenatal corticosteroids for accelerating fetalö lung maturation for women at risk of preterm birth. The Cochrane collaboration. Cochrane Library 4:1–166

Derbyshire WGS (2006) Can fetuses feel pain? BMJ 332(7546):909–912

Fisk NM, Gitau R, Teixeira JM, Giannakoulopoulos X, Cameron AD, Glover VA (2001) Effect of direct fetal opioid analgesia on fetal hormonal and hemodynamic stress response to intrauterine needling. Anesthesiology 95:828–835

Flake AW, Zanjani ED (1999) In utero hematopoietic stem cell transplantation: ontogenic opportunities and biologic barriers. Blood 94:2179–2191

Flake AW, Roncarolo MG, Puck JM et al (1996) Treatment of x-linked severe combined immunodeficiency by in utero transplantation of paternal bone marrow. N Engl J Med 335:1806–1810

Frenkel LM, Brown ZA, Bryson YJ, Corey L, Unadkat JD, Hensleigh PA, Arvin AM, Prober CG, Connor JD (1991) Pharmacokinetics of acyclovir in the term human pregnancy and neonate. Am J Obstet Gynecol 164(2):569–576

Giannakoulopoulos X, Sepulveda W, Kourtis P, Glover V, Fisk NM (1994) Fetal plasma cortisol and beta-endorphin response to intrauterine needling. Lancet 344:77–81

Harrison MR, Slotnick RN, Crombleholme TM et al (1989) In-utero transplantation of fetal liver haemopoietic stem cells in monkeys. Lancet 2:1425–1427

Jacquemard F, Yamamoto M, Costa J-M, Romand S, Jaqz-Aigrain E, Dejean A, Daffos F, Ville Y (2007) Maternal administration of valaciclovir in symptomatic intrauterine cytomegalovirus infection. BJOG 114(9):1113–1121

Jaeggi ET, Fouron JC, Silverman ED et al (2004) Transplacental fetal treatment improves the outcome of prenatally diagnosed complete atrioventricular block without structural heart disease. Circulation 110:1542–1548

Juchau MR, Dyer DC (1972) Pharmacology of the placenta. Pediatr Clin North Am 19:65–69

Krapp M, Kohl T, Simpson JM et al (2003) Review of diagnosis, treatment, and outcome of fetal artrial flutter compared with supraventricular tachycardia. Heart 89:913–917

Lagercrantz H, Changeux J-P (2009) The emergence of human consciousness: from fetal to neonatal life. Pediatr Res 65(3):255–260

Lanari M, Lazzarotto T, Venturi V, Papa I, Gabrielli L, Guerra B et al (2006) Neonatal cytomegalovirus blood load and risk of sequelae in symptomatic and asymptomatic congenitally infected newborns. Pediatrics 117:76–83

Lazzarotto T, Varani S, Guerra B, Nicolosi A, Lanari M, Landini MP (2000) Prenatal indicators of congenital cytomegalovirus infection. J Pediatr 137:90–95

Le Blanc K, Gotherstrom C, Ringden O et al (2005) Fetal mesenchymal stem-cell engrafment in bone after in utero transplantation in a patient with severe osteogenesis imperfect. Transplantation 79:1607–1614

Leeder JS (2009) Developmental pharmacogenetics a general paradigm for application to neonatal pharmacology and toxicology. Clin Pharmacol Ther 86(6):678–682

Liggins GC (1969) Premature delivery of fetal lambs infused with glucocorticoids. J Endocrinol 45:515–523

Liggins GC, Howie RN (1972) A controlled trial of antepartum glucocorticoid treatment for prevention of the respiratory distress syndrome. Pediatrics 50:515–525

Liley AW (1963) Intrauterine transfusion of foetus in haemolytic disease. Br Med J ii: 1107–1109

Mitsuda N, Tamaki H, Amino N, Hosono T, Miyai K, Tanizawa O (1992) Risk factors for developmental disorders in infants born to women with Graves' disease. Obstet Gynecol 80 (3 Pt 1):359–364

Myllynen P, Immonen E, Kummu M, Vähäkangas K (2009) Developmental expression of drug metabolizing enzymes and transporter proteins in human placenta and fetal tissues. Expert Opin Drug Metab Toxicol 5(12):1483–1499

Nigro G, Stuart P, La Torre R, Best A (2005) Passive immunization during pregnancy for congenital cytomegalovirus infection. N Engl J Med 353:13–21

Oudijk MA, Michon MM, Kleinman CS et al (2000) Sotalol in the treatment of fetal dysrhythmias. Circulation 101:2721–2726

Rodeck CH, Kemp JR, Holman CA, Whitmore DN, Karnicki J, Austin MA (1981) Direct intravascular fetal blood transfusion by fetoscopy in severe Rhesus isoimmunisation. Lancet 1:625–627

Simpson JM, Sharland GK (1998) Fetal tachycardias: management and outcome of 127 consecutive cases. Heart 79:576–581

Söderberg-Nauclér C (2008) HCMV microinfections in inflammatory diseases and cancer. J Clin Virol 41(3):218–223

Stone KM, Reiff-Eldridge R, White AD, Cordero JF, Brown Z, Alexander ER, Andrews EB (2004) Pregnancy outcomes following systemic prenatal acyclovir exposure: conclusions from the international acyclovir pregnancy registry, 1984–1999. Birth Defects Res A Clin Mol Teratol 70(4):201–207

Strandberg L, Winqvist O, Sonesson SE, Mohseni S, Salomonsson S, Bremme K, Buyon JP, Julkunen H, Wahren-Herlenius M (2008) Antibodies to amino acid 200–239 (p200) of Ro52 as serological markers for the risk of developing congenital heart block. Clin Exp Immunol 154 (1):30–37

Strumper D, Durieux ME, Gogarten W, Van Aken H, Hartleb K, Marcus MA (2003) Fetal plasma concentrations after intraamniotic sufentanil in chronically instrumented pregnant sheep. Anesthesiology 98:1400–1406

Teixeira JM, Glover V, Fisk NM (1999) Acute cerebral redistribution in response to invasive procedures in the human fetus. Am J Obstet Gynecol 181:1018–1025

Tiblad E, Westgren M (2008) Fetal stem-cell transplantation. Best Pract Res Clin Obstet Gynaecol 22(1):189–201

Touraine JL, Raudrant D, Royo C et al (1989) In-utero transplantation of stem cells in bare lymphocyte syndrome. Lancet I:1382

Van de Velde M, Van Schoubroech D, Lewi LE, Marcus MAE, Jani JC, Missant C et al (2005) Remifentanil for fetal immobilization and maternal sedation during fetoscopic surgery: a randomized double blind comparison with diazepam. Anesth Analg 101:251–258

Van de Velde M, Jani J, De Buck F, Deprest J (2006) Fetal pain preception and pain management. Semin Fetal Neonatal Med 11(4):232–236

Weiner CP, Williamson RA, Wenstrom KD, Sipes SL, Widness JA, Grant SS et al (1991) Management of fetal hemolytic disease by cordocenteses. II. Outcome of treatment. Am J Obstet Gynecol 165:1302–1307

Westgren M (2009) Intrauterine transplantation. Blood 113(19):4484

Westgren M, Jabbar F, Larsen JF, Rahman F, Selbing A, Stangeberg M (1988) Introduction of a programme for intravascular transfusions at severe rhesus isoimmunization. J Perinat Med 16:417–422

Westgren M, Ringden O, Eik-Nes S et al (1996) Lack of evidence of permanent engraftment after in utero fetal stem cell transplantation in congenital hemoglobinopathies. Transplantation 61:1176–1179

Westgren M, Ringden O, Bartmann P et al (2002) Prenatal t-cell reconstitution after in utero transplantation with fetal liver cells in a patient with x-linked severe combined immunodeficiency. Am J Obstet Gynecol 187:475–482

Yaffe SJ (1980) Clinical implications of perinatal pharmacology. Eur J Clin Pharmacol 18(1):3–7

Zanjani ED, Ascensao JL, Flake AW et al (1992) The fetus as an optimal donor and recipient of hemopoietic stem cells. Bone Marrow Transplant 10(Suppl 1):107–114

Fetal Risks of Maternal Pharmacotherapy: Identifying Signals

Gideon Koren

Contents

Abstract Pregnant women may be exposed to a variety of medications that may exert toxic or teratogenic effects on the fetus. Since the thalidomide disaster, physicians and pregnant women tend to withhold medications during pregnancy, although the risk of teratogenic effect from most drugs in therapeutic doses is nonexistent. This chapter will review the principles of teratology and the pharmacoepidemiological evidence for drug safety/risk in human gestation.

Keywords Teratology • Fetal safety • Fetus • Drugs • Teratogenicity • Bias

G. Koren (✉)
The Motherisk Program, Division of Clinical Pharmacology and Toxicology, Hospital for Sick Children, University Avenue 555, Toronto M5G 1X8, ON, Canada
e-mail: gidiup_2000@yahoo.com

H.W. Seyberth et al. (eds.), *Pediatric Clinical Pharmacology*,
Handbook of Experimental Pharmacology 205,
DOI 10.1007/978-3-642-20195-0_14, © Springer-Verlag Berlin Heidelberg 2011

1 Principles of Teratology

Congenital defects occur in 1–3% of the general population. Of the major defects, about 25% are of genetic origin (genetically inherited diseases, new mutations and chromosomal abnormalities) and 65% are of unknown etiology (multifactorial, polygenic, spontaneous errors of development and synergistic interactions of teratogens). Only 2–3% of malformations are thought to be associated with drug treatment (Table 1). The remaining defects are related to other environmental exposures including infectious agents, maternal disease states, mechanical problems, and irradiation (Koren et al. 1998).

The importance of *timing of drug exposure* is critical; the effect produced by a teratogenic agent depends upon the developmental stage in which the conceptus is exposed. The following phases in human development must be recognized:

- The *"all or none" period*, the time from conception until somite formation. Insults to the embryo in this phase are likely to result in death and miscarriage or intact survival. The embryo is undifferentiated, and repair and recovery are possible through multiplication of the still totipotential cells. Exposure to teratogens during the presomitic stage usually does not cause congenital malformations unless the agent persists in the body beyond this period.
- The *embryonic period*, from 18 to 60 days after conception when organogenesis occurs. This is the period of maximum sensitivity to teratogenicity since tissues are differentiating rapidly and damage becomes irreparable. Exposure to teratogenic agents during this period has the greatest likelihood of causing a structural anomaly. Critically because half of all pregnancies are unplanned, many women taking drugs at that stage are not aware of their risks.
- The *fetal phase*, from the end of the embryonic stage to term, when growth and functional maturation of formed organs and systems occurs. The only organ that continues to differentiate until birth is the brain and hence ethanol and drugs of abuse may adversely affect the fetal brain at any stage. Teratogen exposure in this period will affect fetal growth (e.g., intrauterine growth restriction) and the size or function of an organ, rather than cause gross structural anomalies.

Many organ systems continue structural and functional maturation long after birth. Most of the adenocarcinomas associated with first trimester exposure to diethylstilbestrol occurred many years later.

Teratogens must reach the developing fetus in sufficient amounts to cause their effects. Large molecules with a molecular weight greater than 1,000 (e.g., heparin) do not easily cross the placenta into the embryonic–fetal bloodstream. Other factors influencing the rate and extent of placental transfer of drugs include polarity, lipid solubility, and the existence of a specific protein carrier (e.g., P-glycoprotein).

Every year scores of new pharmaceuticals enter the market, almost never with human fetal safety data. Such data typically accumulate during the first years of clinical use, in the form of case reports, case series, prospective and retrospective cohorts, and case control studies. All of these methods suffer from serious sources

Table 1 Teratogenic drugs and chemicals in humans

Drug	Adverse effects
Angiotensin converting enzyme inhibitors (ACEI) and angiotensin II antagonists	Adverse effects related to hemodynamic effects of ACEI and angiotensin II antagonists on the fetus. In late pregnancy, ACEI fetopathy: intrauterine renal insufficiency, neonatal hypotension, oliguria with renal failure, hyperkalemia, complications of oligohydramnios (i.e., fetal limb contractures, lung hypoplasia, and craniofacial anomalies), prematurity, intrauterine growth restriction and fetal death. Questionable teratogenic risk with first trimester exposure of cardiovascular and CNS malformations
Antineoplastic agents	A significant increase in the incidence of various fetal malformations and early miscarriages following first trimester exposure
Carbamazepine	First trimester exposure: 1% risk of neural tube defects (10× baseline risk) and an increased risk of cardiovascular malformations. A pattern of malformations similar to the fetal hydantoin syndrome has also been associated
Cocaine	Abruptio placenta, prematurity, fetal loss, decreased birth weight, microcephaly, limb defects, urinary tract malformations, and poorer neurodevelopmental performance. Methodological problems make the findings difficult to interpret. Cocaine abuse is often associated with poly-drug abuse, alcohol consumption, smoking, malnutrition, and poor prenatal care. Human epidemiology indicates the risk of major malformation from cocaine is probably low, but the anomalies may be severe
Corticosteroids (systemic)	Increased risk of oral cleft
Coumarin anticoagulants	First trimester exposure (6–9 week gestation): fetal warfarin syndrome (nasal hypoplasia and calcific stippling of the epiphyses). Intrauterine growth restriction and developmental delay (CNS damage), eye defects and hearing loss. Warfarin embryopathy is found in up to ½ of the cases where a coumarin derivative was given throughout pregnancy. Associated with high rate of miscarriage. Risk of CNS damage due to hemorrhage after the first trimester
Diethylstilbestrol	Vaginal clear cell adenocarcinoma in offspring exposed in utero before 18th week (>90% of the cancers occurred after 14 years of age). High incidence of benign vaginal adenosis. Increased miscarriage rate and preterm delivery. In males exposed in utero: no signs of malignancy but genital lesions in 27% and pathologic changes in spermatozoa in 29%. The drug is not currently available in Canada
Ethanol	Fetal alcohol syndrome: growth impairment, developmental delay, and dysmorphic facies. Cleft palate and cardiac anomalies may occur. Full expression of the syndrome occurs with chronic daily ingestion of 2 g alcohol per kg (8 drinks/day) in about ½ and partial effects in of offspring
Folic acid antagonists: aminopterin and methotrexate	Fetal aminopterin–methotrexate syndrome: CNS defects, craniofacial anomalies, abnormal cranial ossification, abnormalities in first branchial arch derivatives, intrauterine growth restriction, and mental retardation after first trimester exposure. Maternal dose of methotrexate needed to induce defects is probably above 10 mg/week with a critical period of 6–8 week postconception

(continued)

Table 1 (continued)

Drug	Adverse effects
Hydantoins (phenytoin)	Fetal hydantoin syndrome: craniofacial dysmorphology, anomalies and hypoplasia of distal phalanges and nails, growth restriction, mental deficiency, and cardiac defects
Lithium	Small increase in risk for cardiac teratogenesis in early gestation (1%). The risk of Ebstein's anomaly exceeds spontaneous rate of occurrence. Fetal echocardiography if exposed in first trimester
Misoprostol	First trimester exposure: limb defects and Moebius sequence. Absolute teratogenic risk: probably low. Uterine contraction inducing activity
Retinoids (acitretin, isotretinoin) and megadoses of vitamin A	Systemic exposure: potent human general and behavioral teratogen. Retinoic acid embryopathy: craniofacial anomalies cardiac defects, abnormalities in thymic development and alterations in CNS development. Risk for associated miscarriage: 40%
Tetracyclines	Discoloration of the teeth after 17-week gestation when deciduous teeth begin to calcify. Close to term: crowns of permanent teeth may be stained. Oxytetracycline and doxycycline associated with a lower incidence of enamel staining
Thalidomide	Malformations limited to tissues of mesodermal origin, primarily limbs (reduction and defects), ears, cardiovascular system and gut musculature. Critical period: 34th–50th day after the beginning of the last menstrual period. A single dose of <1 mg/kg has produced the syndrome. Embryopathy found in about 20% of pregnancies exposed in the critical period
Valproic acid	First trimester exposure: neural tube defects with 1–2% risk of meningomyelocele, primarily lumbar or lumbosacral, cardiovascular malformations and hypospadias. Fetal valproate syndrome: craniofacial dysmorphology, cardiovascular defects, long fingers and toes, hyperconvex fingernails and cleft lip, has been delineated by some investigations. Neurobehavioral teratogen

of challenges, often leading to alarming signals of teratogenicity, only to be found later to be false.

Because randomized controlled trials are very rarely available in pregnancy, and almost never during the first trimester of pregnancy, understanding the methodological difficulties is critical in an attempt to evaluate teratogenic risk and in being able to counsel effectively pregnant women exposed to pharmaceuticals.

2 Confounding Effects

Hence, the safety of drugs in pregnancy is almost entirely dependent on observational studies. Such studies, either prospective or retrospective cohorts, or case control studies, involve collecting exposed and unexposed mothers (in cohort studies), or infants with or without a given adverse event (in case-control studies). These designs are subject to a large list of potential pitfalls; leaving them unrecognized can lead to serious error in interpretations, as will be documented herein.

The following are major sources of confounders and bias typical of observational studies.

2.1 Sample Size

Major birth defects are relatively rare, accounting on average to 1–3% of all births. Hence large numbers are needed to show excess risk at alpha of 5% and beta of 80%. For example, 800 women are needed in a two arm study to show a doubling of major malformations. The situation is much more complex in trying to quantify major malformation (rather than all of them lumped together). For example, neural tube defects occur in 1:1,000 births. Valproic acid increases that risk to 20:1,000. Hence, hundreds of cases of maternal exposure to valproic acid during the first 28 days post conception may be needed to be able to document a difference from baseline risk.

The vast majority of cohort studies published to date are underpowered to show significant differences, a problem acknowledged by many of their authors. A common way to overcome this issue is synthesizing similar studies into meta-analysis, thus gaining a large sample size. As would be expected, lumping studies together into meta-analysis introduces its own set of issues, some of which will be addressed herein, including heterogeneity among studies, not being able to control for confounders, and under-reporting of negative studies [i.e., those showing no excess in adverse effects (Einarson et al. 1988)].

2.2 Bias by Indication

Women taking medications during and after conception often suffer from conditions which, per se, may affect pregnancy outcome. For example, chronic hypertension in pregnancy is associated with high risk of prematurity, unrelated to which drug is used to treat the hypertension. We have recently shown that hypertensive women have above 20% rates of prematurity in their offspring, whether treated with labetolol or methyldopa, as compared to only 4% among healthy controls (Nulman et al. 2010).

This source of bias can often be corrected by having, in addition to the drug exposed group and healthy control groups, an additional group with the same condition, treated with another pharmaceutical.

2.3 Time of Enrollment as a Bias

Prospective cohort studies pride themselves that by enrolling women in early pregnancy, (i.e., before the outcome of pregnancy is known), they avoid the serious bias of retrospective data collection. However, most miscarriages occur during the first trimester of pregnancy. Hence, the later one recruits pregnant women, the less likely they are to find cases of miscarriage. For example: if a group of women exposed to paroxetine is recruited at 5 weeks of gestation and followed up, whereas women exposed to other drugs recruited at 10 weeks of gestation, clearly there is a chance for more miscarriages to be detected and reported in the paroxetine cohort. There are two possible ways to overcome this type of bias:

1. By matching women in all arms of the study to be recruited in the same week of gestation.
2. By post-hoc statistical adjustment for the time of enrollment.

2.4 Bias in Retrospective Studies

A large number of studies attempting to associate pharmaceutical exposure with malformation rates are retrospective in nature, that is, the cases were collected *after* pregnancy outcome is known. It is conceivable that women having malformed children would more likely report them to drug companies or to regulatory agencies. This hypothesis was proven in 1999 by Bar Oz and colleagues, who compared a retrospective registry to a prospective one of the same drug (itraconazole) (Bar-Oz et al. 1999).

In the prospectively collected group there was a 3% malformation rate suggesting no increased teratogenic risk. In contrast, there was a more than fourfold a (14%) malformation rate in the retrospectively ascertained cohort (Bar-Oz et al. 1999). Acknowledging this serious source of bias is critical. Yet, there is also a "positive" message here: If, despite this bias, a retrospectively collected cohort *does not* exhibit a higher malformation rate than expected in the general population, it is conceivable that the drug is safe.

2.5 Recall Bias

Case-control studies typically enroll children with a specific malformation (e.g., spina bifida) and a healthy control group, and ask the mothers what pharmaceutical products they had used during pregnancy, and specifically, during the first trimester of pregnancy.

It has been argued that mothers of malformed children may have a different pattern of recall than mothers of healthy children. Specifically, the malformation may facilitate memory in an attempt to find a pregnancy-related cause. This source of bias can be remedied by collecting group of children with a different malformation, unrelated to the hypothesis in question. For example, Pastuszak et al. ascertained that Brazilian women giving birth to children with the Möbius sequence had a much higher likelihood to use misoprostol in an attempt to terminate pregnancy than women giving birth to children with spina bifida (Pastuszak et al. 1988).

A typical prospective cohort study in pregnancy recruits women exposed to pharmaceuticals before the outcome of pregnancy is known, and this is why the term "prospective" is used. However, at a later follow-up, women are asked about their health after the first interview and up till now. It is important to recognize that this part of the study is retrospective and hence open to recall bias. This becomes very important in trying to correlate, for example, the severity of the disease with outcome.

One of the most cited advantages of prescription databases linked to neonatal registries is that the dose of drug and length of treatment are not dependent on maternal recall. The trade-off is that prescription record does not yet prove that the pharmaceutical was taken by the pregnant mother. The seriousness of this source of error was acutely exhibited when Jick and colleagues correlated maternal prescription of spermicides with congenital malformation (Jick et al. 1981). It was argued that prescription of spermicides before conception did not yet mean that the women took them. Indeed, in a follow-up study of the malformed cases in this study, Watkins showed that almost none of the mothers took spermicides into pregnancy (Watkins 1986).

2.6   *Bias in Not Including Elective Abortion Data*

Many administrative database studies do not have data on findings among women who had elected to have an abortion. Rather, they report of "liveborn infants." Levy and colleagues hypothesized that a significant number of elective abortions are performed to date due to a major malformation diagnosed in utero. By not having such data, one takes the risk of missing a signal. Using the example of antifolates in pregnancy, known to increase the risk of neural tube defects, Levy et al. have showed that in their cohort such an association was apparent only when elective abortion data were considered too, but not when only live births were counted (Levy et al. 2009).

2.7   *Bias in Retrospective Ascertainment of Maternal Lifestyle*

Alcohol, maternal smoking and other drugs of abuse may increase fetal risks, both in terms of birth defects, as well as in terms of prematurity, intrauterine growth retardation, miscarriage, still birth, and developmental teratogenicity.

Due to shame, guilt, and fear of losing custody of a child, it is conceivable that women experiencing adverse effects in their offspring may underreport on drugs and alcohol abuse. This hypothesis was proven by Wong et al., studying a cohort of women who were counseled by a teratology information service during the first trimester of pregnancy. In particular, their reports on cigarette smoking were probed. When re-interviewed after the birth of the child, women who had healthy babies reported again very similar patterns of smoking as they had done originally. In contrast, women giving birth to offspring experiencing adverse outcome tended to minimize the numbers of cigarettes consumed when compared to their original reports (Wong and Koren 2001). This type of bias may seriously impair studies on the effect of alcohol, cigarettes, and drugs of abuse by introducing misclassification, i.e., women who smoked are erroneously classified as non smokers.

2.8 Bias Against the Null Hypothesis

Bias against the null hypothesis occurs when "positive" studies (e.g., showing a drug to be teratogenic) are more likely to be submitted for scientific meetings and journals, to be presented, published, and publicized than "negative" studies (e.g., those suggesting the pharmaceutical is safe). The seriousness and pervasiveness of this bias has been shown at each step of the act of reporting results.

Investigating the fate of studies submitted to the Oxford University ethics committee, Easterbrook and colleagues have shown that "negative" studies were significantly less likely to be submitted or published in peer reviewed journals. Of interest, this was not only due to the journals rejecting them more (Easterbrook et al. 1991), but also due to the perception of the investigators that their studies are less likely to be accepted. More related to adverse pregnancy outcome, we have shown that abstracts failing to identify reproductive risks of cocaine were less likely to be accepted by the Society for Pediatric Research than "positive" studies, despite the negative studies being overall of better quality (Koren et al. 1989).

The bias against the null is further augmented by the lay media, which tends to publicize significantly more "positive" studies than "negative" ones. This grim reality was documented unequivocally in the case of two studies published back to back by the Journal of the American Medical Association. In 1992, JAMA published two studies dealing with the risk of radioactive exposure (Koren and Klein 1991). A study on the fate of several thousand workers in Oakridge developing the American Atomic bomb in the 1940s has shown increased risk of leukemia. In contrast, a study investigating whether residing near nuclear energy plants failed to show excess of cases of cancer. Despite similar exposure in the journal, the "positive" study was cited by the lay media significantly more often (Koren and Klein 1991).

It is now evident that the bias against the null hypothesis is pervasive and encompasses every step of the production of new knowledge, starting with the authors not believing in their chances of publishing, continuing with medical meetings not selecting them for presentation.

Because of the confidential nature of the editorial process of selecting peer review papers for publication, it is impossible to verify whether the editorial process also results in bias against the null hypothesis.

3 Conclusions

Due to the inability to collect safety fetal data of sufficiently high quality, assessment of pharmaceutical molecules is one of the most challenging areas of pharmacoepidemiology.

It will be important to continue and refine the methodology involved in this quest for critical data, to avoid misinformation, which may lead to both unwarranted anxiety, as well as unjustified sense of safety.

It is critical to remember that physicians and patients, alarmed by an impression or perception of teratogenic risk may take extreme measures of either terminating an otherwise wanted pregnancy (Koren and Pastuszak 1990), or avoiding treatment even in life-threatening situations (Cohen et al. 2006). We must facilitate a new climate, where this practice is evidence based.

References

Bar-Oz B, Moretti ME, Mareels G, Van Tittelboom T, Koren G (1999) Reporting bias in retrospective ascertainment of drug-induced embryopathy. Lancet 354:1700–1701
Cohen LS, Altshuler LL, Harlow BL, Nonacs R, Newport DJ, Viguera AC, Suri R, Burt VK, Hendrick V, Reminick AM, Loughead A, Vitonis AF, Stowe ZN (2006) Relapse of major depression during pregnancy in women who maintain or discontinue antidepressant treatment. JAMA 295:499–507
Easterbrook PJ, Berlin JA, Gopalan R, Matthews DR (1991) Publication bias in clinical research. Lancet 337:867–872
Einarson TR, Leeder SJ, Koren G (1988) A method for meta-analysis of epidemiological studies. Drug Intell Clin Pharm 22:813–823
Jick H, Walker AM, Rothman KJ, Hunter JR, Holmes LB, Watkins RN, D'Ewart DC, Danford A, Madsen S (1981) Vaginal spermicides and congenital disorders. JAMA 245:1329–1332
Koren G, Klein N (1991) Bias against negative studies in newspaper reports of medical research. JAMA 266:1824–1826
Koren G, Pastuszak A (1990) Prevention of unnecessary pregnancy terminations by counseling women on drug, chemical, and radiation exposure during the first trimester. Teratology 41:657–661
Koren G, Graham K, Shear H, Einarson T (1989) Bias against the null hypothesis: the reproductive hazards of cocaine. Lancet 2:1440–1442
Koren G, Pastuszak A, Ito S (1998) Drugs in pregnancy. N Engl J Med 338:1128–1137
Levy A, Matok I, Gorodischer R, Koren G (2009) Bias toward the null hypothesis by not including abortion data. European Society of Development Pediatric and Perin Pharmacology, France

Nulman L, Chan WS, Koren G, Bamora M, Rezvanl M, Knittel-Keren D (2010) Neurocognitive development of children following in-utero exposure to labetalol for maternal hypertension a cohort study using a prospectively collected database. Hypertens Pregnancy 28(3):271–83

Pastuszak AL, Schüler L, Speck-Martins CE, Coelho KE, Cordello SM, Vargas F, Brunoni D, Schwarz IV, Larrandaburu M, Safattle H, Meloni VF, Koren G (1988) Use of misoprostol during pregnancy and Möbius' syndrome in infants. N Engl J Med 338:1881–1885

Watkins RN (1986) Vaginal spermicides and congenital disorders: the validity of a study. JAMA 256:3095–3096

Wong M, Koren G (2001) Bias in maternal reports of smoking during pregnancy associated with fetal distress. Can J Public Health 92:109–112

Antiepileptic Treatment in Pregnant Women: Morphological and Behavioural Effects

Torbjörn Tomson and Dina Battino

Contents

Abstract It is well established that children exposed to antiepileptic drugs (AEDs) in utero have an increased risk of adverse pregnancy outcomes including foetal growth retardation, major congenital malformations and impaired postnatal cognitive development. However, due to the significant maternal and foetal risks associated with uncontrolled epileptic seizures, AED treatment is generally maintained during pregnancy in the majority of women with active epilepsy.

The prevalence of major malformations in children exposed to AEDs has ranged from 4 to 10%, 2–4 times higher than in the general population. More recent studies

T. Tomson (✉)
Department of Clinical Neuroscience, Karolinska Institutet, S-171 76 Stockholm, Sweden
e-mail: torbjorn.tomson@karolinska.se

D. Battino
Department of Neurophysiopathology and Epilepsy Centre, IRCCS Foundation Carlo Besta, Neurological Institute, Milan, Italy

H.W. Seyberth et al. (eds.), *Pediatric Clinical Pharmacology*,
Handbook of Experimental Pharmacology 205,
DOI 10.1007/978-3-642-20195-0_15, © Springer-Verlag Berlin Heidelberg 2011

suggest a smaller increase in malformation rates. Malformation rates have consistently been higher in association with exposure to valproate than with carbamazepine and lamotrigine. Some prospective cohort studies also indicate reduced cognitive outcome in children exposed to valproate compared to carbamazepine and possibly lamotrigine. Information on pregnancy outcomes with newer generation AEDs other than lamotrigine are still insufficient.

Keywords Antiepileptic drugs • Teratogenicity • Congenital malformations • Pregnancy • Epilepsy

1   Introduction

The first report on possible human teratogenic effects of antiepileptic drugs (AEDs) was published more than 40 years ago (Meadows 1968). Meadows reported six children with orofacial clefts, some with additional abnormalities of the heart and face, all of whom had been exposed to AEDs in utero. Treatment was mainly different combinations of phenobarbital, phenytoin and primidone. In a subsequent retrospective survey of more than 400 pregnancies with epilepsy Speidel and Meadow (Speidel and Meadow 1972) found a twofold increase in malformation rate among children of mothers with epilepsy exposed to AEDs. A specific association between trimethadione and a very high prevalence of malformations was also reported early (German et al. 1970). Since then numerous studies with different methodologies have reported increased rates of teratogenic outcomes in mothers with epilepsy (Harden et al. 2009; Meador et al. 2008; Tomson and Battino 2005; Tomson and Hiilesmaa 2007). These adverse outcomes include major congenital malformations, minor anomalies and dysmorphism, growth retardation, and impaired cognitive development. In addition to trimethadione, all of the major old generation AEDs such as phenobarbital, phenytoin, valproate and carbamazepine, have been reported to be associated with increased risks for major congenital malformations, while less is known about the teratogenic potential of the newer generation AEDs that have been introduced to the market during the last 20 years.

Epilepsy is a condition characterised by the occurrence of recurrent epileptic seizures, with potentially serious consequences. Uncontrolled seizures significantly affect the quality of life of the patient with epilepsy, and major convulsive seizures could be harmful and occasionally even fatal (Tomson et al. 2004a). In addition to these harmful effects on the person with epilepsy, maternal seizures during pregnancy may also adversely affect the foetus (Tomson and Hiilesmaa 2007). Hence, the potential adverse outcomes in the offspring due to maternal use of AEDs need to be weighed and balanced against the risks associated with the underlying disease itself. In epilepsy, the maternal and foetal risks with uncontrolled major convulsive seizures are generally considered to outweigh the teratogenic risks with AEDs. Treatment is therefore maintained also during pregnancy in women with active epilepsy aiming at complete control of generalized tonic-clonic seizures (Tomson and Hiilesmaa 2007).

Women with epilepsy have been estimated to account for 0.3% up to 0.7% of all pregnancies (Gaily 1991; Viinikainen et al. 2006). The proportion of pregnancies with exposure to AEDs is probably even higher considering the increasing use of AEDs for other indications than epilepsy (Spina and Perugi 2004). The vast majority of these women will have uneventful pregnancies and give birth to perfectly normal children. However, the medical management during pregnancy is a matter of special concern since maternal epilepsy and AED treatment are associated with an increased risk for an abnormal pregnancy outcome.

2 Teratogenic Effects of AEDs: Methodological Issues

Many different methods have been used to assess the foetal risks associated with exposure to AEDs. The first years after the initial report on possible teratogenic effects of AEDs saw many publications of case-series of adverse pregnancy outcomes collected in individual centres or regions. A slightly more systematic method is spontaneous reporting of pregnancy outcome to the manufacturers, to drug agencies or surveillance programmes. Such methods can be useful in providing signals. However, reporting is selective, and since information on the denominator (total number of pregnancies exposed to the drug) is missing, these methods cannot be used for a proper risk assessment.

Case–control designs are generally considered useful for assessment of uncommon outcomes, such as birth defects. Cases with malformations are compared to controls regarding exposure to AEDs in foetal life. The method has been used to study the association between some specific malformations and exposure to individual AEDs, e.g. neural tube defects and exposure to valproate and oral clefts and lamotrigine. Case–control studies have also been utilised to analyse exposure to different AEDs and congenital abnormalities in general (Kjaer et al. 2007). A drawback of case–control studies is the risk of recall bias. Mothers of children with malformations are more likely to report drug intake during pregnancy.

Other studies have utilised existing general registries. Information on exposure could be obtained from a national drug prescription database (Artama et al. 2005) or from other registries that systematically and prospectively obtain information on drug intake in early pregnancy. The Swedish and Norwegian Medical Birth Registries are examples of the latter. These can be crosslink with registries of birth defects to assess the association between use of AEDs in early pregnancy and adverse outcome (Veiby et al. 2009; Wide et al. 2004). Such registries can have the advantage of recording exposure before pregnancy outcome is known and in addition being population-based, nationwide and thus representative. Contrarily, they often lack details on important information such as drug dosage, indication for treatment and classification of epilepsy, seizure control during pregnancy and on other factors that could contribute to the outcome. Furthermore, the teratogenic outcome might not be classified according to uniform criteria and the assessor of the child might be influenced by information on drug intake during pregnancy.

Another common approach is cohort studies of pregnancies in women with epilepsy. Retrospective cohort studies (where women are included at a time when pregnancy outcome might be known) are associated with a risk of selection bias. This is avoided in prospective studies where women ideally are identified and enrolled in early pregnancy before any information on pregnancy outcome is known. Such studies have traditionally often been hospital based and many studies based on cohorts from single hospitals or epilepsy centres or from several collaborating clinics were published in the 1980s and 1990s (Tomson et al. 2004b). Additional advantages with such prospective cohort studies is that they usually have a reliable classification and details on the mothers' epilepsy, the course of the epilepsy during pregnancy and on other potential risk factors. The major disadvantage is that they represent selected epilepsy populations, probably more severe cases under specialist care. A further major limitation has been in the number of included pregnancies, often a few hundred and at best a thousand pregnancies (Tomson and Battino 2005).

Special types of cohort studies, antiepileptic drugs and pregnancy registries, were established in the late 1990s and have thus now been operational for more than a decade (Tomson et al. 2010). These registries are prospective observational studies enrolling women with epilepsy early in pregnancy collecting information on drug exposure and other potential risk factors before outcome of the pregnancy is known. Women are followed throughout pregnancy and the outcome in terms of occurrence of birth defects in the offspring is recorded. The advantage of such studies is that they may collect high numbers of pregnancies, the type of drug exposure is recorded in an unbiased way without prior knowledge of teratogenic outcome, and detailed data on other relevant patient characteristics could be obtained. They share the limitations of many previous cohort studies in being based on selected patients, which hampers the possibilities to generalize from the results and although they share many methodological features, there are also significant differences between them (Tomson et al. 2010).

The aforementioned studies are designed primarily to evaluate the risk of major congenital malformations. Assessment of postnatal cognitive development poses further difficulties and challenges. An extended follow-up is necessary. By this, however, environmental factors such as psycho-social factors, including maternal education, cognitive status and epilepsy may all affect the child's performance. The assessor needs to be blinded and appropriate controls included.

Even results of prospective studies of teratogenic effects of AEDs may be difficult to interpret. For obvious reasons, women considering pregnancy have not been randomised to different types of treatment. The selection of a particular treatment depends on individual environmental and genetic factors that could be linked to the risk of adverse pregnancy outcome. An association between exposure to a certain AED and occurrence of adverse pregnancy outcome in an observational study is thus not evidence of a causal relationship. The impact of possible confounders, such as type of epilepsy, seizure frequency, family history of birth defects and exposure to additional risk factors needs to be assessed, which requires large sample sizes. It is thus important to pay attention to methodological issues such as statistical power, reliability of collected data, and attempts to control for appropriate confounding factors in the analyses, rather than to just compare rates of adverse pregnancy outcome in published studies.

3   Growth Retardation

Reduced birth weight, body length and head circumference in the offspring of women treated with phenytoin was reported already in the 1970s (Hanson et al. 1976). Such reductions in body dimensions were confirmed in subsequent studies of larger cohorts (Battino et al. 1992, 1999; Dessens et al. 2001; Hiilesmaa et al. 1981; Wide et al. 2000). In general, more pronounced effects were found in infants exposed to polytherapy, whereas the association between reduced body dimensions and specific AEDs in monotherapy varies. Phenobarbital and primidone have been implicated, whereas others have reported carbamazepine to be most strongly associated with small head circumference. A population-based Swedish study spanning 25 years, found a clear trend towards normalization of the head circumference in parallel with a shift from polytherapy towards monotherapy despite an increasing use of carbamazepine (Wide et al. 2000). Other more recent studies also suggest that, with present treatment strategies, microcephaly may no longer be more common among infants of mothers treated for epilepsy during pregnancy (Choulika et al. 1999). A very recent populations-based nationwide Norwegian study found low birth weight, small for gestational age, and small head circumference to be significantly more common in infants of mothers with epilepsy compared to the general population (Veiby et al. 2009). However, small for gestational age was more common in the offspring of mothers with epilepsy whether the mothers were taking AEDs or not.

A committee of the American Academy of Neurology and the American Epilepsy Society recently reassessed the evidence related to the care of women with epilepsy during pregnancy (Harden et al. 2009). The committee concluded that neonates of women with epilepsy taking AEDs probably have an increased risk of small for gestational age about twice the expected rate.

4   Minor Anomalies and Dysmorphisms

Minor anomalies are structural variations without medical, surgical or cosmetic importance. Discrete minor anomalies are frequently found in normal infants, but combinations of several anomalies can form a pattern, a dysmorphic syndrome, which may indicate a more severe underlying dysfunction. The term "foetal anti-convulsant syndrome" has been used to describe an AED-associated embryopathy variably characterised by microcephaly, growth retardation, hypertelorism, depressed nasal bridge, low set ears, micrognathia and distal digital hypoplasia, other anomalies, and sometimes developmental delay (Dean et al. 2002; Holmes et al. 2001; Moore et al. 2000). More distinctive phenotypes have also been claimed to be associated with specific AEDs, most notably phenytoin, carbamazepine and valproate. Valproate exposure has been claimed to cause a somewhat different dysmorphic syndrome characterised by thin arched eyebrows with medial deficiency, broad nasal bridge, short anteverted nose, and a smooth long filtrum with thin upper lip. Such features have been suggested to be associated with, and indicative of, impaired cognitive development (Dean et al. 2002; Kini et al. 2006). The overlap in the various dysmorphisms is considerable and their drug specificity has therefore been questioned as has their predictive significance vs. cognitive development (Perucca and Tomson 2006). In addition, the pathogenesis is still somewhat controversial. Gaily et al. (1988) attributed most of the minor anomalies to genetic factors rather than drug exposure, although most studies suggest that there is an association between minor anomalies and exposure to AEDs. Indeed one study of infants of untreated mother with epilepsy failed to find any features of the foetal antiepileptic drug syndrome in the offspring (Holmes et al. 2000). It should, however, be underlined that minor anomalies are much more difficult to assess objectively than major malformations, and that the incidence of minor anomalies in exposed infants varies markedly between studies.

5 Major Congenital Malformations

5.1 Overall Malformation Rates with AEDs

Major congenital malformations are commonly defined as a structural abnormality with surgical, medical or cosmetic importance. Numerous studies from the 1980s and 1990s have confirmed increased rates of birth defects in children of mothers with epilepsy. The prevalence of major congenital malformations in children exposed to AEDs has ranged from 4 to 10%, corresponding to a two- to fourfold increase from the expected in the general population (Harden et al. 2009; Meador et al. 2008; Tomson and Battino 2005, 2009; Tomson and Hiilesmaa 2007). A few more recent studies, however, have not demonstrated increased risks in infants exposed to AEDs in utero compared to offspring of women with epilepsy not taking AEDs (Morrow et al. 2006; Veiby et al. 2009). In a prospective observational study from the UK, the relative risk of major congenital malformations among children of mothers with epilepsy taking AEDs during pregnancy vs. women with untreated epilepsy was 1.19 (0.59–2.40) (Morrow et al. 2006). In a nationwide population-based Norwegian registry study, the frequency of major malformations was 3.3% in children of mothers with treated epilepsy, not significantly different from the 2.5% among controls in the general population (Veiby et al. 2009).

Much of the variation in reported outcomes could be explained by differences in study methodology including study populations, in selection of control populations and in criteria for malformations. A possible decrease in recent years in the prevalence of malformations in offspring of women with epilepsy might also be related to changes in treatment strategies. It is possible that more frequent use of AED monotherapy as opposed to polytherapy, use of lower doses, changes in AED preferences, and pre-conceptional counselling has contributed to a more optimal management with reduced foetal risks. Nevertheless, it is still debated whether the usually reported increase in malformation rates is entirely caused by AEDs or if to some extent this could be linked to the underlying epilepsy disorder, or to seizures. The available data, however, strongly suggest that AED exposure is the major factor. In 26 cohort studies that included pregnancies of women with treated as well as untreated epilepsy, the average malformation rate among children exposed to AEDs in utero was 6.1% compared to 2.8% among children of mothers with untreated epilepsy and 2.2% in infants of healthy controls (Tomson and Battino 2009). These observations have been confirmed in a meta-analysis of the evidence of epilepsy per se as a teratogenic risk (Fried et al. 2004). Ten studies reporting rates of congenital malformations in offspring of untreated women with epilepsy were included. The malformation rate in this group was not higher than among offspring of non-epileptic healthy controls, odds ratio (OR) 1.92 (0.92–4.00). The OR was 0.99 (0.49–2.01) after removal of some small studies likely to be affected by publication bias.

Although obviously, untreated women with epilepsy are different in many respects from those who are under treatment during pregnancy, the available evidence strongly suggests that treatment is the major cause of increased risk of adverse pregnancy outcomes. Further support for a drug effect comes from the observation of greater risks with polytherapy compared to monotherapy with AEDs. Polytherapy was associated with a malformation rate of 6.8 vs. 4.0% in monotherapy in a recent pooled analysis (Tomson and Battino 2009).

5.2 Specific Malformations

The pattern of malformations associated with AEDs as a group is mostly similar to that seen in the general population. Cardiac defects are the most common followed by facial clefts, and hypospadia (Battino and Tomson 2007). There may, however, be an association between certain individual AEDs and some specific malformations. Neural tube defects and hypospadia are more common among offspring of mothers who used valproate during pregnancy (Morrow et al. 2006; Samrén et al. 1999), the risk of neural tube defects in association with valproate has been estimated to 1–2% (Lindhout and Schmidt 1986). An increased risk of neural tube defects of 0.5–1% has also been reported after carbamazepine exposure (Kallen 1994; Rosa 1991). Valproate has also been associated with facial clefts (Morrow et al. 2006) and phenytoin and carbamazepine with cleft palate

(Puho et al. 2007). Recent data from the North American AED Pregnancy Registry suggested a tenfold increase in risk of oral clefts among lamotrigine exposed infants (Holmes et al. 2008a), but this specific association has not been confirmed in other registries (Dolk et al. 2008; Holmes et al. 2008a). Exposure to phenobarbital has been suggested to increase the risk of cardiac malformations (Canger et al. 1999).

5.3 Comparative Malformation Rates with Different AEDs

For reasons discussed above, women with active epilepsy will need continued treatment throughout pregnancy. The relative safety during pregnancy is therefore a major criterion for selection of an AED for a woman with epilepsy who is of child-bearing potential. Large studies are needed to draw conclusions on the relative teratogenic potential of different AEDs as the prevalence of birth defects with AEDs fortunately is no more than 4–10%. However, surprisingly few studies in the past have comprised more than 500 pregnancies in total. Clearly much larger cohorts are needed to permit a meaningful assessment of individual AEDs. During the last decade, some different strategies have been applied to achieve this.

One method, which has been used in the Nordic countries, is to utilise different existing national registries and databases for the purpose of assessing the safety of AED use in pregnancy. One example is the Swedish Medical Birth Registry, a nationwide population-based health registry compiled from antenatal maternal health clinic records, and those of the delivery and maternity wards. Drug exposure is recorded at the first visit to the maternity health clinics (typically gestational week 9). Pregnancy outcome is assessed based on registries of birth defects. A report from this registry was based on 1,398 pregnancies with exposure to AEDs (Wide et al. 2004). The odds ratio (OR) for having a malformation in the AED-exposed offspring, compared with the expected estimate from all infants born, was 1.86 (1.42–2.44) overall. OR in monotherapy exposed was 1.61 (1.18–2.19), and in polytherapy 4.20 (2.42–7.49). The OR was higher after exposure to valproate monotherapy compared with carbamazepine monotherapy 2.59 (1.43–4.68).

Another nationwide population-based study utilized the Finnish drug prescription database and the National Medical Birth Registry to identify all women who were prescribed AEDs during pregnancy (Artama et al. 2005), including 1,411 pregnancies with AED exposure. Congenital malformations were more common among offspring of these women (4.6%) than among offspring of untreated patients with epilepsy (2.8%). Compared with untreated patients, the risk of malformations was higher in foetuses exposed to valproate monotherapy (malformation rate 10.7%; OR = 4.18; 2.31–7.57) or valproate as part of polytherapy (malformation rate 9.2%; OR = 3.54; 1.42–8.11). In contrast, the risk of malformations was not elevated in association with exposure to carbamazepine, oxcarbazepine, or phenytoin monotherapy.

A third example is a recent study from Norway. The nationwide compulsory Medical Birth Registry of Norway was surveyed from 1999 to 2005 (Veiby et al.

2009). A total of 961 pregnancies with AED exposure were identified. An increased risk for major congenital malformations compared to unexposed could be demonstrated only for valproate monotherapy (5.6 vs. 2.5% in the general population) and AED polytherapy (6.1%).

The advantage of these studies is that they are population based and the results are likely to be representative. However, they lack detail concerning other potential risk factors, e.g. the indication for treatment and type of epilepsy, seizure control during pregnancy, AED dosage and other. Pregnancies ending in elective abortions are also not included even if the indication was foetal abnormalities. Most importantly, although nationwide, the number of included pregnancies on different specific AEDs is too small to permit a more precise comparison of their teratogenic potential.

In order to facilitate enrolment of greater numbers of pregnancies with AED exposure, and thus more meaningful comparisons, different groups established specific Epilepsy and Pregnancy Registries in the late 1990s (Tomson et al. 2010). Some were set up by pharmaceutical companies and collect data on the manufacturers' own product (e.g. GlaxoSmithKline's International Lamotrigine Registry) (Cunnington et al. 2007). Others have been established by independent research groups and include information on all AED exposures. These are national, regional (e.g. Australia, UK, North America, Kerala, India) or broadly international (European and International Registry of Antiepileptic Drugs in Pregnancy, EURAP). Many of the registries have now been operational for more than 10 years and are beginning to release results.

Malformation rates reported from pregnancy registries and from some other larger and contemporary studies are presented for the five most frequently used AEDs (valproate, carbamazepine, lamotrigine, phenobarbital and phenytoin) in Table 1.

In the absence of a comparator, the results from the company-sponsored registries are difficult to interpret. However, GlaxoSmithKline's International Lamotrigine Pregnancy Registry reported a malformation rate of 2.9% based on 802 monotherapy exposures (Cunnington et al. 2007).

The largest independent AED and pregnancy registries are The North American Antiepileptic Drugs and Pregnancy Registry (NAAPR), the United Kingdom Epilepsy and Pregnancy Register, and EURAP, an international registry enrolling pregnancies from more than 40 countries, in Europe, Australia, Asia, Oceania and South America (Tomson et al. 2010). These registries have enrolled 6,000–14,000 pregnancies and two of them, NAAPR and the UK register, have published results on teratogenic outcome. These three registries are slightly different in their scope and differ significantly in their methodologies, which should be kept in mind when malformation rates are compared across the registries.

NAAPR has reported increased malformation rates in comparison with the general population with phenobarbital monotherapy (6.5%), relative risk (RR) 4.2 (1.5–9.4) (Holmes et al. 2004), and valproate (10.7%) RR 7.3 (4.4–12.2) (Wyszynski et al. 2005). The malformation rate was 2.8% with lamotrigine monotherapy (Holmes et al. 2008a), 2.5% ($n = 873$) with carbamazepine and

Table 1 Rates of malformations,% and (number of monotherapy exposures) with antiepileptic drugs in monotherapy in some major studies

Study/registry	Valproate	Carbamazepine	Lamotrigine	Phenobarbital	Phenytoin
Samrén et al. (1997)	8.7% (184)	7.9% (280)		10.4% (48)	6.4% (141)
Samrén et al. (1999)	5.7% (158)	3.7% (376)		2.9% (172)	0.7% (151)
Kaneko et al. (1999)	11.1% (81)	5.7% (158)		5.1% (79)	9.1% (132)
GlaxoSmithKline (Cunnington et al. 2007)			2.9% (802)		
Finnish Drug prescription (Artama et al. 2005)	10.6% (263)	2.7% (805)			
Swedish Medical Birth Registry (http://www.janusinfo.org/)	7.7% (507)	5.4% (1,199)	4.9% (400)		7.6% (145)
UK Register (Morrow 2007, data on file of the UK Epilepsy Pregnancy Registry, personal communication)	6.2% (715)	2.2% (900)	3.2% (647)		3.7% (82)
North American Registry (Hernandez-Diaz et al. 2007; Holmes et al. 2004, 2008a, b; Wyszynski et al. 2005)	10.7% (149)	2.5% (873)	2.8% (684)	6.5% (77)	2.6% (390)
Australian Register (Vajda et al. 2007)	13.3% (166)	3.0% (234)	1.4% (146)		3.2% (31)
Norwegian Birth Registry (Veiby et al. 2009)	5.9% (204)	2.6% (454)	2.7% (260)	0% (14)	0% (19)

2.6% ($n = 390$) with phenytoin monotherapy (Hernandez-Diaz et al. 2007), not significantly increased from the background rate of 1.6%.

The UK register published their first report based on 3,607 cases (Morrow et al. 2006). The rate of major congenital malformations for pregnancies exposed to valproate monotherapy was 6.2% (4.6–8.2%) compared with 2.2% (1.4–3.4%) for carbamazepine. The malformation rate with lamotrigine monotherapy was 3.2% (2.1–4.9%) based on 647 pregnancies. Interestingly, the malformation rate in offspring of 227 untreated women with epilepsy was 3.5% (1.8–6.8%), very similar to the 3.7% (3.0–4.5%) among the monotherapy exposures in general ($n = 2,468$).

It is evident from Table 1 that malformation rates across studies vary considerably for the same AED in monotherapy. Carbamazepine exposure was associated with rates ranging from 2.2 to 7.9%, lamotrigine from 1.4 to 4.9%, phenytoin from 0.7 to 9.1%, and valproate from 5.7 to 13.3% (Table 1). The wide ranges in malformation rates reflect differences in study populations, criteria and methodology. Prevalences of malformations with different AEDs should therefore not be compared across studies. However, there appears to be a consistent pattern within studies with higher rates with valproate and lower rates with carbamazepine and lamotrigine (Table 1). Even within-study comparisons should be made with caution considering the possible effects of confounding factors.

There is very limited published data on pregnancy outcome with other new generation AEDs than lamotrigine. Malformation rates in reports based on prospective pregnancies with monotherapy exposure to newer generation AEDs other than lamotrigine, such as gabapentin, topiramate, levetiracetam, oxcarbazepine and zonisamide, are shown in Table 2. Even when pregnancies from all available studies are added up, the total number of monotherapy exposures for each of gabapentin, topiramate, levetiracetam, oxcarbazepine is limited to approximately 250–300 pregnancies, and much less for zonisamide. Clearly these numbers are too small for a reliable assessment of the risks.

In their recent evidence-based review, the American Academy of Neurology and the American Epilepsy Society Committee concluded that it is highly probable that valproate exposure during the first trimester is associated with higher risk of major congenital malformations compared to taking carbamazepine, and possibly

Table 2 Monotherapy exposures to some newer generation antiepileptic drugs in different published studies, number of exposures (number of pregnancies with major malformations)

References	GBP	TPM	LEV	OXC	ZNS
Kondo et al. (1996)					4 (0)
Samrén et al. (1999)				2 (0)	
Fonager et al. (2000)	1 (0)			14 (0)	
Hvas et al. (2000)				7 (0)	
Long (2003)			3 (0)		
Montouris (2003)	16 (1)				
Kaaja et al. (2003)				9 (1)	
Meischenguiser et al. (2004)				35 (0)	
Swedish Medical Birth Registry (http://www. janusinfo.org/)	68(5)			4 (0)	
Artama et al. (2005)				99 (1)	
UK Registry 2007 (Hunt et al. 2006; Hunt et al. 2008; Morrow 2007, data on file of the UK Epilepsy Pregnancy Registry, personal communication)	31(1)	42(1)	39(0)		
Ornoy et al. (2008)		29(1)			
Ten Berg et al. (2005)			11 (0)		
Holmes et al. (2008a, b)	127(1)	197(8)	197(4)	121(2)	
Veiby (2010, personal communication)	7(0)	16(1)	15(1)	30(1)	
TOTAL	250 (8)	284(11)	265 (5)	321(5)	4 (0)

compared to phenytoin or lamotrigine (Harden et al. 2009). Other newer generation AEDs are not mentioned in this report.

6 Postnatal Cognitive Development

During the past 3 decades, several studies with different designs have aimed at assessing whether exposure to AEDs in utero could also adversely affect the cognitive development of the child after birth. Such studies are complicated to perform, requiring long-term follow-up. But they are also difficult to interpret because of confounding (e.g. parental cognitive function, socio-economic circumstances, maternal epilepsy) and in particular since environmental factors become more important with increasing age of the child. Few studies have been published, and mostly based on small cohorts. Studies from the 1980s and 1990s have aimed at assessing phenobarbital and more often phenytoin and carbamazepine, the most frequently used AEDs at that time. A prospective population-based study from Helsinki, Finland found no influence of AED (mainly phenytoin and carbamazepine) exposure on global IQ (Gaily et al. 1990). Observed cognitive dysfunction was attributed to maternal seizures and educational level of the parents rather than to the treatment. A Swedish population-based prospective study found no difference in psychomotor development in children exposed to carbamazepine compared with control children of healthy mothers, but a trend for phenytoin exposed children to do slightly worse in some tests of motor coordination (Wide et al. 2002). Scolnik et al. (1994) reported lower global IQ in children exposed to phenytoin but not in those exposed to carbamazepine.

A Cochrane Review from 2004 concluded that at that time there was little evidence about which drugs carry more risks than others to the development of children exposed (Adab et al. 2004b). Some subsequent studies, however, have suggested that exposure to valproate might carry a particular risk of adverse developmental effects (Adab et al. 2001; Meador et al. 2009; Vinten et al. 2005). A retrospective survey from the UK found additional educational needs to be more common among children that had been exposed to valproate than in those exposed to carbamazepine or unexposed control children (Adab et al. 2001). A more detailed investigation revealed lower verbal IQ in those exposed to valproate than in unexposed children and children exposed to carbamazepine or phenytoin (Adab et al. 2004a; Vinten et al. 2005). Multiple regression analysis identified exposure to valproate, frequent tonic-clonic seizures in pregnancy and low maternal IQ to be associated with lower verbal IQ also after adjustment for confounding factors.

Given the retrospective design, small numbers and poor participation rate, the results need to be interpreted with some caution. However, some subsequent prospective studies report similar observations concerning valproate. Hence, a small population-based prospective study from Finland found a lower verbal IQ in children exposed in utero to valproate monotherapy ($n = 13$) and to polytherapy in general compared with non-exposed children or children exposed to carbamazepine (Gaily et al. 2004). However, the results were confounded by low maternal education and polytherapy. Another small prospective population-based Finnish study signals a similar trend for worse outcome in children exposed to valproate but also points to the problem of confounding factors as the mothers using valproate in pregnancy scored lower on IQ than other groups (Eriksson et al. 2005).

A larger, prospective observational study from Kerala, India, evaluated mental and motor development in children of mothers with epilepsy, but already at 15 months of age (Thomas et al. 2008). Children exposed to polytherapy had lower developmental quotients than those exposed to monotherapy. Compared with those exposed to carbamazepine monotherapy ($n = 101$), children exposed to valproate monotherapy ($n = 71$) had significantly lower mental and motor developmental quotients, whereas there was no significant difference between children exposed to other AEDs (mainly phenobarbital or phenytoin) compared with valproate. Of note is that this study did not analyse the possible influence of maternal cognitive function and outcome in the children.

The first reasonably powered truly prospective study of long-term cognitive effects of foetal exposure to AEDs recently published interim results (Meador et al. 2009). Between 1999 and 2004, women from USA and the UK on monotherapy with valproate, carbamazepine, lamotrigine or phenytoin were enrolled in early pregnancy in this observational study. The primary analysis in this study is a comparison of neurodevelopmental outcomes at 6 years of age, but interim results at 3 years of age have been released (Meador et al. 2009). In this carefully designed study, children exposed to valproate ($n = 53$) on average had an IQ score nine points lower than the score of those exposed to lamotrigine ($n = 84$), seven points lower than those exposed to phenytoin ($n = 48$) and six points lower than children exposed to carbamazepine ($n = 73$). IQ scores did not differ significantly among children exposed to the other three AEDs (lamotrigine, phenytoin, carbamazepine). These differences were obtained after adjustment for maternal IQ, infant's gestational age and some other potential confounding factors (Meador et al. 2009). It should, however, be noted that the IQ was within the normal range also among children exposed to valproate. There was also a significant correlation between the valproate dose in pregnancy and the child's IQ. In fact children exposed to valproate doses <1,000 mg/day did not differ in IQ from those exposed to other AEDs.

A few retrospective studies have suggested a specific association between exposure to valproate and the risk of developing autistic disorder (Rasalam et al. 2005), but this also needs further investigations.

The Committee of American Academy of Neurology and the American Epilepsy Society concluded that cognitive outcomes are probably reduced in children exposed to valproate compared to carbamazepine and possible also compared with phenytoin (Harden et al. 2009).

7 Dose-Dependency

A dose–effect relationship has so far been shown most consistently for teratogenicity in association with valproate. Dosages above 800–1,000 mg/day have thus been associated with significantly greater risks than lower dosages (Artama et al. 2005; Kaneko et al. 1999; Morrow et al. 2006; Samrén et al. 1997, 1999; Vajda et al. 2007). Data on cognitive outcome reveal a similar pattern. The retrospective study from Liverpool found that verbal IQ was no different from unexposed controls among children exposed to valproate doses <800 mg/day (Vinten et al. 2005). Likewise, the prospective NEAD study found IQ of children whose mothers took valproate in doses <1,000 mg/day to be similar to IQs in those exposed to other AEDs (Meador et al. 2009).

The UK Epilepsy and Pregnancy Register reported a positive dose response for major congenital malformations also for lamotrigine. Doses above 200 mg/day were associated with higher risks (Morrow et al. 2006). This pattern was, however, not found in the International Lamotrigine Registry of GlaxoSmithKline, nor did the North American pregnancy registry find lamotrigine doses to be significantly higher in mothers to children with malformations than in mothers to healthy children (Cunnington et al. 2007).

The American Academy of Neurology and the American Epilepsy Society Committee concluded that there is probably a relationship between the dose of valproate and lamotrigine and the risk of major congenital malformations (Harden et al. 2009).

8 Mechanisms of Teratogenesis

The mechanisms for the developmental toxicity of AEDs are likely to be multiple and also to partly vary with different AEDs. There is clearly an individual susceptibility as only a fraction of those exposed to the same treatment show signs of teratogenic effects. This is further supported by clinical observations of greater risks of AED-related embryopathy among siblings exposed to the same drug (Malm et al. 2002). A similar variability in the frequency and pattern of adverse pregnancy outcomes has been related to strain differences in experimental studies in mice (Buehler et al. 1990; Dean et al. 1999; Finnell 1991; Lindhout and Omtzigt 1992; Raymond et al. 1995; Strickler et al. 1985; Volcik et al. 2003). The outcome likely depends on gene–environment interactions and susceptible embryos probably carry genetic factors determining their susceptibility to AED-induced adverse foetal effects (Zhu et al. 2009).

A favoured hypothesis for many years suggests that the developmental toxicity of AEDs is related to their interference with folate metabolism. Folates are co-factors involved in the biosynthesis of nucleic acids and in the re-methylation of homocysteine to methionine. Many AEDs, including phenobarbital, phenytoin, primidone and carbamazepine, are known to reduce folate levels. Some clinical studies have reported an association between low maternal serum folate levels and risk of malformations (Dansky et al. 1987; Ogawa et al. 1991), although this has not been a consistent finding. In humans, extra periconceptional supplementation with folate has been demonstrated to reduce the risk of neural tube defects and at higher doses also the risk of recurrence in high-risk groups (MRC 1991). It is, however, important to understand that women with epilepsy were excluded from these studies. Observational data from epilepsy and pregnancy registries have unfortunately not demonstrated any protective effect against adverse pregnancy outcomes of periconceptional folate supplementation to women with epilepsy (Morrow et al. 2009).

The 5,10 methylene tetrahydrofolate reductase (MTHFR) gene has been suggested as one candidate to explain genetic susceptibility to folate sensitive malformations (Dean et al. 1999). MTHFR is involved in the biotransformation of folate and is highly polymorphic. Some mutations have been associated with increased risks of malformations such as neural tube defects, cleft palate and congenital heart disease that are often seen in relation to exposure to AEDs.

Bioactivation of AEDs to toxic reactive intermediate metabolites has been another suggested mechanism for the teratogenic effects (Amore et al. 1997; Bennett et al. 1996; Buehler et al. 1994; Finnell et al. 1995; Finnell and Dansky 1991; Lillibridge et al. 1996; Lindhout et al. 1984; Martz et al. 1977; Pantarotto et al. 1982; Rane and Peng 1985; Roy and Snodgrass 1990; Strickler et al. 1985). Reactive epoxides could be the result of CYP450 mediated oxidation of phenytoin, carbamazepine or phenobarbital. Individual differences in rates of their formation and in their elimination could contribute to the individual susceptibility to adverse outcomes. This could be genetically determined as well as affected by interactions between different AEDs. However, some of the most potent teratogenic AEDs such as trimethadione lack the premises to form epoxides. Additionally, the CYP450 activity in the embryo during the sensitive periods is very low.

Another postulated bio-activating pathway is co-oxidation of AEDs to free radical intermediates. These could release reactive oxygen species (ROS), which may cause oxidative stress and thus teratogenicity. Deficiency of free radical scavenging enzymes, responsible for eliminating ROS, has been associated with malformations in the offspring of epileptic mothers exposed to AEDs (Parman et al. 1998; Wells et al. 1997; Wells and Winn 1996).

A more recent hypothesis suggests that many AEDs, such as phenytoin, trimethadione, carbamazepine, phenobarbital, and possibly lamotrigine may exert their teratogenic effects by inducing embryonic cardiac arrhythmia during specific sensitive restricted periods (Danielsson et al. 2000). These effects on the embryonic heart have been linked to the drugs' ability to block the rapid component of the delayed rectifying K ion current, Ikr (Azarbayjani and Danielsson 2002). It is postulated that the embryonic arrhythmia will cause temporary hypoxia followed by re-oxygenation and generation of ROS, which will cause tissue damage. Orofacial clefts, heart defects, distal digital defects and growth retardation could be hypoxia related and thus explained by such mechanisms.

A different proposed mechanism postulates that the teratogenic effects of AEDs may be explained by induction of neural apoptosis. Animal experiments have demonstrated apoptotic neurodegeneration in the developing brain induced by therapeutic concentrations of AEDs such as valproate, phenytoin, and phenobarbital (Bittigau et al. 2002; Kluger and Meador 2008).

It is clear that the mechanisms behind developmental toxicity of AEDs are presently far from completely understood. They are likely to be multiple and differ between individual AEDs and it is even conceivable that each individual AED can exert its adverse effects through more than one mechanism.

9 Conclusions

It has been known for more than 40 years that children of mothers with epilepsy have an increased risk of adverse pregnancy outcomes. Although multifactorial, the greater risk is mainly due to teratogenic effects of the AEDs. However, due to the significant maternal and foetal risks associated with uncontrolled epileptic seizures, AED treatment is generally maintained during pregnancy in the majority of women with active epilepsy.

Adverse pregnancy outcomes that have been associated with AED exposure include foetal growth retardation, major congenital malformations and impaired postnatal cognitive development. In earlier publications, the prevalence of major malformations in children exposed to AEDs has been 2–4 times higher than in the general population. More recent studies suggest a smaller increase in malformation rates. This seemingly more favourable outcome may be relating new treatment strategies with less polytherapy, lower AED dosages and different AED selection. Recent data from large prospective pregnancy registries have revealed differences between AEDs in their teratogenic potential. Malformation rates have consistently been higher in association with exposure to valproate than with carbamazepine and lamotrigine. Other, albeit more limited, prospective cohort studies also indicate reduced cognitive outcome in children exposed to valproate compared to carbamazepine and possibly lamotrigine. Information on pregnancy outcomes with newer generation AEDs other than lamotrigine are still insufficient.

References

Adab N, Jacoby A, Smith D et al (2001) Additional educational needs in children born to mothers with epilepsy. J Neurol Neurosurg Psychiatry 70:15–21

Adab N, Kini U, Vinten J et al (2004a) The longer term outcome of children born to mothers with epilepsy. J Neurol Neurosurg Psychiatry 75:1575–1583

Adab N, Tudur SC, Vinten J et al (2004b) Common antiepileptic drugs in pregnancy in women with epilepsy (Cochrane Review) The Cochrane Library. Wiley, Chichester

Amore BM, Kalhorn TF, Skiles GL et al (1997) Characterization of carbamazepine metabolism in a mouse model of carbamazepine teratogenicity. Drug Metab Dispos 25:953–962

Artama M, Auvinen A, Raudaskoski T et al (2005) Antiepileptic drug use of women with epilepsy and congenital malformations in offspring. Neurology 64:1874–1878

Azarbayjani F, Danielsson BR (2002) Embryonic arrhythmia by inhibition of HERG channels: a common hypoxia-related teratogenic mechanism for antiepileptic drugs? Epilepsia 43:457–468

Battino D, Tomson T (2007) Management of epilepsy during pregnancy. Drugs 67:2727–2746

Battino D, Granata T, Binelli S et al (1992) Intrauterine growth in the offspring of epileptic mothers. Acta Neurol Scand 86:555–557

Battino D, Kaneko S, Andermann E et al (1999) Intrauterine growth in the offspring of epileptic women: a prospective multicenter study. Epilepsy Res 36:53–60

Bennett GD, Amore BM, Finnell RH et al (1996) Teratogenicity of carbamazepine-10, 11-epoxide and oxcarbazepine in the SWV mouse. J Pharmacol Exp Ther 279:1237–1242

Bittigau P, Sifringer M, Genz K et al (2002) Antiepileptic drugs and apoptotic neurodegeneration in the developing brain. Proc Natl Acad Sci USA 99:15089–15094

Buehler BA, Delimont D, van Waes M et al (1990) Prenatal prediction of risk of the fetal hydantoin syndrome. N Engl J Med 322:1567–1572

Buehler BA, Rao V, Finnell RH (1994) Biochemical and molecular teratology of fetal hydantoin syndrome. Neurol Clin 12:741–748

Canger R, Battino D, Canevini MP et al (1999) Malformations in offspring of women with epilepsy: a prospective study. Epilepsia 40:1231–1236

Choulika S, Harvey E, Holmes LB (1999) Effect of antiepileptic drugs (AED) on fetal growth: assessment at birth. Teratology 59:388

Cunnington M, Ferber S, Quartey G (2007) Effect of dose on the frequency of major birth defects following fetal exposure to lamotrigine monotherapy in an international observational study. Epilepsia 48:1207–1210

Danielsson B, Skold AC, Azarbayjani F et al (2000) Pharmacokinetic data support pharmacologically induced embryonic dysrhythmia as explanation to Fetal Hydantoin Syndrome in rats. Toxicol Appl Pharmacol 163:164–175

Dansky LV, Andermann E, Rosenblatt D et al (1987) Anticonvulsants, folate levels, and pregnancy outcome: a prospective study. Ann Neurol 21:176–182

Dean JC, Moore SJ, Osborne A et al (1999) Fetal anticonvulsant syndrome and mutation in the maternal MTHFR gene. Clin Genet 56:216–220

Dean JC, Hailey H, Moore SJ et al (2002) Long term health and neurodevelopment in children exposed to antiepileptic drugs before birth. J Med Genet 39:251–259

Dessens AB, Cohen-Kettenis PT, Mellenbergh GJ et al (2001) Association of prenatal phenobarbital and phenytoin exposure with genital anomalies and menstrual disorders. Teratology 64:181–188

Dolk H, Jentink J, Loane M et al (2008) Does lamotrigine use in pregnancy increase orofacial cleft risk relative to other malformations? Neurology 71:714–722

Eriksson K, Viinikainen K, Monkkonen A et al (2005) Children exposed to valproate in utero-population based evaluation of risks and confounding factors for long-term neurocognitive development. Epilepsy Res 65:189–200

Finnell RH (1991) Genetic differences in susceptibility to anticonvulsant drug-induced developmental defects. Pharmacol Toxicol 69:223–227

Finnell RH, Dansky LV (1991) Parental epilepsy, anticonvulsant drugs, and reproductive outcome: epidemiologic and experimental findings spanning three decades; 1: animal studies. Reprod Toxicol 5:281–299

Finnell RH, Bennett GD, Slattery JT et al (1995) Effect of treatment with phenobarbital and stiripentol on carbamazepine-induced teratogenicity and reactive metabolite formation. Teratology 52:324–332

Fonager K, Larsen H, Pedersen L et al (2000) Birth outcomes in women exposed to anticonvulsant drugs. Acta Neurol Scand 101:289–294

Fried S, Kozer E, Nulman I et al (2004) Malformation rates in children of women with untreated epilepsy: a meta-analysis. Drug Saf 27:197–202

Gaily E (1991) Development and growth in children of epileptic mothers. A prospective controlled study. Acta Obstet Gynecol Scand 70:631–632

Gaily E, Granstrom ML, Hiilesmaa V et al (1988) Minor anomalies in offspring of epileptic mothers. J Pediatr 112:520–529

Gaily E, Kantola-Sorsa E, Granstrom ML (1990) Specific cognitive dysfunction in children with epileptic mothers. Dev Med Child Neurol 32:403–414

Gaily E, Kantola-Sorsa E, Hiilesmaa V et al (2004) Normal intelligence in children with prenatal exposure to carbamazepine. Neurology 62:28–32

German J, Ehlers KH, Kowal A et al (1970) Possible teratogenicity of trimethadione and paramethadione. Lancet 2:261–262

Hanson JW, Myrianthopoulos NC, Harvey MA et al (1976) Risks to the offspring of women treated with hydantoin anticonvulsants, with emphasis on the fetal hydantoin syndrome. J Pediatr 89:662–668

Harden CL, Meador KJ, Pennell PB et al (2009) Management issues for women with epilepsy – focus on pregnancy (an evidence-based review): II. Teratogenesis and perinatal outcomes: report of the Quality Standards Subcommittee and Therapeutics and Technology Subcommittee of the American Academy of Neurology and the American Epilepsy Society. Epilepsia 50:1237–1246

Hernandez-Diaz S, Smith CR, Wyszynski DF et al (2007) Risk of major malformations among infants exposed to carbamazepine during pregnancy. Birth Def Res 79:357

Hiilesmaa VK, Teramo K, Granstrom ML et al (1981) Fetal head growth retardation associated with maternal antiepileptic drugs. Lancet 2:165–167

Holmes LB, Rosenberger PB, Harvey EA et al (2000) Intelligence and physical features of children of women with epilepsy. Teratology 61:196–202

Holmes LB, Harvey EA, Coull BA et al (2001) The teratogenicity of anticonvulsant drugs. N Engl J Med 344:1132–1138

Holmes LB, Wyszynski DF, Lieberman E (2004) The AED (antiepileptic drug) pregnancy registry: a 6-year experience. Arch Neurol 61:673–678

Holmes LB, Baldwin EJ, Smith CR et al (2008a) Increased frequency of isolated cleft palate in infants exposed to lamotrigine during pregnancy. Neurology 70:2152–2158

Holmes LB, Smith CR, Herndandez-Diaz S (2008b) Pregnancy registries: larger sample sizes essential. Birth Def Res A 82:307

Hunt S, Craig J, Russell A et al (2006) Levetiracetam in pregnancy: preliminary experience from the UK Epilepsy and Pregnancy Register. Neurology 67:1876–1879

Hunt S, Russell A, Smithson WH et al (2008) Topiramate in pregnancy: preliminary experience from the UK Epilepsy and Pregnancy Register. Neurology 71:272–276

Hvas CL, Henriksen TB, Ostergaard JR et al (2000) Epilepsy and pregnancy: effect of antiepileptic drugs and lifestyle on birthweight. BJOG 107:896–902

Kaaja E, Kaaja R, Hiilesmaa V (2003) Major malformations in offspring of women with epilepsy. Neurology 60:575–579

Kallen AJ (1994) Maternal carbamazepine and infant spina bifida. Reprod Toxicol 8:203–205

Kaneko S, Battino D, Andermann E et al (1999) Congenital malformations due to antiepileptic drugs. Epilepsy Res 33:145–158

Kini U, Adab N, Vinten J et al (2006) Dysmorphic features: an important clue to the diagnosis and severity of fetal anticonvulsant syndromes. Arch Dis Child Fetal Neonatal Ed 91:F90–F95

Kjaer D, Horvath-Puho E, Christensen J et al (2007) Use of phenytoin, phenobarbital, or diazepam during pregnancy and risk of congenital abnormalities: a case-time-control study. Pharmacoepidemiol Drug Saf 16:181–188

Kluger BM, Meador KJ (2008) Teratogenicity of antiepileptic medications. Semin Neurol 28:328–335

Kondo T, Kaneko S, Amano Y et al (1996) Preliminary report on teratogenic effects of zonisamide in the offspring of treated women with epilepsy. Epilepsia 37:1242–1244

Lillibridge JH, Amore BM, Slattery JT et al (1996) Protein-reactive metabolites of carbamazepine in mouse liver microsomes. Drug Metab Dispos 24:509–514

Lindhout D, Omtzigt JG (1992) Pregnancy and the risk of teratogenicity. Epilepsia 33:S41–S48

Lindhout D, Schmidt D (1986) In-utero exposure to valproate and neural tube defects. Lancet 1:1392–1393

Lindhout D, Hoppener RJ, Meinardi H (1984) Teratogenicity of antiepileptic drug combinations with special emphasis on epoxidation (of carbamazepine). Epilepsia 25:77–83

Long L (2003) Levetiracetam monotherapy during pregnancy: a case series. Epilepsy Behav 4:447–448

Malm H, Kajantie E, Kivirikko S et al (2002) Valproate embryopathy in three sets of siblings: further proof of hereditary susceptibility. Neurology 59:630–633

Martz F, Failinger C 3rd, Blake DA (1977) Phenytoin teratogenesis: correlation between embryopathic effect and covalent binding of putative arene oxide metabolite in gestational tissue. J Pharmacol Exp Ther 203:231–239

Meador K, Reynolds MW, Crean S et al (2008) Pregnancy outcomes in women with epilepsy: a systematic review and meta-analysis of published pregnancy registries and cohorts. Epilepsy Res 81:1–13

Meador KJ, Baker GA, Browning N et al (2009) Cognitive function at 3 years of age after fetal exposure to antiepileptic drugs. N Engl J Med 360:1597–1605

Meadow SR (1968) Anticonvulsant drugs and congenital abnormalities. Lancet 2:1296

Meischenguiser R, D'Giano CH, Ferraro SM (2004) Oxcarbazepine in pregnancy: clinical experience in Argentina. Epilepsy Behav 5:163–167

Montouris G (2003) Gabapentin exposure in human pregnancy: results from the Gabapentin Pregnancy Registry. Epilepsy Behav 4:310–317

Moore SJ, Turnpenny P, Quinn A et al (2000) A clinical study of 57 children with fetal anticonvulsant syndromes. J Med Genet 37:489–497

Morrow J, Russell A, Guthrie E et al (2006) Malformation risks of antiepileptic drugs in pregnancy: a prospective study from the UK Epilepsy and Pregnancy Register. J Neurol Neurosurg Psychiatry 77:193–198

Morrow JI, Hunt SJ, Russell AJ et al (2009) Folic acid use and major congenital malformations in offspring of women with epilepsy: a prospective study from the UK Epilepsy and Pregnancy Register. J Neurol Neurosurg Psychiatry 80:506–511

MRC Vitamin Study Research Group (1991) Prevention of neural tube defects: results of the Medical Research Council Vitamin Study [see comments]. Lancet 338:131–137

Ogawa Y, Kaneko S, Otani K et al (1991) Serum folic acid levels in epileptic mothers and their relationship to congenital malformations. Epilepsy Res 8:75–78

Ornoy A, Zvi N, Arnon J et al (2008) The outcome of pregnancy following topiramate treatment: a study on 52 pregnancies. Reprod Toxicol 25:388–389

Pantarotto C, Arboix M, Sezzano P et al (1982) Studies on 5,5-diphenylhydantoin irreversible binding to rat liver microsomal proteins. Biochem Pharmacol 31:1501–1507

Parman T, Chen G, Wells PG (1998) Free radical intermediates of phenytoin and related teratogens. Prostaglandin H synthase-catalyzed bioactivation, electron paramagnetic resonance spectrometry, and photochemical product analysis. J Biol Chem 273:25079–25088

Perucca E, Tomson T (2006) Prenatal exposure to antiepileptic drugs. Lancet 367:1467–1469

Puho EH, Szunyogh M, Metneki J et al (2007) Drug treatment during pregnancy and isolated orofacial clefts in Hungary. Cleft Palate Craniofac J 44:194–202

Rane A, Peng D (1985) Phenytoin enhances epoxide metabolism in human fetal liver cultures. Drug Metab Dispos 13:382–385

Rasalam AD, Hailey H, Williams JH et al (2005) Characteristics of fetal anticonvulsant syndrome associated autistic disorder. Dev Med Child Neurol 47:551–555

Raymond GV, Buehler BA, Finnell RH et al (1995) Anticonvulsant teratogenesis: 3. Possible metabolic basis. Teratology 51:55–56

Registry SMB http://www.janusinfo.org/. Accessed 2009

Rosa FW (1991) Spina bifida in infants of women treated with carbamazepine during pregnancy. N Engl J Med 324:674–677

Roy D, Snodgrass WR (1990) Covalent binding of phenytoin to protein and modulation of phenytoin metabolism by thiols in A/J mouse liver microsomes. J Pharmacol Exp Ther 252:895–900

Samrén EB, van Duijn CM, Koch S et al (1997) Maternal use of antiepileptic drugs and the risk of major congenital malformations: a joint European prospective study of human teratogenesis associated with maternal epilepsy. Epilepsia 38:981–990

Samrén EB, van Duijn CM, Christiaens GC et al (1999) Antiepileptic drug regimens and major congenital abnormalities in the offspring. Ann Neurol 46:739–746

Scolnik D, Nulman I, Rovet J et al (1994) Neurodevelopment of children exposed in utero to phenytoin and carbamazepine monotherapy. JAMA 271:767–770

Speidel BD, Meadow SR (1972) Maternal epilepsy and abnormalities of fetus and the newborn. Lancet 2:839–843

Spina E, Perugi G (2004) Antiepileptic drugs: indications other than epilepsy. Epileptic Disord 6:57–75

Strickler SM, Dansky LV, Miller MA et al (1985) Genetic predisposition to phenytoin-induced birth defects. Lancet 2:746–749

ten Berg K, Samrén EB, van Oppen AC et al (2005) Levetiracetam use and pregnancy outcome. Reprod Toxicol 20:175–178

Thomas SV, Ajaykumar B, Sindhu K et al (2008) Motor and mental development of infants exposed to antiepileptic drugs in utero. Epilepsy Behav 13:229–236

Tomson T, Battino D (2005) Teratogenicity of antiepileptic drugs: state of the art. Curr Opin Neurol 18:135–140

Tomson T, Battino D (2009) The management of epilepsy in pregnancy. In: Shorvon S, Pedley TA (eds) The epilepsies 3: blue books of neurology. Saunders Elsevier, Philadelphia, pp 241–264

Tomson T, Hiilesmaa V (2007) Epilepsy in pregnancy. BMJ 335:769–773

Tomson T, Beghi E, Sundqvist A et al (2004a) Medical risks in epilepsy: a review with focus on physical injuries, mortality, traffic accidents and their prevention. Epilepsy Res 60:1–16

Tomson T, Perucca E, Battino D (2004b) Navigating toward fetal and maternal health: the challenge of treating epilepsy in pregnancy. Epilepsia 45:1171–1175

Tomson T, Battino D, Craig J et al (2010) Pregnancy registries: differences, similarities, and possible harmonization. Report of a working group of the Commission on Therapeutic Strategies of the International League Against Epilepsy. Epilepsia 51:909–915

Vajda FJ, Hitchcock A, Graham J et al (2007) The Australian Register of Antiepileptic Drugs in Pregnancy: the first 1002 pregnancies. Aust N Z J Obstet Gynaecol 47:468–474

Veiby G, Daltveit AK, Engelsen BA et al (2009) Pregnancy, delivery, and outcome for the child in maternal epilepsy. Epilepsia 50:2130–2139

Viinikainen K, Heinonen S, Eriksson K et al (2006) Community-based, prospective, controlled study of obstetric and neonatal outcome of 179 pregnancies in women with epilepsy. Epilepsia 47:186–192

Vinten J, Adab N, Kini U et al (2005) Neuropsychological effects of exposure to anticonvulsant medication in utero. Neurology 64:949–954

Volcik KA, Shaw GM, Lammer EJ et al (2003) Evaluation of infant methylenetetrahydrofolate reductase genotype, maternal vitamin use, and risk of high versus low level spina bifida defects. Birth Defects Res A Clin Mol Teratol 67:154–157

Wells PG, Winn LM (1996) Biochemical toxicology of chemical teratogenesis. Crit Rev Biochem Mol Biol 31:1–40

Wells PG, Kim PM, Laposa RR et al (1997) Oxidative damage in chemical teratogenesis. Mutat Res 396:65–78
Wide K, Winbladh B, Tomson T et al (2000) Body dimensions of infants exposed to antiepileptic drugs in utero: observations spanning 25 years. Epilepsia 41:854–861
Wide K, Henning E, Tomson T et al (2002) Psychomotor development in preschool children exposed to antiepileptic drugs in utero. Acta Paediatr 91:409–414
Wide K, Winbladh B, Kallen B (2004) Major malformations in infants exposed to antiepileptic drugs in utero, with emphasis on carbamazepine and valproic acid: a nation-wide, population-based register study. Acta Paediatr 93:174–176
Wyszynski DF, Nambisan M, Surve T et al (2005) Increased rate of major malformations in offspring exposed to valproate during pregnancy. Neurology 64:961–965
Zhu H, Kartiko S, Finnell RH (2009) Importance of gene-environment interactions in the etiology of selected birth defects. Clin Genet 75:409–423

Preventive Medicines

Vaccination, Prophylaxis of Infectious Diseases, Disinfectants

Ulrich Heininger

Contents

Abstract Immunizations belong to the most successful interventions in medicine. Like other drugs, vaccines undergo long periods of pre-clinical development, followed by careful clinical testing through study Phases I, II, and III before they receive licensure. A successful candidate vaccine will move on to be an investigational vaccine to undergo three phases of pre-licensure clinical trials in a stepwise fashion before it can be considered for approval, followed by an optional fourth phase of post-marketing assessment. The overall risk–benefit assessment of a

U. Heininger (✉)
Universitäts-Kinderspital beider Basel (UKBB), Postfach, CH-4005 Basel, Switzerland
e-mail: Ulrich.Heininger@ukbb.ch

H.W. Seyberth et al. (eds.), *Pediatric Clinical Pharmacology*,
Handbook of Experimental Pharmacology 205,
DOI 10.1007/978-3-642-20195-0_16, © Springer-Verlag Berlin Heidelberg 2011

candidate vaccine is very critical in making the licensure decision for regulatory authorities, supported by their scientific committees. It includes analyses of immunogenicity, efficacy, reactogenicity or tolerability, and safety of the vaccine. Public trust in vaccines is a key to the success of immunization programs worldwide. Maintaining this trust requires knowledge of the benefits and scientific understanding of real or perceived risks of immunizations.

Under certain circumstances, pre- or post-exposure passive immunization can be achieved by administration of immunoglobulines. In terms of prevention of infectious diseases, disinfection can be applied to reduce the risk of transmission of pathogens from patient to patient, health-care workers to patients, patients to health-care workers, and objects or medical devices to patients.

Keywords Vaccination • Immunization • Vaccine efficacy • Vaccine safety • Disinfection

1 Vaccination

Immunizations belong to the most successful interventions in medicine. During the last few decades, impressive success has been achieved worldwide with population-based immunization programs against several serious infectious diseases such as tetanus, diphtheria, pertussis, poliomyelitis, measles, rubella embryopathy, and – more recently – invasive bacterial infections caused by *Haemophilus influenzae type b*, *Neisseria meningitidis*, *Streptococcus pneumoniae*, and Human Papilloma Viruses (Gessner and Adegbola 2008; CDC 2008; De Wals et al. 2004). Table 1 presents a historical overview of major developments of vaccines for use in humans.

Like other drugs, vaccines undergo long periods of pre-clinical development, followed by careful clinical testing through study Phases I, II, and III before they receive licensure for marketing. After a vaccine has been licensed by regulatory authorities, national and international committees may formulate recommendations on their use in the broad population. Frequently, reimbursement by health insurances accompanies these recommendations and thereby supports successful implementation. An integral part of implemented vaccines is continuous surveillance of their effectiveness (mainly by means of epidemiological studies) and safety (mainly by mandatory reporting of serious "Adverse Events Following Immunization", AEFI). While in the safety assessment of drugs other than vaccines the term "Adverse Drug Reaction" is commonly used, the term "Adverse Events Following Immunization" is internationally preferred in the context of vaccines and will therefore be used here.

Unfortunately, success of immunizations is continuously being threatened today by a phenomenon coined as "vaccines shovelling their own grave" (Heininger 2004). This means, as the incidence of previously frequent, potentially devastating diseases will decrease due to successful immunization programs, public focus may

Table 1 Milestones in the development of vaccines for use in humans

Year[a]	Live-attenuated vaccines	Inactivated whole organism vaccines	Component vaccines (inactivated)	Gene technology
1885	Rabies			
1896		Typhoid fever		
1896		Cholera		
1897		Plague		
1923			Diphtheria toxoid	
1926		Pertussis		
1927	Tuberculosis		Tetanus toxoid	
1935	Yellow fever			
1936	Influenza			
1955		Poliomyelitis		
1960	Poliomyelitis			
1967	Mumps			
1968	Measles			
1969	Rubella			
1971			Influenza (reassortant)	
1971		FSME		
1974	Varicella			
1975	Typhoid			
1977			Pneumococcal polysaccharides (14-valent)	
1980			Tick-borne encephalitis	
1981			Hepatitis B surface antigen (plasma derived)	
1981			Pertussis (acellular)	
1982			Meningococcal polysaccharides (tetravalent)	
1984			Pneumococcal polysaccharides (23-valent)	
1985			Hib (polysaccharide)	
1986			Hepatitis B surface antigen	Yeast derived
1987			Hib (protein conjugated)	
1992		Hepatitis A		
1998	Rotavirus			Rhesus assortant
1999			Meningococcal group C (protein conjugated)	
2000			Pneumococcal (protein conjugated, 7-valent)	
2003	Influenza			Cold adapted, intranasal (trivalent)
2005	MMR-V combination vaccine			
2005	Rotavirus			Bovine, assortant (pentavalent) Humane, assortant (monovalent)

(continued)

Table 1 (continued)

Year[a]	Live-attenuated vaccines	Inactivated whole organism vaccines	Component vaccines (inactivated)	Gene technology
2006			Meningococcal groups A, C,W135,Y (protein conjugated)	
2006/2007		Human papilloma virus (HPV)		HPV-6, -11, -16, -18 (quadrivalent), HPV-16, -18 (bivalent)
2007	Herpes zoster			
2009			Pneumococcal (protein conjugated, 10-valent and 13-valent)	

[a]First used routinely in humans

shift towards true and alleged "side effects" of vaccines. This can lead to the dilemma of waning public confidence in the necessity, tolerability, and safety of vaccinations (Guillaume and Bath 2008). It is therefore important to continuously evaluate risks and benefits of vaccines and results of these evaluations need to be openly communicated to health professionals and the public in order to strengthen the confidence in existing and new immunization programs.

1.1 Development of Vaccines

There are several prerequisites for successful and meaningful vaccine development which include the following:

- The microorganism (or its specific mediators of disease, such as toxins and other major virulence factors) that causes an infectious disease needs to be identified
- Characteristics of the causative agent that leads to disease in the human host should be explored in order to determine the optimal composition of the vaccine to be designed against it
- Protective immune responses against the targeted microorganism in the human host need to be explored in order to identify the optimal route of delivery (mucosal, systemic) of the vaccine antigen(s)
- The disease is severe enough, i.e. life threatening or even potentially fatal, leading to significant complications and/or the disease is frequent enough to cause a significant health or economic burden in the population. This requires precise description of the overall (or regional) distribution and frequency of the disease by age groups and characterization of complications caused by the targeted disease. Frequently this is required on a national basis, if possible, as immunization recommendations will usually also be formulated nationally
- Lack of successful and rational alternatives to prevent and/or treat the targeted disease
- Incentives for investment in the development of a new vaccine by research groups and/or manufacturers should be secured

- Public perception of the infectious disease against which a vaccine is to be developed should be such that prevention by immunization is warranted

The microorganism against which a vaccine is to be developed has to be characterized in great detail and needs to be multiplied, harvested, and worked up under "Good Laboratory Practice" principles to fulfill the requirements of the final product. This includes strict safety and quality control measurements.

In the case of live-attenuated vaccines, safety of the attenuated live organisms has to be guaranteed and proven. In the case of inactivated vaccines, a decision has to be made whether the whole organism should serve as the immunological target (e.g. hepatitis A) or one (e.g. tetanus toxin) or more specific virulence factors (e.g. pertussis toxin, filamentous haemagglutinin, and pertactin in the case of acellular pertussis vaccines) will serve this purpose. The decision on this depends mainly on basic scientific work on the pathogenesis of the microorganism and the mechanisms of the human host's immune response.

This work may require years, sometimes decades, of continuous basic research which is frequently initiated in academic or private research laboratories before the pharmaceutical industry takes over the task of developing a vaccine. This requires significant investment and carries the risk of failure at any step of the vaccine's development.

1.2   Preclinical Vaccine Trials

Preclinical vaccine trials are being performed under the principles of "Good Manufacturing Practices", as established by major regulatory and scientific authorities such as the US Food and Drug Administration (FDA) and the European Medicines Agency (EMA, formerly called EMEA). Specifically, EMA has developed guidelines for the development of medicines for paediatric use, including vaccines   (http://www.ema.europa.eu/pdfs/human/qwp/13893108en.pdf)   which specify the particular needs for such products in infants and children, including pre-term infants.

For preclinical testing of a candidate vaccine, adequate preparations are first tested in cell culture or tissue culture systems. If results are promising, the candidate will then enter the phase of testing in animals such as mice, rats, guinea pigs or sometimes even primates (usually monkeys). More recently, three-dimensional visualization of vaccine compounds by use of sophisticated computer technology has entered preclinical testing. This technology can assist researchers to predict how a candidate vaccine will interact with the host's immune system.

Further, preclinical tests comprise

- Proof of non-toxicity:
  Local and systemic toxicity is first assessed in appropriate animal models and in vitro settings before clinical testing in humans can be initiated. Further, mutagenicity needs to be assessed as some chemical compounds included in

vaccines may potentially act as base analogs and get inserted into the DNA strand during replication instead of the natural substrates. Other compounds may react with DNA and cause structural changes that can lead to miscopying of the template strand when the DNA is replicated. Similarly, carcinogenicity of vaccine compounds may be of concern, especially when the microorganism against which the vaccine is directed can lead to cancer, for example, human papilloma virus. Carcinogens alter the cellular metabolism or directly damage DNA in cells by inducing uncontrolled cell division, inhibiting the programmed cell death, leading to malignant cell expansion and finally the development of tumours.

- Pharmacodynamic and pharmacokinetic vaccine trials:
The main purpose of these early steps in preclinical testing in animal models is to estimate the appropriate content of vaccine antigens (dose) and schedule of administration (number of doses, intervals). This is followed by secondary vaccine trials on the dose effect, tolerability, and distribution of vaccine antigens in different organs of the immunized host (=primary safety assessment).
- Product characteristics:
After a candidate vaccine has successfully passed non-toxicity and pharmacodynamic and pharmacokinetic vaccine trials, the next step before entering clinical vaccine trials is demonstration of a reliable production process. This requires demonstration of genetic stability of the seed microorganism (which is repeatedly used to produce consecutive batches of vaccine), stability and purity (i.e., absence of substances introduced during the manufacturing process which are neither needed nor accepted to be present in the final product) of the vaccine formulation, and characterization of its shelf life under defined storing conditions (e.g. cold temperature, room temperature conditions etc.).

If the vaccine candidate performs to the researchers' satisfaction during these preclinical evaluations, it will be called "investigational vaccine" and can finally be used in human volunteers in Clinical Vaccine Trials.

Traditionally, most inactivated vaccines have been supplemented by chemicals called adjuvants which support the host's immune response to vaccine antigens. This is frequently necessary to allow a sufficient immune response without increasing the antigen content to a magnitude which would cause significant intolerability due to side effects (e.g. large local injection site swelling or febrile reactions). In the past, most adjuvants have been chemical formulations based on aluminium, mainly in the form of aluminium hydroxide (AlOH) and phosphate ($AlPO_4$). More recently, new (modern) adjuvants have entered clinical testing and proven successful by means of better immunogenicity and similar tolerability in terms of local and systemic reactions in the immunized human host including young children, immunocompromised individuals, and elderly people (Pichichero 2008).

An overview of selected promising or proven to be successful new adjuvants is shown in Table 2.

- The adjuvant system 02 (AS02) is included in the currently most advanced anti-malaria vaccine, undergoing clinical testing in Phase III vaccine trials in children and adults in several African countries (Sacarlal et al. 2009; Abdulla et al 2008).

Table 2 New adjuvants in vaccines for use in humans

Adjuvant	Characteristics	Vaccine (manufacturer)	Stage of clinical testing	References
AS02	Oil-in water emulsion: monophosphoryl lipid (MPL A) and saponin-type detergent (QS21)	*P. falciparum*, malaria (GlaxoSmithKline)	Phase II/III (Africa)	Cooper et al. (2004) and De Wals et al. (2004)
AS04	Oil-in water emulsion: monophosphoryl lipid (MPL A) and aluminium hydroxide	Hepatitis B; Human papilloma virus, cervical and other cancers (GlaxoSmithKline)	Licensed	De Stefano et al. (2004), Dettenkofer and Daschner (1997) and Didierlaurent et al. (2009)
CpG 7907	24-mer B-Class CpG Oligodeoxynucleotide	Hepatitis B; *P. falciparum*, malaria (GlaxoSmithKline)	Phase I/II	Ellebedy and Webby (2009) and Gessner and Adegbola (2008)
AS03	Oil-in water emulsion: Squalen, Tocopherol (Vitamine E) and Polysorbat 80 in a phosphate buffer	Influenza, novel H1N1 vaccine (GlaxoSmithKline)	Licensed	Giannini et al. (2006)
MF59	Oil-in water emulsion: Squalen, polysorbat (Tween 80), and Sorbitantrioleat (Span 85)	Influenza, including novel H1N1 vaccine (Novartis)	Licensed	Grüber et al. (2003), Guillaume and Bath (2008) and Heininger (2003)

It induces strong immune-specific responses and the vaccine has proven successful in Phase II vaccine trials.

- The adjuvant system 04 (AS04) combines the TLR4 agonist MPL (3-O-desacyl-4′-monophosphoryl lipid A) and aluminium salt. It has first been used in hepatitis B conventional vaccine non-responders and immunocompromised hosts (Boland et al. 2004). Its further inclusion in novel anti-human papilloma virus vaccines, aimed at precancerous lesions and cancer primarily in the female genital tract (cervical cancer and others), has led to the development of successful and licensed vaccines for women 9–26 years of age (Giannini et al. 2006; Didierlaurent et al 2009).
- CpG 7907 is an adjuvant that directly activates B-lymphocytes and plasmacytoid dendritic cells and indirectly activates macrophages and other monocytes by inducing the secretion of Th1-like cytokines and chemokines. It also facilitates a Th1-type immune response via cytotoxic T-lymphocytes and has been successfully tested in hepatitis B vaccines and malaria caused by *Plasmodium falciparum* (Cooper et al. 2004, Sagara et al 2009) in Phase II and III trials.
- Finally, oil-in-water adjuvants such as MF59 and adjuvant system 03 (AS03) have recently been used to develop antigen sparing influenza vaccines against the novel H1N1 subtype, also called "swine-flu" (www.emea.europa.eu/humandocs/PDFs/.../pandemrix/H-832-de1.pdf; Ellebedy and Webby 2009; Keitel et al. 2010). With the help of these adjuvants, vaccine antigen content could be reduced by as much as sixfold compared to conventional, non-adjuvanted influenza vaccines. Further, these adjuvanted vaccines induced very potent immune responses after even a single dose administration. They have been licensed and used worldwide during the winter in 2009/2010. Moreover, an MF59 adjuvanted seasonal influenza vaccine has been licensed and made available for use in elderly individuals in Europe for several years and was recently also shown to be of use in children (Vesikari et al 2009).

1.3   Clinical Vaccine Trials

Like any other drug, a successful candidate vaccine will move on to be an investigational vaccine to undergo three phases of pre-licensure clinical trials in a stepwise fashion before it can be considered for approval, followed by an optional fourth phase of post-marketing assessment (Table 3).

Pre-licensure vaccine trials rely upon

- Dedicated basic and clinical research teams (usually in collaboration between the manufacturer and one or more principal investigators from academic research centers or other clinical trial units);
- Motivated and engaged local field investigators (frequently in multi-centre study design, including hospital based and/or physicians in private practices);

Table 3 Phases of clinical testing of vaccines for use in humans

Phase I	Assessment of tolerability and immunogenicity in a limited study population ($<$100 healthy adult volunteers)
Phase II	Testing of lot consistency; confirmation of acceptable tolerability; potentially assessment of efficacy and reactogenicity and safety profile in extended study populations (target age group or groups and/or targeted patient population; $>$1,000 to $>$10,000 study subjects)
Phase III	Confirmation of efficacy and/or safety (target age group or groups and/or targeted patient population; $>$10,000 study subjects)
Phase IV	Post-licensure assessment of safety and/or effectiveness (whole population or representative sample of the population)

- The participation of hundreds to ten thousands of volunteers to be immunized under study conditions;
- And professional clinical study organizations acquainted with the multiple legal and logistic requirements in performing and monitoring such vaccine trials.

Post-marketing assessment of vaccines relies upon immunizing physicians and a motivated study population (vaccinees), willing to assess a licensed vaccine under further study conditions.

Further, continuous effectiveness and safety assessment of a given vaccine should be undertaken after licensure, unlimited in time. This requires functional national and international pharmacovigilance systems, implementation of epidemiological surveillance systems, and ideally a mandatory reporting system for adverse events following immunization (safety) but also for vaccination failures (effectiveness).

Clinical vaccine trials nowadays have to be registered in international databases (e.g. www.clinicaltrials.gov). A typical volunteer in a vaccine study (called "vaccinee") formally agrees to be vaccinated, to make frequent visits to a clinic or study centre for evaluation, to participate in medical testing, and to provide blood or tissue samples that are used to assess the vaccine's performance in terms of tolerability, immune response in the host (immunogenicity), safety, and efficacy. Research staff counsel volunteers about the study, and volunteers must sign an informed consent document, indicating their understanding of the study and their willingness to participate.

Close collaboration of vaccine manufacturers, research teams, clinicians, regulatory authorities and study subjects or the broad population is needed for successful performance of clinical vaccine trials throughout Phases I–IV.

The 3 phases of pre-licensure clinical vaccine trials fulfill the following purposes:

- Phase I
  Dose finding (antigen content or amount of attenuated vaccine microorganisms) and dose schedule (numbers of doses required and optimal intervals from dose to dose); determination of acceptable local and systemic tolerability of the candidate vaccine and absence of toxicity in the human host.
- Phase II

Lot consistency testing; confirmation of Phase I findings in terms of local and systemic tolerability and absence of toxicity; preliminary determination of efficacy and confirmation of Phase I immunogenicity results. Importantly, study subjects will be recruited from the future target population for the vaccine (age group or groups, possibly patients with specific conditions).

- Phase III
  Critical ("pivotal") phase with sufficient numbers of study subjects to confirm Phase II findings and to proof efficacy or immunogenicity and safety of the candidate vaccine in the target population.

Planning and conduction of Phase III vaccine trials is challenging. Depending on the specific vaccine and clinical as well as epidemiological characteristics of its targeted disease, different endpoints for proof of efficacy are required:

- If a serological (i.e., serum antibody level) correlate of immunity or protection is known for a disease, proof of immunogenicity by demonstration that a predetermined percentage of trial subjects (e.g. 99%) do reach the minimal antibody level after immunization will be sufficient. Vaccine efficacy will then be inferred from its immunogenicity. In this case, the number of trial participants can be comparatively small (e.g. 100–200 per targeted age group). Examples for vaccine preventable diseases with known serological correlates of protection are hepatitis B, diphtheria, and tetanus.
- If there is no known correlate of immunity, clinical endpoints need to be defined to assess a vaccine's efficacy. If ethical circumstances allow, double-blind and controlled prospective trials are the ideal design for calculation of vaccine efficacy by comparing the incidence of disease (=the clinical endpoint) in the control group with that of the vaccine group. The percent reduction of disease incidence in the vaccinated cohort will then define the vaccine's efficacy. If the clinical endpoint is a comparatively frequent disease (e.g. acute otitis media), statistical power calculation will reveal a comparatively low number of trial participants and/or short duration of the trial. If, however, the disease is rare (e.g. meningitis), the number of trial participants has to be high and/or the duration of the trial has to be sufficiently long to reach the number of cases in the control group that will be needed for demonstration of vaccine efficacy.
- If there is no known correlate of immunity and the clinical endpoint is difficult to assess, another level of complexity is added. This was the case with acellular pertussis vaccine efficacy trials in the 1990s, where various endpoints for "pertussis" depending on duration of cough illness and microbiological proof of Bordetella pertussis infection were assessed in various trials (Stehr et al 1998). Similarly, if a vaccine protects from different disease manifestations as clinical endpoints, different estimates of vaccines efficacy will result as is the case with pneumococcal conjugate vaccines. Their efficacy against invasive disease (meningitis, sepsis) is significantly higher than efficacy against pneumonia or acute otitis media (Heininger 2003).
- If long-term efficacy and/or the need for booster doses of a specific vaccine have to be determined, prolonged follow up of trial cohorts or sub-cohorts is

necessary in order to monitor persistence of immunity. Again, this will be done by use of clinical endpoints and/or longitudinal testing of serum antibody values.

After completion of the clinical tests in pre-licensure vaccine trials, the candidate vaccine may be submitted to regulatory authorities for licensure.

Later on, Phase IV vaccine trials after licensure of the vaccine are designed to investigate vaccine-specific issues that may have become apparent during pre-licensure testing and which need specific attention in a large enough number of vaccines. Some Phase IV vaccine trials will become necessary as specific issues related to efficacy, safety, or tolerability of the vaccine only arise when the product has already been used for a while in the population.

For these reasons, after licensure, further continuous assessment of the vaccine may be requested by regulatory authorities. Justifications for performing such Phase IV vaccine trials include determination of effectiveness (i.e., preventing the targeted disease or some of its manifestations under field conditions rather than under stringent study conditions) and further proof of safety beyond the limited experience obtained during pre-licensure vaccine trials. This has become increasingly important over the last several years as also very rare side effects (<1 per 10'000 doses) have been become of interest among the public and health professionals recently. Especially when signals of potential safety problems were detected in pre-licensure vaccine trials, the manufacturers are forced to perform Phase IV vaccine trials to elucidate the issues which arose.

For example, an oral rotavirus vaccine (Rotashield®) was licensed in the US in 1998. During pre-licensure vaccine trials more cases of intussusception (defined as the invagination of a proximal segment of intestine into a distal segment of intestine, usually ileo-colic) occurred in rotavirus vaccine recipients compared to controls (Kombo et al. 2001). Although the difference was not statistically significant, for obvious reasons more data were required to draw firm conclusions. This was an important issue, because intussusception results in obstruction of bowel passage, constriction of the mesentery, and obstruction of the venous blood flow which is characterized by sudden onset of colicky abdominal pain and can potentially lead to death. After more than 1.5 million doses of vaccine had been used within less than a year in the USA, an approximately threefold risk for intussusception was discovered after vaccine doses 1 and 2 compared to unvaccinated, age-matched control infants and the vaccine had to be taken off the market. This example demonstrates both the necessity as well as the functionality of post-marketing vaccine safety assessment today.

1.4   Specific Pediatric Aspects in Pre-licensure Vaccine Trials

Specific pediatric needs and requirements in the context of clinical vaccine trials on drugs, including vaccines, have received special attention recently (http://www.ema.europa.eu/htms/human/paediatrics/pips_procedural.htm).

A new pediatric regulation ("The EU Paediatric Regulation") became law in the European Union (EU) on 26 January 2007. It was accompanied by a number of specific regulations which not only provide precise guidelines for researchers and manufacturers throughout the process of clinical testing but also protect the rights of children as active study subjects. This is of special relevance in the context of pre-licensure trials with vaccines as many of those are performed exclusively in children, who are the only target population for a number of specific vaccines such as combination vaccines which include *Haemophilus influenzae* type B polysaccharide conjugate and/or high antigen content of diphtheria toxoid. The development of vaccines in children has to follow a pediatric investigation plan (PIP) by the manufacturers seeking licensure. Of note, all clinical vaccine trials performed with children as participants must be registered in a database called EudraCT if the trial is part of a PIP. This database is publicly accessible (https://eudract.emea.europa. eu/index.html).

If ethical considerations suggest that testing of a specific vaccine in children would pose them at unjustified risks (or if there is no intended application for a specific vaccine in children), the regulation allows a limited "deferral" or even a full exception ("waiver").

1.5   *Licensure of Vaccines*

The overall risk–benefit assessment of a candidate vaccine is very critical in making the licensure decision for regulatory authorities, supported by their scientific committees. It includes analyses of immunogenicity, efficacy, reactogenicity or tolerability, and safety of the vaccine.

Licensure or authorization of a vaccine can be requested by a manufacturer via the "human unit" of EMA ("central approval").

In addition to general authorization of a vaccine, each lot of a vaccine needs to be tested and released. For this purpose, "Official Medicine Control Laboratories, OMCL" have been assigned by the "European Directorate for the Quality of Medicines, EDQM" in Strasbourg, France (http://www.edqm.eu).

1.6   *Vaccine Safety Assessment in Post-marketing Settings*

Public trust in vaccines is a key to the success of immunization programs worldwide. Maintaining this trust requires knowledge of the benefits and scientific understanding of real or perceived risks of immunizations.

The risk–benefit assessment, which vaccine recipients and providers need to make continuously, should be based on evidence of best achievable quality.

In terms of reactogenicity, information on a specific vaccine can be found in the "Summary of product characteristics". By convention, side effects (i.e., events with proven causal relationship to the vaccine) and adverse events following immunization, AEFI (i.e., events which occur in temporal but not necessarily causal relationship after immunization) are categorized by frequency of occurrence following the terminology as proposed by WHO (http://www.who.int/vaccines-documents/DocsPDF05/815.pdf):

Causality assessment is also an integral part of vaccine safety evaluation. Assessment of local reactions after injected vaccines (e.g. swelling, induration, injection site pain) is straight forward: the time interval between immunization and occurrence of the reaction is usually short (several hours to few days) and a causal association with immunization therefore is obvious. Systemic reactions, however, such as fever or malaise may or may not be causally related to previous immunization. Here, the kind of vaccine (inactivated versus live-attenuated) determines the temporal relationship between vaccination and occurrence of causally related side effects. The attributable risk of a systemic event after vaccination has to be determined by comparing the observed rate after vaccination with the background rate to see if and by which magnitude it is increased. Again, this is straightforward in controlled vaccine trials. For example, in a clinical study with an oral rotavirus vaccine, fever, and irritability occurred in more than 50% of study subjects and loss of appetite, diarrhea, vomiting, and cough in 20–60% (Ruiz-Palacios et al. 2007), irrespective of administration of placebo or the vaccine. This example illustrates the difficulty to attribute systemic adverse events after immunization to the vaccine in an individual. Of note, *side effects* after vaccination are therefore a diagnosis of exclusion.

Admittedly, there are many examples of real side effects after vaccination. For example, a nasal influenza vaccine that was available in Switzerland for a short period of time clearly was temporally associated with an increased risk for peripheral facial palsy. The initial hypothesis of a causal relation was based on several reports of facial palsy to the Swiss regulatory authority which had occurred shortly after nasal influenza vaccine administration. In a well-organized post-marketing surveillance system, these observations prompted a prospective controlled study which finally proved that the relation to immunization was causal and not only temporal (Mutsch et al. 2004).

Potential uncertainty about the safety of vaccines – particularly in countries where some vaccine preventable diseases have disappeared from the public awareness due to efficacious vaccines and high immunization rates in well structured immunization programs – is currently aggravated by a large volume of unstructured information of varying quality available to health care professionals and parents, frequently via the worldwide web and other mass media. However, in the obvious absence of perfectly safe health interventions, patients have the right to be objectively advised about benefits and possible risks.

As mentioned, providing evidence of the safety of a given vaccine is of paramount importance. From a health professional's perspective, this can be achieved by individual search of the literature (which is time-consuming and can be cumbersome especially when personal resources are limited) or reliance on information provided by experts specialized in pharmacovigilance, public health, and vaccinology. For these specialists, published information on characteristics of a vaccine and study results is usually more easily accessible. However, scrutinizing and evaluating the information again is cumbersome.

In the past, a major obstacle to compare results of vaccine tolerability and safety as published in scientific journals, has been the lack of standardized case definitions for AEFI (Ioannidis and Lau 2001; Bonhoeffer et al. 2002). In the meantime, a considerable number of standardized adverse event case definitions and guidelines on how to use them has been developed by "The Brighton Collaboration" (http://brightoncollaboration.org), an independent international organization, dedicated to standardizing vaccine safety assessment (Kohl et al. 2007).These case definitions have undergone (Tapiainen et al 2006) or are currently undergoing validation and are increasingly recommended by national and international authorities including WHO, EMA, FDA, and the US Centers for Disease Control (CDC).

The availability and use of standardized case definitions for certain AEFI will improve vaccine safety assessment in the future for the following reasons:

- Clinical vaccine trials can be designed in a way that allows obtaining relevant clinical information depending on the requirements of a given case definition.
- Metaanalyses of vaccine safety issues can be performed over different clinical trials if the same standardized case definitions have been used in the individual trials.
- Also clinical reports of AEFI in surveillance settings (post-marketing) can be verified by use of standardized case definitions.
- Frequencies and incidences of AEFI as obtained from different surveillance systems can be compared in a meaningful way if standardized case definitions have been used.

The importance of alleged vaccine side effects, because of their influence on the public perception of vaccine safety, needs to be stressed, too. After many carefully conducted vaccine trials and plausibility assessments, the great majority of suspected, mostly serious suspected "side effects" of specific vaccinations receiving public attention in the recent past have turned out to be coincidental observations. These events include diabetes mellitus in young children after *Haemophilus influenzae* type b vaccination (Black et al. 2002), autism and inflammatory bowel disease after measles–mumps–rubella (MMR) vaccine (De Stefano et al. 2004), demyelinating diseases in adolescents after hepatitis B immunization (Hocine et al. 2007), asthma after various childhood immunizations (Grüber et al. 2003), and sudden infant death syndrome (SIDS) after pertussis component containing combination vaccines for infants (Stratton et al. 1994).

Differentiation between coincidence and causality therefore is of high importance to maintain public trust in immunization programs.

2 Prophylaxis of Infectious Diseases

In addition to active immunization, prophylaxis of infectious diseases can be achieved by

- Avoidance of exposure

- Pre- or post-exposure passive immunization
- Pre- or post-exposure administration of antivirals or antibiotic administration

2.1 Avoidance of Exposure

Avoidance of exposure is difficult in daily practice, especially as many infections are contagious before manifestation of disease, e.g. as in the case of measles and varicella where contagiousness starts 2 days before the typical rash. Therefore, avoidance of exposure is unrealistic most of the time, especially in close contact persons. An exception is the situation of an outbreak, where transmission may be ongoing for a prolonged period of time and contact isolation may be warranted depending on individual circumstances.

2.2 Pre- or Post-exposure Passive Immunization

Pre- or post-exposure passive immunization can be achieved by administration of immunoglobulines. Immunoglobulines, or antibodies, are proteins in blood and other body fluids produced by specialized B-lymphocytes (plasma cells) which do recognize bacteria, viruses, and other microorganisms invading the human host. They are made of two large heavy chains and two small light chains. There are different types of heavy chains which allow grouping of antibodies into different isotypes. The different human antibody isotypes are called IgA, IgD, IgE, IgG, and IgM. For prophylactic or therapeutic use, mainly IgG preparations and rarely IgM preparations are being used. Human ("homologous") immunoglobulin preparations are obtained by Cohn fractionation (or ethanol fractionation) from the pooled plasma of large numbers of healthy donors.

The Cohn fractionation primarily aims at extracting and recovering albumin from the donor's blood plasma. This process is based on the differential solubility of albumin and other major plasma proteins depending on pH value, ethanol concentration, temperature, ionic strength, and protein concentration in the solution. Here, albumin has the highest solubility and lowest isoelectric point of all major human plasma proteins. Importantly, during Cohn's fractionation, human proteins such as the immunoglobulins will retain their biological activity. Further, elimination of potential pathogenic microorganisms has to be assured by various methodologies including filtration processes and radiation.

Immunoglobulin donors are selected by manufacturers based on particularly high specific antibody values in their serum against a particular pathogen or its known virulence factors, e.g. toxins, allowing production of a specific immunoglobulin, formerly called hyper-immunoglobulin. Indications for the administration of specific immunoglobulins are:

Table 4 Immunoglobulins[a] for passive immunization

Disease	Product[a]	Indication and dose	Application
Hepatitis A	Beriglobin	Pre- and post-exposure: 0.02 ml/kg body weight (bw)	i.m. or s.c.
Hepatitis B	Hepatitis-B-immunglobulin[b]	Post-exposure: 0.06 ml/kg bw (newborns: 1 ml total dose)	i.m.
	Hepatect CP[b]	Post-exposure: 0.16–0.2 ml/kg bw (newborns: 0.4 ml/kg bw)	i.v.
Tetanus	Tetagam P[b] oder Tetanobulin S/D[b]	Post-exposure: 1 (−2) ml (independent of age). Therapeutic dose: 12–24 ml	i.m.
Rabies	Berirab[b] or Tollwutglobulin Mérieux® P[b]	Post-exposure: 0.14 ml/kg bw	i.m.
Varicella	Varitect CP	Post-exposure: 1 (−2) ml/kg bw	i.v.
Cytomegaly	Cytotect CP	Pre-exposure: 1 ml/kg bw (at least 6× every 2–3 weeks)	i.v.

[a]Available in Germany

[b]Simultaneously with active immunization

- Pre-or post-exposure prophylaxis of certain infectious diseases in susceptible individuals for whom the respective disease would pose specific risks
- Pre-or post-exposure prophylaxis in rare but dangerous infectious diseases if it is too late for active immunization (e.g. rabies prophylaxis after animal bites)
- Early treatment to neutralize toxin effects (such as those caused by diphtheria or tetanus)

Typical indications, available products (in Germany), dosage and route of administration are shown in Table 4.

Besides specific immunoglobulins, so-called homologous standard immunoglobulins are available which reflect the whole repertoire of specific IgG antibodies of the respective human donors. They find their applications

- For pre- or post-exposure prophylaxis of certain infectious diseases in susceptible individuals for whom the respective disease would pose a specific health risk (e.g. measles, rubella, varicella)
- As a substitution in primary or secondary immunoglobulin deficiency states
- For the treatment of autoimmune diseases (e.g. idiopathic thrombocytopenia, Rhesus factor incompatibility in the newborn, and Kawasaki syndrome)

In contrast to homologous immunoglobulins, heterologous immunoglobulins against specific toxins are obtained from animals (e.g. horses immunized with the respective toxin) by blood sampling. Since heterologous immunoglobulins can induce severe allergic reactions including anaphylaxis, they are only used for infections or intoxications for which no sufficient amounts of immunoglobulin from homologous donors are available. These indications include protection from or treatment against

- *Corynebacterium diphtheriae* (diphtheria)
- *Clostridium botulinum* (botulism)

- *Clostridium perfringens* (gas gangrene)

Futher, various preparations against snake and scorpion toxins are available. They are rarely used in clinical practice. Unfortunately, immunoglobulins against diphtheria toxin are no longer available in most parts of the world.

Before each administration of heterologous immunoglobulins, a pre-existing allergy has to be ruled out in the individual patient. This is usually done by preparing a 1:100 dilution of the immunoglobulin (0.1 ml in 10 ml 0.9% NaCl solution) and one drop is applied on the volar forearm. Then the skin is punctured though the drop with a small needle or lancet. As a negative control, one drop of 0.9% NaCl solution is used and the same procedure is repeated. In the case of sensitization, a blister with a red court appears within 10–20 min at the site of the immunogloblin whereas no such reaction occurs at the site of the negative control. In this case, the heterologous immunoglobulin may only be used after desensitization, for example by following one of the two alternative procedures recommended by the American Academy of Pediatrics (American Academy of Pediatrics 2009): via the *intravenous* route, 1:1,000 dilutions of the immunoglobulin are administered with increasing volumes (0.1, 0.3 and 0.6 ml) followed by 1:100 and 1:10 dilutions with the same escalating volumes and finally the undiluted immunoglobulin with increasing volumes of 0.1, 0.3, 0.6 and 1.0 ml. The interval from injection to injection is 15 min during which the patient is monitored closely for immediate allergic reactions which – if serious in nature (generalized urticaria or arterial hypotonia or dyspnoea) – require appropriate treatment and termination of the desensitization procedure. The alternative procedure, with the same escalating dilutions and volumes but sequentially switching from intradermal to subcutaneous to intramuscular applications, is less preferable as it is less safe in terms of standardization of the absorbed antigen content.

3 Disinfectants

Disinfectants are antimicrobial agents that are frequently used in medical settings with the goal to reduce the load of pathogenic or facultative pathogenic microorganisms (pathogens) on body surfaces (mainly hands) and objects in the environment of patients or medical devices (Dettenkofer and Daschner 1997). The ultimate goal of disinfection is to reduce the risk of transmission of pathogens from patient to patient, health-care workers to patients, patients to health-care workers, and objects or medical devices to patients. Usually, a reduction of 3–5 log of the pathogens at the site of application (i.e., by 99.9–99.999%) is achieved by disinfection. In contrast to disinfection, sterilization describes the process of complete elimination of pathogenic microorganisms.

Disinfection can be achieved by means of

- Heat
- Physical treatment

- Chemical treatment

Heat is frequently used to disinfect heat-resistant objects. Before disinfection, thorough cleaning is required to eliminate biologic (blood, phlegm, other excretions) and non-biologic material. Afterwards, decontamination by residing pathogens is achieved by exposing the objects to 75°C for at least 10 min. This procedure can be standardized and programmed by use of disinfection machines. Heat acts by disrupting membranes and denaturing proteins and nucleic acids.

Physical disinfection can be attempted by ultraviolet light at 260 nm. Application of UV light leads to the formation of pyrimidine dimers in DNA which then lead to genetic damage to cells. Theoretically, ultraviolet irradiation is an effective method of reducing the amount of pathogens on surfaces and in the air, but it does not penetrate glass. Its effect, however, is questionable among hygiene experts and it is not frequently used.

Use of chemicals is the preferred method of disinfection in medical settings. The properties, modes of action, advantages, disadvantages, and indications of chemicals most widely used now or in the past are discussed here.

3.1 Alcohol

Alcohols (ethanol or isopropanol at concentrations of 50–80%, plus purified water) are frequently used as a disinfectant on living tissue, mainly hands, and on nonliving surfaces. As alcohols evaporate quickly, there is only limited residual activity resulting in short contact times. They are effective against a wide spectrum of bacteria and lipid-enveloped viruses (e.g. hepatitis B and C, HIV). However, alcohols have limited efficacy against non-enveloped viruses (e.g. rotavirus, norovirus, enteroviruses, hepatitis A) and is ineffective against fungi and bacterial spores.

3.2 Aldehydes

Aldehydes, such as formaldehyde and glutaraldehyde, have a broad disinfectious activity (bacteria, viruses, fungi) and are also effective against bacterial spores. They are partly inactivated by organic material and have only little residual activity. They are mainly used for disinfection of non-living surfaces and medical devices (e.g. endoscopes).

Of note, mycobacteria can be resistant against aldehydes.

3.3 Phenolics

Phenolics are active ingredients in some disinfectant soaps, e.g. used for handwashing in medical settings. They are active against bacteria and fungi, but not against bacterial spores and enveloped and non-enveloped viruses. Therefore, they should only be used in combination with other disinfectants.

Due to their potential toxicity to sensitive individuals and also for reasons of environment protection (toxicity to newborns, accumulation in water and food, slow natural degradation) phenolics are less frequently used today than previously.

3.4 Quaternary Ammonium Compounds

Quaternary ammonium compounds, such as benzalkonium chloride, dimethyl-distearyl-ammonium chloride, and cetylpyridinium chloride are surface active compounds. Their spectrum of disinfection activity covers mainly gram-positive bacteria whereas their activity against gram-negative bacteria, fungi, and viruses is minimal or absent. This limits their usefulness in the clinical setting and usually requires additional use of other disinfectants.

3.5 Oxidizing Agents

Oxidizing agents destroy the structure of cell membranes of microorganisms leading to cell lysis. They have broad disinfection activity against bacteria, bacterial spores, fungi, and enveloped and non-enveloped viruses. They are mainly used for disinfection of laundry, medical devices and instruments.

Chloramine is mostly used for wound disinfection as is hydrogen peroxide.

3.6 Iodine

Povidone (PVP)-iodine preparations are used to disinfect skin and mucosal surfaces, primarily in treatment and prophylaxis of wound infections. It is broadly active against bacteria, bacterial spores, fungi, and enveloped and non-enveloped viruses. Due to interference with the thyroid gland, PVP-iodine is contraindicated in newborns and infants and in patients with thyroid gland dysfunction.

References

Abdulla S, Oberholzer R, Juma O et al (2008) Safety and immunogenicity of RTS, S/AS02D malaria vaccine in infants. N Engl J Med 359:2533–2544

American Academy of Pediatrics (2009) Passive immunization. In: Pickering LK, Baker CJ, Kimberlin DW, Long SS (eds) Red book: 2009 report of the committee on infectious diseases, 28th edn. American Academy of Pediatrics, Elk Grove Village, IL

Black SB, Lewis E, Shinefield HR et al (2002) Lack of association between receipt of conjugate *haemophilus influenzae* type B vaccine (HbOC) in infancy and risk of type 1 (juvenile onset) diabetes: long term follow-up of the HbOC efficacy trial cohort. Pediatr Infect Dis J 21:568–569

Boland G, Beran J, Lievens M et al (2004) Safety and immunogenicity profile of an experimental hepatitis B vaccine adjuvanted with AS04. Vaccine 23:316–320

Bonhoeffer J, Kohl K, Chen R et al (2002) The Brighton Collaboration: addressing the need for standardized case definitions of adverse events following immunization (AEFI). Vaccine 21:298–302

Centers for Disease Control and Prevention (CDC) (2008) Invasive pneumococcal disease in children 5 years after conjugate vaccine introduction–eight states, 1998–2005. MMWR Morb Mortal Wkly Rep 57:144–148

Cooper CL, Davis HL, Morris ML et al (2004) CPG 7909, an immunostimulatory TLR9 agonist oligodeoxynucleotide, as adjuvant to Engerix-B HBV vaccine in healthy adults: a double-blind phase I/II study. J Clin Immunol 24:693–701

De Stefano F, Bhasin TK, Thompson WW, Yeargin-Allsopp M, Boyle C (2004) Age at first measles-mumps-rubella vaccination in children with autism and school-matched control subjects: a population-based study in metropolitan Atlanta. Pediatrics 113:259–266

De Wals P, Deceuninck G, Boulianne N, De Serres G (2004) Effectiveness of a mass immunization campaign using serogroup C meningococcal conjugate vaccine. JAMA 292:2491–2494

Dettenkofer M, Daschner F (1997) Umweltschonende Sterilisation und Desinfektion. In: Daschner F (ed) Praktische Krankenhaushygiene und Umweltschutz, 1st edn. Springer, Heidelberg

Didierlaurent AM, Morel S, Lockman L et al (2009) AS04, an aluminum salt- and TLR4 agonist-based adjuvant system, induces a transient localized innate immune response leading to enhanced adaptive immunity. J Immunol 183:6186–6197

Ellebedy AH, Webby RJ (2009) Influenza vaccines. Vaccine 27(Suppl 4):D65–D68

Gessner BD, Adegbola RA (2008) The impact of vaccines on pneumonia: key lessons from *Haemophilus influenzae* type b conjugate vaccines. Vaccine 26(Suppl 2):B3–B8

Giannini SL, Hanon E, Moris P et al (2006) Enhanced humoral and memory B cellular immunity using HPV16/18 L1 VLP vaccine formulated with the MPL/aluminium salt combination (AS04) compared to aluminium salt only. Vaccine 24:5937–5949

Grüber C, Illi S, Lau S et al (2003) Transient suppression of atopy in early childhood is associated with high vaccination coverage. Pediatrics 111:e282–e288

Guillaume L, Bath PA (2008) A content analysis of mass media sources in relation to the MMR vaccine scare. Health Inform J 14:323–334

Heininger U (2003) Prävention von Pneumokokkeninfektionen. Monatsschr Kinderheilkd 151:391–396

Heininger U (2004) The success of immunization – shoveling its own grave? Vaccine 22:2071–2072

Hocine MN, Farrington CP, Touzé E et al (2007) Hepatitis B vaccination and first central nervous system demyelinating events: reanalysis of a case-control study using the self-controlled case series method. Vaccine 25:5938–5943

Ioannidis JPA, Lau J (2001) Completeness of safety reporting in randomized trials. An evaluation of 7 medical areas. JAMA 285:437–443

Keitel W, Groth N, Lattanzi M et al (2010) Dose ranging of adjuvant and antigen in a cell culture H5N1 influenza vaccine: safety and immunogenicity of a phase 1/2 clinical trial. Vaccine 28:840–848

Kohl KS, Gidudu J, Bonhoeffer J et al (2007) The development of standardized case definitions and guidelines for adverse events following immunization. Vaccine 25:5671–5674

Kombo LA, Gerber MA, Pickering LK et al (2001) Intussusception, infection, and immunization: summary of a workshop on rotavirus. Pediatrics 108(2):E37

Mutsch M, Zhou W, Rhodes P et al (2004) Use of the inactivated intranasal influenza vaccine and the risk of Bell's palsy in Switzerland. N Engl J Med 350:896–903

Pichichero ME (2008) Improving vaccine delivery using novel adjuvant systems. Hum Vaccin 4:262–270

Ruiz-Palacios GM, Guerrero ML, Bautista-Márquez A et al (2007) Dose response and efficacy of a live, attenuated human rotavirus vaccine in Mexican infants. Pediatrics 120:e253–e261

Sacarlal J, Aide P, Aponte JJ et al (2009) Long-term safety and efficacy of the RTS, S/AS02A malaria vaccine in Mozambican children. J Infect Dis 200:329–336

Sagara I, Ellis RD, Dicko A (2009) A randomized and controlled Phase 1 study of the safety and immunogenicity of the AMA1-C1/Alhydrogel + CPG 7909 vaccine for *Plasmodium falciparum* malaria in semi-immune Malian adults. Vaccine 27:7292–7298

Stehr K, Cherry JD, Heininger U et al (1998) A comparative efficacy trial in Germany in infants who received either the Lederle/Takeda acellular pertussis component DTP (DTaP) vaccine, the Lederle whole-cell component DTP vaccine or DT vaccine. Pediatrics 101:1–11

Stratton KR, Howe CJ, Johnston RB Jr (1994) Adverse events associated with childhood vaccines other than pertussis and rubella. Summary of a report from the Institute of Medicine. JAMA 271:1602–1605

Tapiainen T, Bar G, Bonhoeffer J, Heininger U (2006) Evaluation of the Brighton Collaboration case definition of acute intussusception during active surveillance. Vaccine 24:1483–1487

Vesikari T, Groth N, Karvonen A, Borkowski A, Pellegrini M (2009) MF59-adjuvanted influenza vaccine (FLUAD) in children: safety and immunogenicity following a second year seasonal vaccination. Vaccine 27:6291–6295

Postmarketing Surveillance

Vera Vlahović-Palčevski and Dirk Mentzer

Contents

Abstract Postmarketing drug surveillance refers to the monitoring of drugs once they reach the market after clinical trials. It evaluates drugs taken by individuals under a wide range of circumstances over an extended period of time. Such surveillance is much more likely to detect previously unrecognized positive or negative effects that may be associated with a drug.

The majority of postmarketing surveillance concern adverse drug reactions (ADRs) monitoring and evaluation. Other important postmarketing surveillance components include unapproved or off-label drug use, problems with orphan drugs,

V. Vlahović-Palčevski (✉)
Department for Clinical Pharmacology, University of Rijeka Medical School, University Hospital Center Rijeka, Krešimirova 42, 51000 Rijeka, Croatia
e-mail: vvlahovic@inet.hr

D. Mentzer
Paul-Ehrlich-Institut, Referate Arzneimittelsicherheit, Paul-Ehrlich-Str. 51-59, 63225 Langen, Germany

H.W. Seyberth et al. (eds.), *Pediatric Clinical Pharmacology*,
Handbook of Experimental Pharmacology 205,
DOI 10.1007/978-3-642-20195-0_17, © Springer-Verlag Berlin Heidelberg 2011

and lack of paediatric formulations, as well as issues concerning international clinical trials in paediatric population.

The process of evaluating and improving the safety of medicines used in paediatric practice is referred to as paediatric pharmacovigilance. It requires special attention. Childhood diseases and disorders may be qualitatively and quantitatively different from their adult equivalents. This may affect either benefit or risk of therapies (or both), with a resulting impact on the risk/benefit balance. In addition, chronic conditions may require chronic treatment and susceptibility to ADRs may change throughout the patient's lifetime according to age and stage of growth and development. Therefore, paediatric pharmacovigillance aspects need to be tailored to a number of variables based on heterogeneity of paediatric population. This chapter will summarize and discuss the key issues.

Keywords (MeSH) Pharmacoepidemiology • Child • Drug Surveillance • Postmarketing • Clinical Trial • Phase IV • Drug Approval • Off-label Prescribing • Unlabeled Indication • Drug Formulation

1   General background

1.1   *The Importance of Postmarketing Surveillance in Paediatric Practice*

Postmarketing drug surveillance refers to the monitoring of drugs once they reach the market after three phases of clinical trials that are designed to test safety and efficacy of drugs. Postmarketing drug surveillance using interventional or non-interventional clinical trial aims to evaluate drugs taken by individuals under a wide range of circumstances in real-world conditions over an extended period of time. Such surveillance is much more likely to detect any undiscovered positive or negative effects, which may be associated with a drug. Postmarketing drug surveillance is critical to ensuring that a medication is safe for use by a wide variety of people (i.e. varying ages, genders, races, lifestyles, etc.) under different circumstances (i.e., people with comorbidities or on multiple drugs, with varying nutritional status, taking over-the-counter supplements, etc.). The majority of postmarketing surveillance encompasses adverse drug reaction (ADRs) monitoring and evaluation.

Postmarketing surveillance in paediatric population denotes surveillance of approved drugs used by persons aged 0–18. Many medicines are prescribed to paediatric patients on an unlicensed or "off-label" basis because they have not been adequately tested and/or formulated and authorized for use in appropriate paediatric age group. Thus, additional important postmarketing surveillance components involve unapproved or off-label drug use, problems with orphan drugs and lack of paediatric formulations, the issues of conduction international clinical trials.

1.2   Off-Label and Unlicensed Drug Use in Children

The term off-label relates to the use of a medicine in a manner different from that recommended by the manufacturers in their product license i.e., on a trial and error basis. It may result either in benefit, no therapeutic effect, or adverse reaction.

The assumption that children with diseases or conditions similar to that of adults respond similarly has perpetuated the use of medications approved in adults to treat children, frequently without the appropriate studies in paediatric population. Only one third of drugs used to treat children have been studied adequately in the population in which they are being used and have appropriate use information on the product label. For the other two thirds of drugs, information regarding safety and efficacy for paediatric patients is insufficient or absent. The younger the patient's age group, the more likely the lack of information. It is estimated that 80–97% of infants in neonatal wards receive at least one off-label or unlicensed drug (Pandolfini and Binati 2005; Grégoire and Finley 2007). Typically, labels for new medications provide physicians with no guidance regarding a product's effectiveness, dosing or safety among paediatric patients. For most drug classes, there exists almost no information on use in patients less than 2 years of age (Roberts et al. 2003; Clark et al. 2006). The problem of off-label use is international and affects hospitalized or non-hospitalized children. Those who administer drugs to children are forced to deviate from the established labeling indications, for example, by manipulating a drug's formulation to obtain a "paediatric" dose (e.g. splitting tablets into pieces), or by changing the indicated route of administration (e.g. to avoid intramuscular injections in young patients) (Pandolfini and Binati 2005). Paediatric patients may also be deprived of potentially effective medication because of the prescriber's reluctance to use a medication for an off-label use.

Not all off-label drug use is inappropriate. A distinction should be made between "well-founded" and "ill-founded" (disputable) off-label prescriptions. In contrast to "ill-founded", "well-founded" off-label prescriptions are recommended in clinical practice guidelines or pharmcotherapeutic handbooks. These recommendations are based on systematic examination of the published literature. The efficacy of "ill-founded" off-label prescription is often questionable and adverse drug reactions and unjustified healthcare costs may result (Gijsen et al. 2009).

Unlicensed is the use of drugs that do not have a product license, most often those whose formulation is modified, that are prepared as extemporaneous preparations, are imported or used before a license is granted, or that are chemicals used for therapeutic purposes (Kimland et al. 2007). The reasons for a drug being unlicensed in children are many. It occurs often because a drug has not been tested in children, and this may be due to financial constraints or because of the apparent difficulties with trial design and ethics of testing drugs in children.

The extent to which drugs are prescribed to children in an off-label manner vary among different countries and settings. Data from UK suggest that in primary care about 11% of drugs prescribed for children are used off-label (McIntyre et al. 2000). In a retrospective cohort study analysing 1.74 million prescriptions in primary care in Germany, 13% were found to be prescribed off-label (Bücheler et al. 2002). Similarly, another German study has shown that 87% of drugs prescribed to children were prescribed in accordance with their license, but only 3% were rated as off-label, and for the rest the licensing status could not be established within the drug information supplied by the manufacturers (Mühlbauer et al. 2009). Higher figures have been found in the Netherlands (29%) ('tJong et al. 2002) and France (33%) (Chalumeau et al. 2000). A survey on unlicensed and off-label drug use in paediatric wards in European countries has shown that as much as 46% of drug prescriptions were either unlicensed (39%) or off label (7%), and that 67% of patients received an unlicensed or off-label drug prescription. The most common reason for off-label use were that the medicine was prescribed at a different dose or frequency, in a different formulation, or in an age group for which it had not been licensed (Conroy et al. 2000). Furthermore, neonatologists do not have another choice but to use drugs in an unauthorized way because their patients are rarely entered into trials of new preparations. Eighty percent of infants in an Australian neonatal intensive care unit received an off-label or unlicensed preparation (O'Donnell et al. 2002).

1.3   Orphan Drugs

Orphan drugs are usually defined as drugs that have been abandoned or "orphaned" by major drug companies. However, this definition can be extended to medications that could be useful to a minority of population (i.e. orphan group), such as children, physically or cognitively disabled patients, or the elderly if the medications were available and approved for those groups.

According to European Medicines Agency (EMA), a medicinal product is designated as an orphan medicinal product if: it is intended for the diagnosis, prevention or treatment of a life-threatening or chronically debilitating condition affecting no more than five in 10,000 persons in the European Union at the time of submission of the designation application (prevalence criterion), or it is intended for the diagnosis, prevention, or treatment of a life-threatening, seriously debilitating or serious and chronic condition and without incentives it is unlikely that expected sales of the medicinal product would cover the investment in its development, and no satisfactory method of diagnosis, prevention, or treatment of the condition concerned is authorized, or, if such method exists, the medicinal product will be of significant benefit to those affected by the condition (EMA 2010, http://www. ema.europa.eu, accessed 27 Jan 2010).

2   Pharmacovigilance for Paediatric Medicines

The purpose of postmarketing adverse drug event surveillance is to obtain information on rare, latent, long-term adverse drug events or changes in drug-effect frequencies not identified during premarket testing. However, knowledge of risks associated with drug use in children is limited due to few paediatric drug safety studies. At registration, little information on adverse drug reactions in children is available since many drugs have not been tested in children. Risk–benefit analyses of drugs for children are dependent on observations of adverse drug reactions and effects from clinical use. The limited available information regarding adverse drug events in paediatric population is based on medication errors such as overdosing or accidental exposure (Fortescue et al. 2003; Kaushal et al. 2001). The potential for adverse drug reactions among children is greater than that in adults. Young children have immature metabolizing mechanisms, which decreases their ability to process drugs and metabolites. In addition, drug doses must be adjusted individually for a significantly broader range of body sizes and weights.

Paediatric pharmacovigilance is therefore the process of evaluating and improving the safety of medicines used in paediatric patients of all ages (Choonara 2006). Most investigations concerning ADRs in children have focused on hospitalized patients. In a meta-analysis of nine prospective studies among hospitalized children, Impicciatore and colleagues calculated an overall incidence of ADRs of 9.5%, of which 12.3% was regarded as severe. ADRs in hospitalized children require attention because they often involve serious illnesses, advanced drugs, and complicating factors such as concomitant medication and comorbidity (Impicciatore et al. 2001). However, ADRs outside the hospital should not be overlooked. Not only do many children in primary care continue drug therapy that has been initiated in the hospital, but also the number of drug-using children in primary care is much larger than the number of hospitalized patients. Based on the few prospective studies, it has been estimated that 1–1.5% of the drugs used by children outside the hospital result in an ADR (Impicciatore et al. 2001; Sanz and Boada 1987; Cirko-Begovic et al. 1989). In reported suspected paediatric adverse drug reactions (ADRs) in Sweden using data from a nation-wide ADR reporting system during a period of 15 years, it was found that the proportion of children suffering from a serious ADR was 13.0% and that for drug related deaths was 0.14% (Kimland et al. 2005). In a report from the US, 6% of the total ADR reports in a 5-year period concerned individuals aged less than 18 years (Johann-Liang et al. 2009).

2.1 *Pharmacovigillance for Off-Label and Unlicensed Drug Use and Orphan Drugs*

Off-label and unlicensed drug use in children has resulted in questions to drug information centers and has been reported to be extensive, and, as reported, has resulted in an increased risk of adverse drug reactions. A French study that involved more than 1,400 children has shown that 42% of outpatients were exposed to at least one off-label prescription, and the incidence of adverse drug reactions was 1.4 in the whole population and 2.0% in patients exposed to at least one off-label prescription (Horen et al. 2002). An observational analysis of spontaneous adverse drug reaction reported in 1 year in Sweden investigated the extent and characteristics of off-label prescribing for paediatric outpatients among drugs reported to have caused an adverse reaction. Of all the adverse reactions, 42.4% were related to the use of drugs that had been prescribed outside the terms of the product licence. It was more frequently associated with serious than non-serious ADRs and mostly due to a non-approved age or dose (Ufer et al. 2004).

Orphan drugs must go through the same development process as any other drug and must be shown to meet the same standards for effectiveness and safety as a drug for a common condition. Indeed, because of the small number of patients available to be enrolled in clinical trials of orphan drugs, these products must be even more effective than the average drug if a statistically significant benefit is to be established. Since 85–90% of known rare diseases are serious or life threatening, patients and physicians may be willing to accept a slightly higher level of risk than they would from a treatment for a less serious disease. But the limited number of patients plays a role here as well: although there have been no reports of serious adverse reactions to any orphan drugs thus far, when a product is tested in a very small population, our knowledge of the safety profile may not be complete as it can be for a treatment for a more prevalent condition (Haffner 2006).

2.2 Paediatric Formulation and Dosing Issues

Today's standards of clinical drug development require clinical trials enrolling several hundred patients, which is in general not practical or possible in a paediatric population. Therefore, drugs are not adequately tested and labeled in children with regard to dosing and formulation, especially not in very young children (Nunn and Williams 2005). Additional constraints may be seen in low prevalent diseases and varying patient phenotypes (e.g. neurometabolic disease).

Incorrect dosing, under- as well as over-dosing, and use of products with improvised formulations or inappropriate drug concentration are known to be responsible for ADRs (Horen et al. 2002; Turner et al. 1999).

Additional problems may arise, if there is a poor knowledge about validity of laboratory parameters and values of diagnostic and clinical endpoints in a clinical trial.

Besides the challenges with logistic and organisation of a clinical trial, special physiology of maturing organs needs to be considered for dose-finding studies as well as for the development of an age appropriate formulation (Kearns et al. 2003).

For instance, much higher extracellular fluid volume, especially in premature babies as compared to full-term infants, older infants or adults is an important example of the need for thorough investigation of the pharmacokinetics of drugs. Conversely, fat content is lowest in premature babies, higher in neonates and even higher in infants and this has to be considered when applying doses on an mg/kg body weight basis to achieve plasma concentrations similar to those of adults. Further on, an initial loading dose may be necessary as a part of the treatment regimen, the dosage interval may need to be increased and the total dose decreased depending on hepatic and renal function. For medicines that are cleared by liver, they may have a longer plasma half-life and thus a longer time to reach steady state. Similarly, for medicines that are entirely eliminated through kidneys, the greater the prematurity, the less are the kidneys able to excrete the substance and consequently the longer will be the half-life.

The lack of reliable pharmacokinetic and pharmacodynamic data in paediatric populations deriving from systematic drug development and clinical trials are claimed to be responsible for some complications and difficulties following treatment in paediatric population. In most cases it has been related to missing information on the right dose and appropriate formulation. These deficiencies need to be reflected according to each of the different age subpopulations in paediatrics in order to strive toward safer medicines for children (Hartford et al. 2006; International Conference on Harmonisation 2000).

Where unlicensed and off-label paediatric use is common, it is important for both the marketing authorization holder and the regulatory authorities to monitor for any consequential safety concerns and to take appropriate measures to address them and include in the Summary of Product Characteristics as a standard risk minimisation measure. The reasons for a relative or absolute contraindication should also be presented in the product information leaflet to appropriately communicate the risk of off-label use (WHO 2007).

2.3 Enhanced Spontaneous Reporting System

The major concern with ADRs is for serious adverse reactions, which are often rare, and will generally not be observed in paediatric clinical trial programme, particularly if there is a latent period before the onset or a trigger such as change in growth or development (Impicciatore et al. 2001). Some serious ADRs may only be diagnosed in a distinct age subgroup of paediatric population (e.g. febrile convulsion, growth retardation). Taking this into account, collection and extrapolation of safety data in paediatric population from data in adults is not always possible due to physiological facts such as metabolism, growth, and mental development.

Therefore, routine pharmacovigilance measures for detecting new safety signals with extensively used drugs in adults may be much less effective in paediatric population. A different, more proactive, approach is needed to conduct pharmacovigilance for these types of low usage products.

Clinical trial protocols should set out actions to be taken and their timing, by category of ADR, if it occurs. For example, if a serious ADR is suspected, a blood, saliva or urine sample (as appropriate) should be taken as soon as possible after the suspected event. Preferably the samples should be frozen for drug and metabolite measurement. For postauthorization safety studies, similar provisions might be appropriate, but then it needs to be understood that including such a provision in a trial protocol would disqualify it from having non-interventional status.

Special consideration should be given to long-term follow up as the susceptibility to ADRs may change throughout the patient's lifetime according to age and the stage of growth and development. This applies especially to chronic conditions, which may require long term, or even life-long, treatment. ADRs related to the central nervous system are often of critical importance in this respect. Open questions concerning long-term safety may be answered by results from additional animal studies, such as juvenile animal toxicology studies. Mutagenicity and carcinogenicity data are also important and may need further scientific investigation through juvenile animal studies (EMA 2005). However, the predictive value of such studies in terms of subsequent effects in paediatric population is currently unknown.

Disease databases and registries as well as active surveillance systems and enhanced reporting may help to monitor event rates. Furthermore, specialist networks and paediatric clinical trial networks may be equally useful in this context.

Several methods have been used to encourage and facilitate reporting by healthcare professionals in different situations, such as in-hospital settings for new products or for limited time periods. Such methods include online reporting of adverse events and systematic enhanced reporting of adverse events based on predefined criteria. While these methods have been shown to improve reporting, the limitations of passive surveillance, especially selective reporting, are well known (Haffner et al. 2005; Neubert et al. 2006).

Active surveillance, in contrast to passive surveillance, seeks to ascertain completely the number of adverse events via continuous pre-organized process. An example of active surveillance is a follow-up of patients treated with a particular drug through a risk management program. In general, it is more feasible to get comprehensive data on individual ADR reports through an active surveillance system than through a passive reporting system. Elaborating surrogate parameters and indicator symptoms for adverse reactions is useful to establish specific case definitions for adverse drug reactions in children (Wong and Murray 2005).

In this respect, different categories of ADRs may need different methods for detection. Routine pharmacovigilance is predominantly based on spontaneous reporting, but other methods may be considered depending on the estimated frequency of the expected ADRs (Table 1) (Meyboom et al. 1997).

To provide evidence-based evaluation of relative frequency of adverse drug reactions or incidence associated with a disease in relation to drug administration, pharmaco-epidemiological studies should be performed. To establish a causal association between treatment and ADR, cohort or case–control studies may be considered; these have been established in adult postmarketing safety studies.

Epidemiological studies using patient databases have been helpful for collecting information on the incidence of a specific event in general population and may be useful for increasing knowledge of particular safety issues (Garcia Rodriguez and Perez Gutthann 1998).

In cases where safety issue is predictable, for example, based on preclinical findings, long-term follow up registries or long-term cohort studies should be considered.

Table 1 Methods to detect ADRs

Methods (−) No relevance (+) Possible supportive (++) Supportive	Frequency of reaction					
	> 1/ 10–1/ 100	1/100–1/ 1,000	1/1,000–1/ 5,000	1/5,000–1/ 10,000	1/10,000–1/ 50,000	<1/ 50,000
Spontaneous reporting (international)	+	++	++	++	++	+/−
Intensified monitoring	+	++	++	+	−	−
Prescription event monitoring	+	++	++	+	−	−
Case–control studies	−	+	++	++	−	−
Post-marketing surveillance studies	+	++	+	−	−	−
Large data resources (+record linkage)	−	++	++	+	+	−
Clinical trials	++	+	−	−	−	−

As detection and monitoring of ADRs is very much depending on the concerned paediatric age groups, it is necessary that specific pharmacovigilance plans, strategies and activities should be tailored accordingly. For example, small children are less able to communicate their complaints verbally and the relevant information concerning ADRs is mainly dependent on the interpretation of their behavior by the parents or healthcare professionals Therefore, the need for an enhanced pharmacovigilance approach in paediatric pharmacovigilance appears more appropriate.

2.4 Signal Detection Methods

By definition a drug safety signal may arise from a previously unrecognized safety issue, a change in the frequency or severity of a known safety issue or identification of a new at risk group. These aspects are all relevant in paediatric population and both Marketing Authorisation Holder and regulatory authorities are responsible for identifying these kinds of signals.

Signal detection and data mining in paediatric population are dependent on detection methods used which needs to be effective for small populations and low numbers of possible cases. Enhanced data capture techniques can increase the completeness and quality of the information obtained (Bate et al. 1998; Evans et al. 2001).

Signal detection should include appropriate stratification for the data collected based on specific needs (for example by age group or specific medicines like vaccines), as this can be helpful to increase the ability to detect signals from spontaneous databases. However, signal detection is an evolving field and the most up-to-date and suitable statistical methods should be considered based on the content of the data and the size of database used (Evans 2008).

The review and interpretation of results coming from signal detection analyses should be at a high and cautious level of suspicion and should have an emphasis on follow-up to obtain essential information before coming to a final conclusion. Even one case report may be enough to trigger further investigation or risk minimisation measures.

In paediatric drug development, the age-related physiological aspects should not only be considered when conducting clinical trials in children and adolescence as it is routine for efficacy-related objectives, but they are also very important for signal detection methods and monitoring of the safety aspect of the product once used in children.

Given these limitations every opportunity should be taken to maximise the information obtained following the occurrence of an ADR during the paediatric development programme.

3   Legislation

Guidance for paediatric pharmacovigilance has recently been emerging. European Medicinal Agency (EMA; former European medicines Evaluation Agency, EMEA) has an entire guidance dedicated to safety-monitoring concepts for paediatric indications in which it is recognised that susceptibility to ADRs with chronic treatment may change throughout a patient's lifetime. It includes a particular focus upon aspects of growth and development. This guidance also recognises that in most cases clinical trials provide limited data regarding safety because of limited patient exposure which makes it difficult to detect rare or delayed events, and therefore it is important to conduct long-term follow up.

New legislation governing the development and authorisation of medicines for use in children aged 0–17 years was introduced in the European Union in January 2007. The new piece of legislation – Regulation (EC) No 1901/2006 as amended (the "Paediatric Regulation") – introduces sweeping changes into the regulatory environment for paediatric medicines, designed to better protect the health of children in the EU. The Paediatric Regulation also brings in many new tasks and responsibilities for the European Medicines Agency, chief of which is the creation and operation of a Paediatric Committee within the Agency to provide objective scientific opinions on any development plan for medicines for use in children.

In 1997, the United States Congress passed the Food and Drug Administration Modernization Act (FDAMA), which encourages studies of certain therapies being used in paediatrics by providing an exclusivity incentive provision.

In 1998 came the Pediatric Rule, a mandatory regulation that requires paediatric studies for those conditions being studied in adults and in which significant use or benefit in paediatrics was expected (Regulations required manufacturers to assess the safety and effectiveness of new drugs and biological products in paediatric patients. 63 Federal Register. 66631 (1998). The Best Pharmaceuticals for Children Act, enacted 4 January 2002, renewed the paediatric exclusivity provision. It aimed to amend the Federal Food, Drug, and Cosmetic Act to improve the safety and efficacy of pharmaceuticals for children (Best Pharmaceuticals for Children Act. Pub L No. 107–109). A fund was created for research and studies on older products devoid of commercial interest. This fund is managed by the National Institutes of Health (NIH) and the Food and Drug Administration (FDA). On 17 October 2002, the Pediatric Rule was enjoined. As a consequence, the Pediatric Research Equity Act of 2003 became a law on 3 December 2003. This Act gave the FDA the authority to require certain research into drugs used in paediatric patients. On September 27, the Food and Drug Administration Amendments Act of 2007, was signed. Among the many components of the law, the Best Pharmaceuticals for Children Act (BPCA) and the Pediatric Research Equity Act (PREA) were reauthorized. Both of these are designed to encourage more research into, and more development of, treatments for children. They cover many issues including the need to strengthen surveillance of adverse events and to define the role of the Paediatric Advisory Committee which now bears the requirement to review all paediatric safety data at least 1 year post approval.

In a meeting on June 14–15, 2007, the US Food and Drug Administration (FDA), the European Commission (EC), and the European Medicines Agency (EMEA) have agreed to expand their current cooperative activities in several important areas, in particular paediatrics (http://www.ema.europa.eu/htms/human/paediatrics/).

4 The Future

As the biological sciences have evolved, pharmacovigilance has slowly shifted toward earlier, proactive consideration of risks and potential benefits of drugs in the pre- and post-approval stages of drug development.

Since the introduction of the EU paediatric regulation in January 2007, the development and the life cycle of a drug in the pre- and post-authorization periods have changed significantly. Pharmacovigilance science has traditionally been a discipline focused on the post-marketing or post-authorization period, in particular with attention directed toward pre-clinical safety data, clinical trials, and adverse events. In this respect, the central function in this EU paediatric regulation, the paediatric investigation plan, plays an additional important role for the survey of drug safety in paediatrics.

Despite the new activity of drug development in paediatrics the particular emphasis on monitoring off-label use, medication errors and reports of poisoning needs to continue, as still a large number of established drugs, not jet authorized for the paediatric population, are used. If important safety information relating to off-label use becomes available, this should be included in the Summary of Product Characteristics as a standard risk minimisation measure.

Special consideration should be given to the need for long-term follow up, for example, through treatment registries, including possible effects on skeletal, neural, behavioral, sexual, and immune maturation and development. Specific proposals for prospective monitoring will depend on the size of the target population and expected incidence of ADRs (if available).

The development of drugs for the paediatric population has changed the awareness that both safety and efficacy need to be thoroughly investigated for safe treatment of children. In conjunction with the knowledge about efficacy, pharmacokinetics, pharmacodynamics and the age-appropriate formulation for the concerned drug, the impact on the objective of making available safe medicines for children will steadily improve. Under the umbrella of the proposal for safer medicines for children, a joint effort is needed to carry out clinical research and appropriate drug development.

References

Bate A, Lindquist M, Edwards IR (1998) A Bayesian neural network method for adverse drug reaction signal generation. Eur J Clin Pharmacol 54:315–321

Bücheler R, Schwab M, Mörike K et al (2002) Off label prescribing to children in primary care in Germany: retrospective cohort study. BMJ 324:1311–1312

Chalumeau M, Treluyer J, Salanave B et al (2000) Off label and unlicensed drug use among French office based paediatricians. Arch Dis Child 83:502–505

Choonara I (2006) Paediatric pharmacovigilance. Paed Perinat Drug Ther 7:50–53

Cirko-Begovic A, Vrhovac B, Bakran I (1989) Intense monitoring of adverse drug reactions in infants and preschool children. Eur J Clin Pharmacol 36:63–65

Clark RH, Bloom BT, Spitzer AR et al (2006) Reported medication use in the neonatal intensive care unit: data from a large national data set. Paediatrics 117(6):1979–1987

Conroy S, Choonara I, Impicciatore P et al (2000) Survey on unlicensed and off label drug use in paediatric wards in European countries. BMJ 320:79–82

European Medicines Agency. Guideline on the need for non-clinical testing in juvenile animals of pharmaceuticals for paediatric indication (EMEA/CHMP/SWP/169215/2005), published 24.01.2008

European Medicines Agency. Medicines for children. http://www.ema.europa.eu/pdfs/human/comp/29007207en.pdf. Accessed 27 Jan 27 2010

Evans SJW (2008) Stratification for spontaneous report databases. Drug Saf 31(11):1049–1053

Evans SJW, Waller PC, Davis S (2001) Use of proportional reporting ratios (PRRs) for signal generation from spontaneous adverse drug reaction reports. Pharmacoepidemiol Drug Saf 10(6):483–486

Fortescue EB, Kaushal R, Landrigan CP et al (2003) Prioritizing strategies for preventing medication errors and adverse drug events in paediatric inpatients. Paediatrics 111:722–729

Garcia Rodriguez LA, Perez Gutthann S (1998) Use of the UK general practice research database for pharmacoepidemiology. Br J Clin Pharmacol 45:419–425

Gijsen R, Jochemsen H, vanDijk L et al (2009) Frequency of ill-founded off-label prescribing in Dutch general practice. Pharmacoepidemiol Drug Saf 18:84–91

Grégoire MC, Finley A (2007) Why were we abandoned? Orphan drugs in paediatric pain. Paediatr Child Health 12(2):95–96

Haffner ME (2006) Adopting orphan drugs – two dozen years of treating rare diseases. N Engl J Med 354:445–447

Haffner S, von Laue N, Wirth S et al (2005) Detecting adverse drug reactions on paediatric wards: intensified surveillance versus computerised screening of laboratory values. Drug Saf 28(5):453–464

Hartford CG, Petchel KS, Mickail H et al (2006) Pharmacovigilance during the pre-approval phases: an evolving pharmaceutical industry model in response to ICH E2E, CIOMS VI, FDA and EMEA/CHMP risk-management guidelines. Drug Saf 29(8):657–673

Horen B, Montastruc JL, Lapeyre-Mestre M (2002) Adverse drug reactions and off-label drug use in paediatric outpatients. Br J Clin Pharmacol 54:665–670

Impicciatore P, Choonara I, Clarkson A et al (2001) Incidence of adverse drug reactions in paediatric in/out-patients: a systemic review and meta-analysis of prospective studies. Br J Clin Pharmacol 52:77–83

International Conference on Harmonisation (ICH) (2000) Topic E 11: clinical investigation of medicinal products in the paediatric population. http://www.europa.emea.eu./pdfs/human/ich/271199EN.pdf

Johann-Liang R, Wyeth J, Chen M et al (2009) Paediatric drug surveillance and the food and drug administration's adverse event reporting system: an overview of reports, 2003–2007. Pharmacoepidemiol Drug Saf 18:24–27

Kaushal R, Bates DW, Landrigan C et al (2001) Medication errors and adverse drug events in paediatric inpatients. JAMA 285:2114–2120

Kearns GL, Abdel-Rahman SM, Alander SW et al (2003) Developmental pharmacology–drug disposition, action, and therapy in infants and children. N Engl J Med 349(12):1157–1167

Kimland E, Rane A, Ufer M et al (2005) Paediatric adverse drug reactions reported in Sweden from 1987 to 2001. Pharmacoepidemiol Drug Saf 14:493–499

Kimland E, Bergman U, Lindemalm S et al (2007) Drug related problems and off-label drug treatment in children a seen at a drug information centre. Eur J Pediatr 166:527–532

McIntyre J, Conroy S, Avery A et al (2000) Unlicensed and off-label prescribing of drugs in general practice. Arch Dis Child 83:498–501

Meyboom RH, Egberts AC, Edwards IR et al (1997) Principles of signal detection in pharmacovigilance. Drug Saf 16(6):355–365

Mühlbauer B, Janhsen K, Pichler J et al (2009) Off-label use of prescription drugs in childhood and adolescence. Dtsch Arztebl Int 106(3):25–31

Neubert A, Dormann H, Weiss J et al (2006) Are computerised monitoring systems of value to improve pharmacovigilance in paediatric patients? Eur J Clin Pharmacol 62(11):959–965

Nunn T, Williams J (2005) Formulation of medicines for children. Br J Clin Pharmacol 59(6):674–676

O'Donnell CP, Stone RJ, Morley CJ (2002) Unlicensed and off-label drug use in an Australian intensive care unit. Paediatrics 110:e52

Pandolfini C, Binati M (2005) A literature review on off-label drug use in children. Eur J Pediatr 164:552–558

Roberts R, Rodriguez W, Murphy D et al (2003) Paediatric drug labeling. Improving the safety and efficacy of pediatrc therapies. JAMA 290(7):905–911

Sanz E, Boada J (1987) Adverse drug reactions in paediatric outpatients. Int J Clin Pharmacol Res 7:169–172

'tJong GW, Eland IA, Strukenboom MC et al (2002) Unlicenced and off-label prescription of drugs to children: population based cohort study. BMJ 324:1313–1314

Turner S, Nunn AJ, Fielding K et al (1999) Adverse drug reactions to unlicensed and off label drugs on paediatric wards: a prospective study. Acta Paediatr 88(9):965–968

Ufer M, Kimland E, Bergman U (2004) Adverse drug reactions and off-label prescribing for paediatric outpatients: a one-year survey of spontaneous reports in Sweden. Pharmacoepidemiol Drug Saf 13:47–152

Wong I, Murray ML (2005) The potential of UK clinical databases in enhancing paediatric medication research. Br J Clin Pharmacol 59(6):750–755

World Health Organization Guideline (2007) Promoting safety of medicines for children. www.who.int/medicines/publications/essentialmedicines/Promotion_safe_med_childrens.pdf

Global Aspects of Drug Development

Kalle Hoppu and Hans V. Hogerzeil

Contents

K. Hoppu (✉)
Poison Information Centre, Helsinki University Central Hospital and Hospital for Children and Adolescents, Institute for Clinical Sciences, University of Helsinki, P.O. Box 790 (Tukholmankatu 17), 00029 HUS (Helsinki), Finland
e-mail: kalle.hoppu@hus.fi

H.V. Hogerzeil
Essential Medicines and Pharmaceutical Policies, World Health Organization, 1211 Geneva 27, Switzerland

H.W. Seyberth et al. (eds.), *Pediatric Clinical Pharmacology*,
Handbook of Experimental Pharmacology 205,
DOI 10.1007/978-3-642-20195-0_18, © Springer-Verlag Berlin Heidelberg 2011

Abstract About nine million children die every year before they reach the age of 5 years, of conditions largely amendable with existing medicines. Lack of medicines is not the single most important health problem of children, but work to provide children with better access to appropriate medicines is essential for achievement of the child health goals set. Taking into consideration the global aspect in the development of paediatric medicines the benefits of the regional paediatric initiatives can be spread worldwide. This chapter provides insights in the challenges and opportunities of developing paediatric medicines for health needs of children in the developing world. The Essential Medicines List for children first made available in 2008 serves as an example of the many tools available from WHO to improve children's access to the medicines they need.

Keywords Drug development • Essential medicines • Access to medicines • Quality of medicines • Clinical trials • WHO • Ethics • Developing world • Children

1 Introduction

About 28% of the 2008 world population of 6.7 billion is of less than 15 years of age. In less developed countries children and adolescents less than 15 years of age make out about a third, and in the sub-Saharan Africa about 43% of the population. The trend in childhood mortality has been favourable on the global level and contributes to the increase in life expectancy. However, many countries still have high child mortality, particularly in sub-Saharan Africa and South Asia, and in recent years made little or no progress in reducing the number of child deaths. While lack of medicines is not the single most important health problem of children, it is clear that work to provide children with better access to appropriate medicines is essential for achievement of the child health goals set, like the Millennium Development Goals (MDG) – MDG 4 (Reduce child mortality by two thirds) and MDG 6 (combat HIV/AIDS, malaria, and other major diseases).

The paediatric medicines initiatives launched in the US and the EU, in essence public health interventions to improve child health, have successfully increased interest in study and development of paediatric medicines and already led to positive results. However, the increased research and development of paediatric medicines initiated by these regional initiatives are unlikely to benefit children of the less developed world unless their special needs and requirements are considered in the process. The aim of this chapter is to discuss factors to be considered, challenges but also opportunities of developing paediatric medicines that meet the needs of children in less developed world.

2 Meeting the Health Needs of Children Around the World

It is estimated that about nine million children die every year before they reach the age of 5 years, 70% of them from treatable conditions. More than three million die in the neonatal period. The main causes of death in the first month are preterm birth,

birth asphyxia, and infections. After the age of one month and up until the age of five, the main causes of death are pneumonia (approximately two million/year), diarrhoeal diseases (approximately 1.9 million/year, comprising 18% of all under-five deaths), malaria (estimated one million/year), measles, and HIV/AIDS. Malnutrition contributes to more than one third of under-five deaths.

Effective interventions in the form of medicines exist for many of these conditions, but a significant proportion of the children do not have access to these medicines. Like even in the richest countries of the world, the medicines available for children are often not appropriate for their needs. Many of the medicines that do exist do not exist in appropriate formulations for children. A recent study on the inclusion of key medicines for children in national essential medicines lists (EMLs) and standard treatment guidelines, and to assess the availability and cost of these medicines in 14 countries in central Africa found that the availability of key essential medicines for children was poor (Robertson et al. 2009).

Making medicines available, medicines supply, is part of a functioning health care system. Most health programmes depend on access to affordable medicines; without quality medicines success is not possible. Recognizing that better access to medicines is a prerequisite for improving health outcomes in children, in May 2007 the World Health Assembly passed Resolution WHA60.20 "Better Medicines for Children", which identified key steps for ensuring better medicines for children (World Health Assembly 2007). Key points of the Resolution are summarized in Table 1.

The WHA60.20 resolution set goals and called for action by Member States and WHO to address the global need for children's medicines. One important target for action was the WHO Model List of Essential Medicines (EML), a global standard for 30 years, used by many countries as a model for national lists to guide drug procurement and supply. Although this list has included some paediatric medicines, a children's list had not been systematically developed.

3   The Concept of Essential Medicines

Essential medicines are those that satisfy the priority health care needs of the population. They are selected on the basis of disease prevalence, evidence on efficacy, safety and comparative cost-effectiveness. The selection of essential medicines is one of the core principles of a national medicine policy because it helps to set priorities for all aspects of the pharmaceutical system. This is a global concept, which can be applied in any country, in private and public sectors and at different levels of the health care system.

There is good evidence that clinical guidelines and essential medicines lists, when properly developed, introduced and supported, improve prescribing quality and lead to better health outcomes (Grimshaw and Russell 1993; Kafuko and Bagenda 1994; Woolf et al. 1999; Laing et al. 2001). But there is also an economic

Table 1 Key points of the World Health Assembly resolutionWHA60.20 on Better medicines for children

WHA60.20 urges member states:
To take steps to identify appropriate dosage forms and strengths of medicines for children, and to encourage their manufacture and licensing
To encourage research and development of appropriate medicines for diseases that affect children, and to ensure that high-quality clinical trials for these medicines are conducted in an ethical manner
To facilitate timely licensing of appropriate, high-quality and affordable medicines for children and innovative methods for monitoring the safety of such medicines
To encourage the marketing of adequate paediatric formulations together with newly developed medicines
To promote access to essential medicines for children through inclusion, as appropriate, of those medicines in national medicine lists, procurement and reimbursement schemes, and to devise measures to monitor prices
To collaborate in order to facilitate innovative research and development on, formulation of, regulatory approval of, provision of adequate prompt information on, and rational use of, paediatric medicines and medicines authorized for adults but not approved for use in children
WHA60.20 requests the WHO director-general
To promote the development, harmonization, and use of standards for clinical trials of medicines for children
To revise and regularly update the Model List of Essential Medicines in order to include missing essential medicines for children
To ensure that all relevant WHO programmes, including but not limited to that on essential medicines, contribute to making safe and effective medicines as widely available for children as for adults
To promote the development of international norms and standards for quality and safety of formulations for children, and of the regulatory capacity to apply them
To make available evidence-based treatment guidelines and independent information on dosage and safety aspects of medicines for children, and to work with Member States in order to implement such guidelines

argument. First, in developing countries pharmaceuticals are the second biggest budget line in the health system, after salaries. Secondly, new essential medicines are expensive. For example, even with good differential pricing lumefantrine-artemisinine at the time of its introduction for use in developing countries was 20 times more expensive than chloroquine, the first-line antimalarial it is supposed to replace; atovaquone-proguanil is about 400 times as expensive. Life-saving antiretroviral combinations cost \$80–100 per year while 38 countries have less than \$2 per person per year available for all their medicine needs. The selection of new essential medicines for public supply, subsidy or reimbursement has enormous financial implications for developing countries.

The advantages of limited lists are therefore both medical and economical. From a medical point of view they lead to better quality of care and better health outcomes and help focus quality control, drug information, prescriber training and medical audit. Economically they lead to better value for money, to lower costs through economies of scale and to simplified systems of procurement, supply, distribution and reimbursement. All of this is even more important in resource-poor situations where the availability of medicines in the public sector is often erratic. Under such circumstances measures to ensure a regular supply of essential medicines will result in real health gains and in increased confidence in the health services.

The concept of essential medicines was launched in 1977 with the publication of the first WHO Model List of Essential Medicines. Since then the List was revised every 2 years. Both its content and the process by which it is updated are intended as a model for developing countries. In 2002, WHO completed a rigorous overhaul of the process to update the list. An important change was that affordability changed from a precondition into a consequence of the selection. For example, before 2002 effective but expensive medicines, such as single-dose azithromycin for trachoma, were not listed because of their price. The new definition of essential medicines is:

> Essential medicines are those that satisfy the priority health care needs of the population. They are selected with due regard to disease prevalence, evidence on efficacy and safety, and comparative cost-effectiveness. Essential medicines are intended to be available within the context of functioning health systems at all times, in adequate amounts, in the appropriate dosage forms, with assured quality, and at a price the individual and the community can afford. The implementation of the concept of essential medicines is intended to be flexible and adaptable to many different situations; exactly which medicines are regarded as essential remains a national responsibility (WHO 2003)

Under the new definition, twelve antiretroviral medicines for HIV/AIDS were listed, irrespective of their high cost at that time. Their listing implied that these medicines should become affordable to all patients who need them; and seven years later we can conclude that prices have indeed come down dramatically.

Within a country, market approval of a pharmaceutical product is usually granted on the basis of efficacy, safety and quality, and rarely on the basis of a comparison with other products already on the market, or cost. This regulatory decision defines the availability of a medicine in the country. In addition, most public drug procurement and insurance schemes have mechanisms to limit procurement or reimbursements of drug costs. For these decisions, an evaluation process is necessary, based on a comparison between various drug products and on considerations of value for money. This second step leads to a national list of essential drugs.

A list of essential drugs is best developed for different levels of care, and on the basis of standard treatment guidelines for common diseases and complaints that can and should be diagnosed and treated at that level. National lists of essential medicines are used to guide the procurement and supply of medicines in the public sector, reimbursement schemes, medicine donations and local medicine production; they also help define the training of health workers. In short, essential medicines lists provide the scientific and public health basis for focus and expenditure in the pharmaceutical sector.

In many countries it has taken several years and several editions of treatment guidelines and lists of essential medicines before a more or less stable product was developed which was accepted by most prescribers and actually used for training, procurement and supply. Although time-consuming, the wide involvement of a

large number of prescribers, academic departments, health facilities and professional organizations is crucial. It is also important to stress the point that essential
medicines are not second-rate medicines for poor people, but that they represent the
most cost-effective treatments for a given condition. Over time, prescribers increasingly begin to recognize and trust the value of the clinical guidelines.

At the turn of the century, over 150 countries had official essential medicines
lists, of which 127 had been updated in the previous 5 years. Most developing
countries have national lists and some have provincial or state lists as well.
Many international organizations, including UNICEF and UNHCR, as well as
non-governmental organizations and international non-profit supply agencies,
have adopted the essential medicines concept for their supply systems. Several
developed countries, such as Australia, also use the same approach.

4 WHO Essential Medicines List for Children

Effective treatments exist for many of the priority diseases and conditions of
children, however many of these essential medicines do not exist in formulations
for children. There are many gaps in evidence and knowledge about the use of
existing medicines in children and in identifying what medicines do not exist. The
development of the first WHO Essential Medicines List for children (EMLc) in
2007 was a first step in addressing this knowledge gap.

The first EMLc (WHO 2008a), which was adopted on the day of the 30th
Anniversary of the EML, was developed using the same procedures that are used
to update the main list. Selection of medicines as essential is based on public health
need and evidence of their efficacy and safety. In selecting essential medicines for
children, one of the first difficulties encountered was the relative lack of evidence
about medicines used to treat children with "neglected" diseases such as leishmani-
asis. The first EMLc included about 200 medicines in about 450 dosage forms.
Many were marked as needing further review, or had age restrictions on use
because of lack of data. The meeting report also lists many medicines for which
further evidence is required to confidently assess the benefits and harms of their use
in children. Some of the questions might be answered by systematic reviews of
existing information, but others require more research and drug development. The
published report of the WHO Expert Committee (WHO 2008a) also includes a
listing of Research Priorities for Children's Medicines developed by a group of
experts convened by the WHO in October 2007.

A second EMLc was adopted in March 2009, and included for the first time a
listing of essential medicines that can be used in neonates (WHO 2009b). A
temporary Subcommittee of the WHO Expert Committee on the Selection and
Use of Essential Medicines prepared these first two Essential Medicines Lists for
children. The subcommittee meetings were held from 9 to 12 July 2007 and 29
September to 3 October 2008. In its last meeting, the Subcommittee recommended
that for the foreseeable future, it is essential that the EMLc remain separate from the

WHO Model List of Essential Medicines in order to maintain a critical focus on the needs of children. However, it was considered that a Paediatric Subcommittee as such would not be necessary and that it would be feasible for Expert Committees to update the EMLc if appropriate consideration is given to the constitution of future Expert Committees. Wide paediatric expertise will be necessary in order to meet the needs of children and the demands of United Nations Millennium Goals 4 and 6 to focus on paediatric priorities of Resolution WHA60.20.

The most up-to-date WHO Essential Medicines List for children is available from the WHO Selection of essential medicines – web-site (http://www.who.int/selection_medicines/list/en/) as are the Technical reports of the Expert Committee meetings (WHO 2008a; WHO 2009b).

5 Developing Appropriate Paediatric Formulations for the Different Environments

Many of the essential medicines do not exist in formulations for children, and many of the existing dosage forms of medicines for children are associated with significant problems. Practical experience from the children, their caregivers, and health care professionals from all over the world is that the existing paediatric formulations are not optimal when it comes to dosing, dispensing, and administering the medicines to children. This problem of lack of age-appropriate paediatric formulations has been widely recognized, including by the US and EU paediatric initiatives, which include measures designed to try to alleviate the problem.

The problems of paediatric formulations are even more difficult in resource poor settings, and especially in areas of the world where high temperature and humidity combined with problems of transport make logistics and storage a real challenge. These problems exist at the country level for logistics needed for medicines supply, at the level of local health care delivery and for the end users, the children and their caregivers.

High humidity, present often in combination with high temperature, is detrimental to the quality of medicines and may render them inactive quite rapidly. Access to electricity is not given in areas where temperatures are highest, therefore facilities for cold storage of medicines – common requirement for liquid formulations such as anti-infective agents once reconstituted – may not be reliably available in all health care facilities, and even less so in households. Bulky formulations – liquids are much more bulky than solid dosage forms – pose significant logistical challenges, require more warehouse space, pharmacy space and compel parents to carry home a heavier load of medicines. The transport problems for the end users become even more significant in case of multi-drug treatments, long distances and lack of means of transportation.

Paediatric formulations are most often in a liquid form but at the time of dispensing or before administration may have to be dissolved in water. Water needed to reconstitute medicines has to be clean, and clean water cannot be assumed to be readily available all over the world. If age-appropriate formulations are only available in bulk, containers for repackaging have to be provided, as there is no guarantee that containers the patients/caregivers can provided are suitable (e.g. may not be clean). Preferably medicines should be provided in packages ready for dispensing. If injectable medicines are provided in strengths and vials for adults, and are stable only for a short time after reconstitution, a lot of wastage occurs as one child can use them only – the rest is waste. Appropriate handling of waste may add to the problems.

Successful administration of the right dose of a medicine to a young child is challenging all over the world. Clear instructions on administering medicines for children that can be given to parents/caregivers are helpful. However, illiteracy is common in many areas of the world and good illustrations or drawn instructions have not been developed for paediatric use. The need for non-verbal instructions that can be given to the parents who bring children to hospitals is highlighted when the parents are not the ones who administer the medicines, so that they have to communicate instructions to another caregiver (grandparents, house help, mother in law, school matron, school nurse, teacher, etc). Given that medicine administration in children is often complicated and requires specific directions, mistakes may occur when information is transferred to "third parties".

6   Accounting for Sociocultural Differences

In a global world sociocultural differences still play a major role, also when it comes to paediatric medicines. Colour, form and taste of a medicine may not only affect the success of administration to children but also the assessment people make on the strength and effect of medicines. The preferences and interpretations can have a significant cultural variability. These differences have been noted and for example taste preferences routinely influence development of paediatric medicines for the developed world. When the cultural variability of the less developed world is added to that, the issue becomes even more complicated. A large pill may be interpreted as "stronger" than a small one, and a bitter tasting medicine more powerful than a sweet one. "Western" medicines may be considered too "strong" and with too many "side effects" and traditional (homeopathic or herbal) medicines may be preferred, a phenomenon not unfamiliar in the "western" world either. Pill burden is a pragmatic problem, in any culture. Multiple concomitant diseases increase the pill burden irrespective of geography, but are more common in areas of high disease burden.

Traditional beliefs, misconceptions, irrational use of medicines are not unfamiliar anywhere in the world, but their variability and effect may be more pronounced in resource poor setting where education and other services are available only to a limited extent. The global coverage of data on sociocultural differences is limited, and we do not even know the real relevance of the existing information. While there can be no doubt that sociocultural differences need to be considered in global development of paediatric medicines, we do not yet really know how and to what extent.

7   Paediatric Fixed-Dose Combinations

Combination therapy is necessary for successful treatment of acute infections and for prohibiting resistance to emerge in many of the priority diseases. Fixed dose combinations (FDCs) can reduce the pill burden of combination therapies and improve adherence to treatment. FDCs made their breakthrough in HIV/AIDS treatment of adults and are now considered essential in other diseases such as malaria and TB.

The concept of a FDC is valid for children also. In children the common difficulties in administration and the increased physical mass that has to be carried and stored when liquid formulations are used for long-term combination therapy are additional arguments for use of FDCs. However, developing FDCs for children brings some additional challenges. Developmental disposition of each individual component (active ingredient) of a combination therapy may be different. The ratio of the components providing optimal exposure for efficacy and safety may be different in children when compared to adults, and may change in relation to development. Simple linear scaling down of adult FDCs to lower strength paediatric formulations may not be appropriate and increase in children the risk of treatment failures and development of resistance. The latter may have wide reaching consequences affecting also adults. Scoring of adult FDCs into infinitely small fragments to adjust dosing for use of children cannot be safely done, unless the pharmaceutical specifications of the product guarantee that dose accuracy is maintained.

In practice, dosing children with 1/4 or ½ adult FDCs tablet is often feasible as long as the tablet is suitable for scoring. When developing paediatric FDCs for children needing lower doses than this, it is highly recommended to ascertain whether developmental pharmacokinetic differences require changes of the ratio of the components. Failure to do so has led to rejection of applications for inclusion of newly developed paediatric FDCs on the EMLc.

8   The New Paradigm for Global Paediatric Formulations

The majority of paediatric formulations are in some liquid form – provided as syrups or solutions, or powders that have to be dissolved in water. Liquid FDCs exist, but they are usually more difficult to develop than solid FDCs. Many of the presumed benefits of liquid formulations are not valid. Studies indicate that both parents and children – sometimes unrealistically – in fact prefer tablets to liquids.

The possible benefit of the potentially greater dose accuracy of liquid vs. solid formulations is not always necessary, when the active substance has a broad therapeutic range (e.g. common antimicrobials) or is lost when inaccurate measuring devices (e.g. a tablespoon) are used. Liquids are expensive, less stable than solid forms, difficult to ship and store. As indicated earlier, liquid formulations are particularly problematic in many areas of the developing world.

In the current growing interest and need to develop new paediatric formulations of old and new medicines to benefit from the incentives and fulfil the requirements of the US and EU paediatric legislations, great global benefit could be achieved if one of the development specifications would be appropriateness for global use. An expert meeting was convened by the WHO in December 2008 to identify the dosage forms of medicines most suitable for children with particular attention to conditions prevailing in the developing countries, and to flag future research required in this area (WHO 2008c). The most important proposal was a shift from the traditional paradigm of liquid paediatric formulations to *flexible solid dosage forms*. Many stakeholders have subsequently endorsed this recommendation.

Flexible solid oral dosage forms such as tablets that are oro-dispersible and/or that can be used for preparation of oral liquids (for example, suspension or solution) could potentially be used in very young children (0–6 months) provided the product can be dispersed in breast milk from the mother. This type of product is feasible to manufacture in facilities that have conventional tableting facilities, but requires excipients that ensure stability and palatability. Examples of existing dispersible tablet products suggest that they can be more affordable than standard liquid dosage forms. These dosage forms could be used for many of the medicines necessary to treat the diseases that are the major causes of mortality and morbidity in under five-year-olds (lower respiratory tract infection, malaria, diarrheal diseases).

Some medicines require precise dose measurement or titration. For such oral medicines, the most suitable dosage form should be based on use of a *solid platform technology* (multi particulate solid, including those that could be dispersed to form a liquid dose), rather than oral liquids. This makes possible production of tailored doses and strengths as well as preparation as a range of dosage forms such as tablets or capsules. Examples of currently existing forms are mini-tablets and spherical granules (pellets). These dosage forms are feasible to manufacture and can be produced from standard excipients including those that are pre-mixed and suitable for a range of actives, and they have potential flexibility for constructing appropriate FDCs.

Some chemical substances are "difficult molecules", with problems of permeability and/or solubility (defined using BCS classes). Techniques for these difficult molecules need to be developed/or evaluated, including manipulation (e.g. spray drying, micronization) prior to use with some platform technology that may produce suitable dosage forms for children.

9 Simplified Dosage Regimens Needed: Without Compromising Safety and Efficacy

In resource poor settings, the medicine may be prescribed and dispensed by a community health worker. If administration is not possible by the parents at home, e.g. injections for severe neonatal infections, and treatment as in-patient is not an option, administration of every dose will require a visit by the health care worker to the patient or vice versa. Only a simple, short course of a minimal number of administrations is feasible under such circumstances. Simplicity in dosing and administration is also necessary if the treatment is administered at home by a parent or a caregiver, and particularly if the dosing is to be determined by them. Such challenges are common and unavoidable in programmatic approaches to priority diseases such as malaria.

To adjust for developmental and size differences, drug doses in children are typically calculated according to body weight. However, weight-based dosing may be challenging in less developed countries where priority diseases such as malaria are endemic because functioning weighing scales are scarce, and access to formal health services is limited. The methods used to establish regional age-based dose regimens for the treatment of uncomplicated falciparum malaria have been based on "epidemiological" modelling, carried out to translate weight-based recommendations to age-based dosing regimens for programmatic use in the target population (Taylor et al. 2006). The basic assumption is that the recommended mg/kg starting dose is correct, based on efficacy and safety data and PK data from paediatric populations. This weight-based information is then converted to age-bands, using regional weight-for-age reference curves from compiled country-level, population-representative nutritional data.

For malaria and other diseases where medicines are bought over-the-counter, age-based dosing is appropriate. For treatment and management of diseases such as HIV, weight information is imperative, since ARVs have a narrow therapeutic index, and weight change is used to monitor response to treatment.

Age-based dosing requires a drug with a relatively large therapeutic index, because it considerably increases the variability in dose intake, which will lead to some under- or over-dosing, particularly in drugs with relatively narrow therapeutic indexes. In principle, medicines with a wide therapeutic index could be safely dosed by age. Those with a narrow therapeutic index would need to be dosed by weight.

The determining factors for the accuracy and applicability of age-based dosing include the availability of appropriate tablet that is preferably scorable, and solid knowledge of the therapeutic dose range and therapeutic index (WHO 2009a). The starting point, as with any dosing regimen, is appropriate efficacy, safety, and PK data in the relevant age group.

The lack of data on the optimum target dose and therapeutic dose range for paediatric medicines and the unavailability of appropriate paediatric dosage forms result in children frequently being prescribed medicine doses that are inappropriate. Sub-optimal dosing is a major determinant of treatment failure in individual patients and may drive the development of drug resistance in the population. Overdosing may lead to serious adverse effects in individuals and may negatively affect the reputation of an efficacious medicine in communities, thereby affecting use and compliance.

Population pharmacokinetic modelling (POPPK) and simulations have been undertaken to evaluate some of the recommended ARV and TB treatment regimens (WHO 2009a). The advantages of using POPPK modelling is that a broad spectrum of subjects can be included, and covariates for size, age, genotype, binding proteins, diet, and interacting drugs are incorporated into the model. For many important medicines in use today, paediatric-specific PK data from large, well-conducted clinical trials spanning the continuum of the paediatric age spectrum do not generally exist. Paediatric PK data may be available from only a few published studies, with small subject cohorts that restrict the ability to accurately determine the true variability associated with specific PK parameters for each of the drugs. However, modelling and simulation based on limited PK data in children can be supplemented to a certain extent with information from adult studies and provide valuable information, which ideally should be validated by exposure data collected from subjects of different age ranges. The information from the modelling exercises can also be used to design future studies of these drugs to better eliminate the knowledge gaps.

10 Paediatric Clinical Trials in the Developing World

Many essential medicines have not been properly tested in children for efficacy and safety. Without adequate clinical trials, regulatory authorities cannot approve use of medicines in children. Approval of paediatric medicines by regulatory authorities, even the stringent ones, in earlier times were often based on efficacy and safety data-sets, which would be today considered insufficient. Clinical experience from years of use may strongly indicate that there are no major paediatric safety concerns with the dosage used. However, paediatric dosages tend to be biased towards underdosing as a consequence of conscious or unconscious fear of dose related toxicity and lack of appropriate PK and dose-ranging studies. These problems affecting paediatric drug therapy, well illustrated by the TB medicines, are global and call for additional clinical trials of many medicines having already approval for use in children.

The need for paediatric clinical trials is global. The general ethical and scientific principles for clinical trials are the same all over the world, and are discussed in Section "The Concept of Essential Medicines". However, differences between high and lower income countries lead to problems and challenges, which require some comments.

10.1 Ethical Aspects of Clinical Trials in the developing world

Clinical trials must be done in the developing world for diseases that do not exist elsewhere, and to account for variables, which may affect dosing, safety, or efficacy. These variables include differences in genetic and environmental factors, and health-care provision. Such trials are necessary and provide a direct benefit for the paediatric population from which the trial subjects come. It would be unethical not do the trials, and treat the children without proper knowledge or not treat them at all.

Less developed countries have some characteristics, which make them increasingly attractive for clinical trials not, or at least not primarily, intended to benefit the local paediatric population. These characteristics include high prevalence of diseases, commonly in treatment-naïve form, and lower trial costs. Such trials are usually intended to provide data for regulatory approval of a medicine in the developed countries, and in the case of paediatric medicines especially in the areas providing lucrative incentives for development of medicines for children. These trials are not necessarily inherently unethical, but run the risk of leading to exploitation, if the paediatric population from which the trial subjects come will not have access to the medicine once it is approved.

For an individual child participating in a clinical trial in a developing country, the ethical framework for recruitment and protection of the study subjects is provided by international agreements (Chapter Ethical Considerations in Conducting Pediatric Research). However, also at the individual level the real situation in a resource-poor country may often be significantly different from that of a high-income country child. In the environment the child is living, participation in a clinical trial may be the only real chance to get a treatment that may be life saving, a maximum benefit on individual level. In relation to this, the risk–benefit ratio would be positive even when the risks could be long-term adverse effects not treatable in the local health-care system or risk of relapse when the child has no longer access to the study treatment after the trial ends. Children in resource-poor settings have an increased risk of being exploited. In poor settings almost any form of reimbursement of expenses may run the risk of being an undue inducement for the family to provide consent for the participation of the child. Problematic may also be, if the study offers a big benefit for the local community in the form of an improvement in health-care infrastructure (facility, equipment etc.) that will remain after the study, but the risks are borne by the child. However, a clinical trial may also bring risks to the local community and health-care provision, if it focuses too much of the local resources and captures the best health-care workers for a single disease, and leads to deterioration of care for other health needs.

Principally the ethical framework of the international agreements makes provision to take care of these special challenges of the resource poor settings by the local ethical committees and/or national authorities. In practice, it is not uncommon that even when a system of ethical assessment and approval is in place paediatric expertise may be lacking, or at least expertise on paediatric clinical trials of medicines. A somewhat functional system of ethical assessment lacking appropriate paediatric trials expertise, but recognizing vulnerability and rights of children, tends not to approve applications for paediatric trials, often by not at all or belatedly responding to the applications. While this may protect the children from exploitation, it also denies them the opportunity to have better treatments through research.

10.2 Scientific Aspects of Paediatric Clinical Trials in Developing World

The scientific criteria for planning and performance of a valid paediatric clinical trial are similar all over the world. In the developing world, it may be easier to recruit enough patients to find a significant difference, and to find treatment-naïve patients. On the other hand, normal values or validated scales used to measure end-points may not be available for the population to be studied. Confounding variables may be completely different or have a different scale. For example the capacity to offer concomitant non-medical treatment for a psychiatric condition may not be comparable to other settings and render the results difficult to generalize.

Practical problems in performing trials in developing world settings are numerous, ranging from illiteracy of parents who should give consent, lack of electricity, and problems of logistics to corruption and unforeseeable changes in regulations, which may delay or make it impossible to export collected samples for the planned analysis.

Within the scope of this book it is possible only to give some ideas about the wide variety of ethical, scientific, and practical challenges of paediatric clinical trials in developing world settings. It is clear that the international agreements and conventions on ethics do not go to the level of interpretation needed to handle the increasing redistribution of paediatric clinical trials to the developing world. Support to build competency and capacity for paediatric clinical trials is also needed. It remains to be hoped that the WHO within the tasks set by the WHA 60.20 resolution, and the main profiteers of the trial redistribution, the US and EU, take initiative to fill the gaps in the international ethical framework and provide other support needed.

11   Price, Quality, and Access

Even when appropriate formulations of medicines for the important priority conditions have been developed, they are often in poor supply in low-income countries. This is mainly due to high prices, and weak medicines procurement and supply capacity. Paediatric formulations are often more expensive than formulations for adults. More generally, manufacturers are reluctant to undertake research and development into medicines for children, due to the unpredictable and smaller market size for these products.

Baseline data from a sample of African countries highlight discrepancies between WHO's first Model List of Essential Medicines for Children and national lists and treatment guidelines. Drug regulatory review of medicine for children in these countries is also highly variable.

After new medicines for children have been developed and appropriate formulations and data on dosing, safety, and efficacy have become available, the question comes up how to improve access to these new and better medicines at country level.

11.1 Providing Access to Essential Medicines for Children at Country Level

Any discussion on access to medicines for children has to start with the question: *access to which medicines?* In practice, this implies that every national essential medicines programme must first agree on the clinical guidelines for children, and draw up a list of essential medicines for children. The most sustainable solution is that the clinical guidelines for children be included in the national clinical guidelines used for training and supervision, and that the list of essential medicines for children be included in the national list of essential medicines for supply and reimbursement (Fig. 1). When the national list of essential medicines for children has been defined, focused efforts can start to increase funding for these medicines through government supply, bilateral support, donations, Global Fund grants, World Bank loans, etc.

This explains also why the *selection* of essential medicines for children was also the first and most important step to guide future drug development. In 2006, an analysis of the then current WHO Model List of Essential Medicines showed that over hundred medicines listed by WHO did not include a formulation for children,

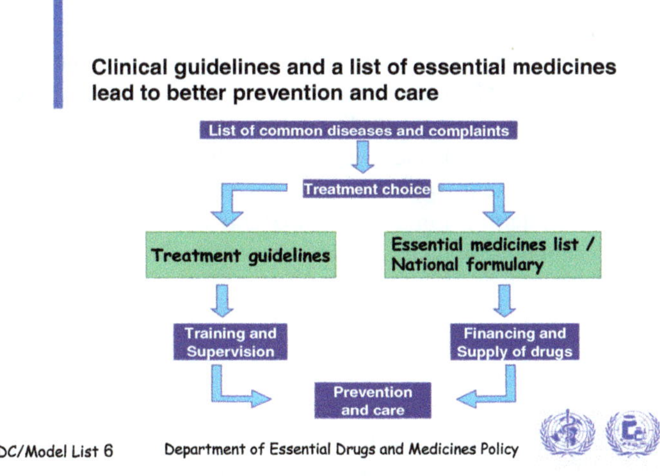

Fig. 1 Link between selection of essential medicines, clinical guidelines and the supply system

either because they were simply forgotten, or because they did not exist in the market. The resulting list of "missing essential medicines for children" added a new dimension to WHO's concept of essential medicines.

When new children's formulations have become available and added to WHO's global Model List of Essential Medicines, it is equally important that national clinicians include the new medicine in their updated national clinical guidelines; and that the national formulary committee includes the new medicine in their new national list. In this regard it may help to prepare and present short clinical update-sheets to make clinicians and formulary committee members aware of the new evidence.

11.2   Quality: A Major Challenge

With regard to *quality*, there is always a tendency to buy the cheapest medicines irrespective of quality. This is a dangerous approach, which needs to be resisted. The product with the lowest price can only be chosen when at least minimum quality standards are guaranteed. Within the UN system (but also used by the Global Fund, World Bank, UNITAID and international NGOs), WHO operates a programme of "*prequalification*" of suppliers and products for the treatment of HIV/AIDS, tuberculosis, malaria (including the paediatric formulations for these diseases) and a few other essential medicines for children (e.g. zinc tablets). This system is based on rigorous international assessments of the product dossiers and manufacturing site inspections (www.who.int/medicines; look under "prequali-fication"). By the end of 2009, 239 products had been prequalified for UN procure-ment, of which 34 are children's formulations.

This prequalification programme is of great practical relevance for all national and international procurement agencies, as it gives clear guidance in which paediatric products available in international commerce have been approved for UN procurement. This also removes the need for each and every national regulatory agency to invest heavily in their own dossier assessments and expensive site inspections in countries such as India, where most of the cheapest generic medicines are produced. But the programme also has a special function in paediatric drug development, by offering a mechanisms by which the quality of newly developed medicines can be assessed and endorsed at the global level, facilitating their regulatory uptake and procurement in developing countries.

11.3   Medicines Have to Be Affordable

Prices of children's medicines are often significantly higher than the cost of adult dosages making procurement and supply a challenge. There are many ways to improve *affordability* of essential medicines, including those for children.

In general, the preferred mechanism is competition. Competition is best guaranteed by the availability of several similar products of assured quality, and price transparency. Globally, whole-sale prices for generic medicines from not-for-profit suppliers are published by WHO and Management Sciences for Health (www. msh.org). In addition, national price surveys can be performed, price negotiations can be started, and pricing policies can be developed, including generic policies. In case of high prices linked to patent protection and failure of price negotiations, voluntary or compulsory licenses can be issued for local production or importation of generic products. Parallel import (import of a registered branded product from another country in which its market price is lower) is not generally recommended as it undermines differential pricing agreements and leads, in the long run, to higher prices for the poorer countries.

12 Rational Use of Medicines

About half of the medicines used are not prescribed in the most cost-effective manner: overprescription, unnecessary prescription, wrong doses, overuse of antibiotics, overuse of injections and prescriptions not in line with clinical guidelines are very common. After that, about half the patients do not adhere to the treatment; many never collect the medicines of the prescription; do not follow the instructions or interrupt the treatment before it is completed. All this leads to enormous medical and economic waste. The situation is not any better in the treatment of children.

There are many proven effective ways to promote *rational and cost-effective prescribing* (WHO 2002), such as the use of clinical guidelines and essential medicines lists, drugs and therapeutic committees in districts and major hospitals, and problem-based undergraduate training in pharmacotherapy. In general a combination of interventions is more effective than isolated measures. In the case of treatment of children, the use of clinical guidelines and standard protocols for use by doctors and other health workers is the best option; especially for the treatment and follow-up in rural clinics. This is also the way to promote the introduction and use of newly developed essential medicines for children.

13 National Medicine Policy

Different aims and objectives of a national pharmaceutical programme are often contradictory. For example, reimbursement restrictions may lead to irrational alternative prescribing, and support to the national pharmaceutical industry usually results in higher domestic medicine prices. A *national medicines policy*, when developed in a consultative way, helps to bring out and resolve such diverging interests (WHO 2001). The policy then becomes the expression of government commitment to a common goal and a framework for action. For example, the 1996 national medicine policy of South Africa (Ministry of Health 1996) strongly focuses on equity. By the turn of the century, 109 developing countries had developed a national medicines policy.

With regard to children, in many developing countries the needs are so great that drastic nation-wide measures are needed. In addition, several aspects of the problem touch upon other departments, such as the medicine regulatory agency (for speedy registration of medicines, quality assurance, licensing of national production), supply and distribution (for inclusion of medicines for children in the regular medicine supply system) and human resources (for clinical guidelines and prescriber training programmes); or other ministries, such as the Ministry of Finance (for additional funding for essential medicines for children, tax reductions, inclusion of paediatric formulations in health insurance and reimbursement schemes), the Ministry of Trade (for international trade agreements, patent legislation, compulsory licenses) and the Ministry of Education (for undergraduate and in-service training).

14   Public Health Approach to Innovation

WHO gives public health-based guidance to innovation in many ways (Table 2). First, the list of "missing essential medicines for children" describes exactly which medicines or formulations are missing. This can help interested companies to choose a certain niche in the market for drug development. Secondly, the published criteria for the Model List of Essential Medicines describe exactly which *clinical and safety data* will be needed for considering the new medicine for inclusion on

Table 2 Useful resources available from WHO

The WHO model list of essential medicines

  The WHO Model List of Essential Medicines is a model for national programmes and reimbursement decisions. It has been updated every 2 years since 1977. The Model List of 2009 (WHO 2009b) contains about 350 active ingredients and is divided into a main list and a complementary list. Drugs are specified by international non-proprietary name (INN) or generic name without reference to brand names or specific manufacturers. The List aims to identify cost-effective medicines for priority conditions, linked to evidence-based clinical guidelines and with special emphasis on public health aspects and considerations of value of money

The WHO model formulary for children

  The WHO Model Formulary (WHO 2008b) presents model formulary information on all medicines on the Model List and is a useful reference to individual prescribers. It is also intended as a starting point for developing national or institutional formularies. A separate WHO Model Formulary for Children is available (WHO 2010)

The WHO medicines web Site: www.who.int/medicines

  All WHO publications on essential medicines, including the Model List, Model Formulary, Essential Medicines Library, guidelines for national drug policies, information on prices, quality, prequalification, patent status, regulatory status are freely available on this website

WHO's Model List of Essential Medicines. This helps companies in designing the necessary studies and also further strengthens the public health approach to innovation. These clinical and safety data, which are public, can later also assist decision-making by national formulary committees. Thirdly, the WHO/UN prequalification programme describes exactly the *quality requirements* for the product application file, again guiding the innovation process and subsequent national regulatory review.

The advantages for the manufacturers are not only that the clinical, safety, and quality requirements of the missing paediatric formulations are clearly described and that the assessment process is predictable. In addition, if the product is indeed prequalified by WHO, most international and national medicine procurement agencies are likely to procure the new product, and an increasing number of national regulatory agencies will fast-track regulatory approval for their private markets. The advantages for public health authorities are that separate in-depth regulatory assessments are no longer needed, and that a fair competition is promoted between "prequalified" products of assured quality, leading to lower prices.

References

Grimshaw JM, Russell IT (1993) Effect of clinical guidelines on medical practice: a systematic review of rigorous evaluations. Lancet 342:1317–1322

Kafuko J, Bagenda D (1994) Impact of national standard treatment guidelines on rational drug use in Uganda health facilities. UNICEF/Uganda, Kampala

Laing R, Hogerzeil H et al (2001) Ten recommendations to improve use of medicines in developing countries. Health Policy Plan 16:13–20

Ministry of Health (1996) National drug policy of South Africa. Pretoria

Robertson J, Forte G et al (2009) What essential medicines for children are on the shelf? Bull World Health Organ 87:231–237

Taylor WR, Terlouw DJ et al (2006) Use of weight-for-age-data to optimize tablet strength and dosing regimens for a new fixed-dose artesunate-amodiaquine combination for treating falciparum malaria. Bull World Health Organ 84:956–964

WHO (2001) How to establish and implement a national drug policy. WHO, Geneva

WHO (2002) Promoting rational use of medicines: core components. WHO Policy Perspectives on Medicines, Geneva

WHO (2003) The selection and use of essential medicines. Report of the WHO Expert Committee, 2002 (including the 12th model list of essential medicines). Technical Report Series, No 914. WHO, Geneva

WHO (2008a) The selection and use of essential medicines. Report of the WHO Expert Committee, October 2007 (including the model list of essential medicines for children). Technical Report Series, No 950. WHO, Geneva

WHO (2008b) The WHO model formulary. WHO, Geneva

WHO (2008c) Report of the informal expert meeting on dosage forms of medicines for children. Available form: http://www.who.int/selection_medicines/committees/expert/17/application/paediatric/Dosage_form_reportDEC2008.pdf

WHO (2009a) Report of the technical consultation on the use of pharmacokinetic analyses for paediatric medicine development. Available form: http://www.who.int/childmedicines/progress/Pharmacokinetic_June2009.pdf

WHO (2009b) The selection and use of essential medicines. Report of the WHO Expert Committee, March 2009 (including the 16th WHO model list of essential medicines and the 2nd model list of essential medicines for children). Technical Report Series, No 958. WHO, Geneva
WHO (2010) WHO model formulary for children 2010. WHO, Geneva
Woolf SH, Grol R et al (1999) Clinical guidelines: potential benefits, limitations, and harms of clinical guidelines. BMJ 318:527–530
World Health Assembly (2007) Resolution WHA60.20 Better medicines for children.

Index

H.W. Seyberth et al. (eds.), *Pediatric Clinical Pharmacology*,
Handbook of Experimental Pharmacology 205,
DOI 10.1007/978-3-642-20195-0. © Springer-Verlag Berlin Heidelberg 2011

Printed in the USA
CPSIA information can be obtained
at www.ICGtesting.com
LVHW020837221023
761324LV00013B/45

9 783642 201943